UNDERSTANDING AND MANAGING

ENDOMETRIOSIS

Advances in Research and Practice

UNDERSTANDING AND MANAGING

ENDOMETRIOSIS

Advances in Research and Practice

Edited by A. Lemay, MD, and R. Maheux, MD
Endocrinology of Reproduction Research Centre,
Pavillon St-François d'Assise, Quebec, Canada

The Parthenon Publishing Group
International Publishers in Medicine, Science & Technology

NEW YORK LONDON

Library of Congress Cataloging-in-Publication Data

World Congress on Endometriosis (6th : 1998 : Quebec, Quebec)
Understanding and managing endometriosis : advances in research and practice : the proceedings of the VIth World Congress on Endometriosis, June 30–July 4, 1998, Quebec City, Canada / edited by Andre Lemay & Rodolphe Maheux.
p. cm.
Includes bibliographical references and index.
ISBN 1-85070-070-2
1. Endometriosis Congresses. 2. Generative organs, Female – Diseases Congresses. I. Lemay, Andre. II. Maheux, Rodolphe. III. Title.
[DNLM: 1. Endometriosis – physiopathology Congresses. 2. Endometriosis – therapy Congresses. 3. Endometriosis – etiology Congresses.
WP 390 W927u 1999]
RG483.E53W69 1998
618.1–dc21
DNLM/DLC
for Library of Congress 98-30330
CIP

British Library Cataloguing in Publication Data

Understanding and managing endometriosis : advances in research and practice : the proceedings of the 6th World Congress on Endometriosis, June 30–July 4, 1998, Quebec, Canada
1. Endometriosis – Congresses
I. Lemay, Andre II. Maheux, Rodolphe III. World Congress on Endometriosis (6th : 1998 : Quebec, Canada)
618.1

ISBN 1-85070-070-2

Published in the UK and Europe by
The Parthenon Publishing Group Limited
Casterton Hall, Carnforth,
Lancs., LA6 2LA, UK

Published in the USA by
The Parthenon Publishing Group Inc.
One Blue Hill Plaza
PO Box 1564, Pearl River,
New York 10965, USA

Typesetting by H&H Graphics, Blackburn, UK
Printed and bound by Bookcraft (Bath) Ltd., Midsomer Norton, UK

Contents

Recurrent endomentriosis

List of contributors

S.K. Agarwal
Department of Obstetrics and Gynecology
Cedars-Sinai Medical Center
Suite 160W
8700 Beverly Boulevard
Los Angeles, CA 90048
USA

A. Akoum
Unit of Endocrinology of Reproduction Research Centre
St Francis of Assissi Hospital
10 rue de l'Espinay
Quebec
Canada GIL 3L5

A. Arici
Department of Obstetrics and Gynecology
Yale University School of Medicine
333 Cedar Street
P.O. Box 208063
New Haven, CT 06520-8063
USA

A.J.M. Audebert
IGF1-35 Rue de Turenne
33000 Bordeaux
France

G. Benagiano
Institute Superiore di Sanità
Viale Regina Elena 299
00161 Rome
Italy

A. Bergqvist
Department of Obstetrics and Gynecology
Karolinska Institute, Huddinge University Hospital
S-141 86 Huddinge
Sweden

J.J. Brosens
Department of Reproductive Sciences and Medicine
Imperial College School of Medicine
Hammersmith Hospital
Du Cane Road
London W12 ONN
UK

W.M. Buckett
Department of Obstetrics and Gynecology
McGill University
Royal Victoria Hospital
Women's Pavilion
687 Pine Avenue West
Montreal
Canada H3A 1A1

S.E. Bulun
Division of Reproductive Endocrinology
Department of Obstetrics and Gynecology
University of Illinois at Chicago
M/C 808
820 S. Wood Street
Chicago, IL 60612
USA

M. Canis
Department of Obstetrics, Gynecology and Reproductive Medicine
Polyclinique de l'Hotel Dieu
13 Bd Charles de Gaulle
63033 Clermont-Ferrand
France

J. Cohen
Sterility Centre
Hospital de Sevres
8 Rue de Marignan
Paris 8
France

J. Collins
Departments of Obstetrics and Gynecology and Clinical Epidemiology and Biostatistics
McMaster University
4D9 - 1200 Main Street West
Hamilton, Ontario
Canada L8N 3Z5

S. Daya
Department of Obstetrics and Gynecology
McMaster University
1200 Main Street West
HSC: 3N52
Hamilton, Ontario
Canada L8N 3Z5

A.H. DeCherney
Office of the Chairman
Department of Obstetrics and Gynecology
UCLA School of Medicine
10833 Le Conte Avenue
Los Angeles, CA 90024-1740
USA

W.P. Dmowski
Institute for the Study and Treatment of Endometriosis
Grant Hospital
550 West Webster Avenue
Chicago, IL 60614
USA

J. Donnez
Department of Gynecology
Catholic University of Louvain
St Luc University Clinics
Avenue Hippocrate 10
1200 Brussels
Belgium

B. Eskenazi
School of Public Health, Maternal and Child Health
University of California, Berkeley
140 Warren Hall
Berkeley, CA 94720-7360
USA

J.L.H. Evers
Department of Obstetrics and Gynaecology
Academishch Ziekenhuis Maastricht and Maastricht University
PO Box 5800
6202 AZ Maastricht
The Netherlands

C. Gargett
Department of Obstetrics and Gynaecology
Monash University
Level 5
Monash Medical Centre
246 Clayton Road
Clayton, Victoria 3168
Australia

M.D. Hornstein
Department of Obstetrics and Gynecology
Brigham and Women's Hospital
75 Francis Street
Boston, MA 02115
USA

I.R. Horowitz
Department of Gynecology and Obstetrics
Emory University School of Medicine
1639 Pierce Drive
Atlanta, GA 30322
USA

P.R. Koninckx
Department of Obstetrics and Gynecology
University Hospital Gasthuisberg
KU Leuven
Herestraat 49
B-3000 Leuven
Belgium

M.R. Laufer
Division of Gynecology
Children's Hospital
300 Longwood Ave
Boston, MA 02115
USA

A. Lemay
Endocrinology of Reproduction Research Centre
Pavillon St-François d'Assise (CHUQ)
10 Rue de l'Espinay
Quebec
Canada G1L 3L5

R. Maheux
Endocrinology of Reproduction Research Centre
Pavillon St-François d'Assise (CHUQ)
10 Rue de l'Espinay
Quebec
Canada G1L 3L5

E. Marbaix
Department of Pathology
ANPS-1712
St Luc University Clinics
Avenue Hippocrate 75
B-1200 Brussels
Belgium

D.C. Martin
Department of Obstetrics and Gynecology
University of Tennessee
Memphis, TN 38163
USA

F. Nezhat
Stanford Endoscopy Center for Training and Technology
Stanford University School of Medicine
300 Pasteur Drive, MSOB X340
Palo Alto, CA 94305-5414
USA

M. Nisolle
Department of Gynecology
Catholic University of Louvain
St Luc University Clinics
Avenue Hippocrate 10
1200 Brussels
Belgium

K.G. Osteen
Department of Obstetrics and Gynecology
Vanderbilt University School of Medicine
1161 21st Ave S
MCN B-1100
Nashville, TN 37232
USA

H. Ota
Department of Obstetrics and Gynecology
Akita University School of Medicine
1-1-1 Hondo
Akita City, Akita-ken
010-8543 Japan

D.B. Redwine
2190 NE Professional Court
Bend, OR 97701
USA

G.L. Schattman
Department of Obstetrics and Gynecology
The Center for Reproductive Medicine and Infertility
The New York Hospital/Cornell Medical Center
505 East 70th Street
New York, NY 10021
USA

R.S. Schenken
Department of Obstetrics and Gynecology
The University of Texas Health Science Center at San Antonio
7703 Floyd Curl Drive
San Antonio, TX 78284-7836
USA

K.W. Schweppe
Department of Gynecology
Womens Clinic Ammerland
Academic Teaching Hospital of the University of Gottingen
Lange Straße 38
D-26655 Westerstede
Germany

K.L. Sharpe-Timms
Department of Obstetrics and Gynecology
University of Missouri
1 Hospital Drive
N 610 Health Sciences Center
Columbia, MO 65212
USA

R.N. Taylor
Reproductive Endocrinology Center
Department of Obstetrics, Gynecology and Reproductive Sciences
University of California
San Francisco, CA 94143-0556
USA

P. Vercellini
First Department of Obstetrics and Gynecology
University of Milan
Via Commenda 12
20122 Milan
Italy

P. Viganò
Second Department of Obstetrics and Gynecology and Istituto Auxologico Italiano
University of Milan
Via Commenda 12
20122 Milan
Italy

K.T. Zondervan
Department of Public Health
Institute of Health Sciences
University of Oxford
Old Road
Headington
Oxford OX3 7LF
UK

Foreword

Endometriosis is an enigmatic disease, it can be asymptomatic in some women yet cause excruciating pain in others. It is also a leading cause of infertility in women. We still do not know the exact cause of this disease and are only just beginning to understand why its clinical manifestations are so widely diverse from one woman to another. We have to acknowledge that the scientific and the medical communities have not made very significant progress in terms of finding a cure for the disease. We still try to ease the pain it causes and, for many women unfortunately, this means hysterectomy. This, of course, may eliminate physical pain but may also heighten the psychological pain for the woman since it does not address the problem of fertility.

It is a challenge to both the scientific and the medical communities to search for answers to this important problem. At the same time we have to be careful that we do not over-treat a condition that may stay asymptomatic in many women for several years. At the present time, it appears the correct answers elude us.

Some of the recent positive findings in this area, however, worthy of mention at this time. More and more randomized clinical trials are effectively providing women with valid therapeutic options. New ethiopathogenic factors have been identified and this may greatly help us in understanding endometriosis. In addition, physicians are now paying more attention to the views of the women who are actually living with endometriosis. However, there are still many areas remaining to be investigated; how to properly identify this disease without laparoscopy? How to identify those who will develop symptoms and those who will stay asymptomatic? How to cure the severe forms without having to rely on hysterectomy?

The VIth World Congress on Endometriosis was held to highlight the current developments in both basic and clinical sciences regarding this disease. This development was encouraged by the priming of the best basic and clinical oral presentations and posters. During the course of the congress there were four premeeting satellite workshops, four plenary sessions, four industry symposia, three parallel sessions and a video presentation. Some 30 oral papers were delivered and more than 200 communications were presented as posters.

Each of the chapters presented in these proceedings has been written by eminent scientists or clinicians in their respective fields. They cover most of the main topics concerning new developments in the ethiopathogeny and management of endometriosis. Although these chapters only give partial answers to the numerous problems related to endometriosis we are confident that the review of recent progress made in various areas will be helpful for the scientist and the clinician dealing with this complex disorder.

It is also important to mention that the VIth World Congress on Endometriosis has been the theater of the foundation of the World Endometriosis Society. The missions of the society include the following:

1. Promote the exchange of clinical experience, scientific thought and investigation among gynecologists, endocrinologists, researchers, biologists and other qualified persons interested in endometriosis.

2. Foster research into the pathogenesis and treatment of endometriosis.

3. Disseminate information about endometriosis.
4. Encourage and support collaboration among national and international societies interested in endometriosis.
5. Organize the World Congresses on Endometriosis.

We felt privileged to host this well attended International meeting in Quebec in 1998 and we look forward to the report and discussion of future progress in the VIIth Biennial World Congress in London in May 2000.

André Lemay, Rodolphe Maheux

Endometriosis is an inflammatory disease 1

A. Arici and D.L. Olive

INTRODUCTION

Endometriosis, defined by the presence of viable endometrial tissue outside the uterine cavity, is among the most common gynecologic disorders affecting women of reproductive age. The pathogenesis of endometriosis involves retrograde dissemination of endometrium and/or development *in situ* by metaplasia and there is evidence suggesting that genetic and hormonal factors may play a role. There is also substantial evidence that immunologic factors namely, peritoneal macrophages, T cells, natural killer cells and soluble products secreted by these cells are involved in the pathogenesis of endometriosis. The immunologic profile of endometriosis is typical of an inflammatory disease.

THEORIES ON THE PATHOGENESIS OF ENDOMETRIOSIS

Numerous theories of the histogenesis of endometriosis have been proposed by many investigators in the field. However, three main theories dominate current thinking. The original theory proposed that endometriosis develops from metaplasia of cells lining the pelvic peritoneum[1]. The basis of the coelomic metaplasia concept derives from the fact that both endometrial and peritoneal cells derive from the same coelomic epithelium. It has never been shown, however, that differentiated peritoneal cells can differentiate further. A second problem with this theory is that if metaplasia of coelomic tissue is the source, all such tissue should contain the same developmental potential. Although the coelomic membrane covers both the abdominal and thoracic cavities, endometriosis occurs primarily in the pelvis. Finally, the incidence of most metaplastic processes increases with advancing age; endometriosis, however, is virtually limited to reproductive-age women. The theory of estrogen-induced metaplasia explains the observed age distribution, but this mechanism is inconsistent with the low observed incidence of endometriosis in anovulatory women with chronically elevated estrogen levels.

A second theory of histogenesis is transplantation of shed uterine endometrium to ectopic locations, as suggested by Sampson in the 1920s[2]. Many mechanisms have been proposed, including lymphatic, vascular, and iatrogenic dissemination and retrograde menstruation. Considerable circumstantial evidence supports the role of retrograde menstruation with subsequent endometrial transplantation as an etiologic factor. Viable endometrial cells have been demonstrated in the lumen of Fallopian tubes and in peritoneal fluid. Recent experiments in animals and in human subjects have shown that the placement of endometrial tissue in ectopic locations results in endometriosis. Finally, the anatomic distribution of endometriotic implants clearly supports this hypothesis, as implants are found much more commonly in dependent areas of the pelvis. Taken together, these pieces of evidence strongly implicate retrograde menstruation in the development of endometriosis[3].

The third theory, also known as the induction theory, is a combination of the first two. It states that unknown substances released from shed endometrium induce undifferentiated mesenchyma to form endometriotic tissue. The demonstration of glands similar to endometrial structures adjacent to areas of subcutaneous deposition of denatured endometrium or implantation of endometrium-containing Millipore chambers in the peritoneal cavity of rabbits supports this theory[4]. But the role of such effects in the induction of complete endometriosis in humans is unclear.

Retrograde menstruation is a well-established phenomenon consistent with either the transplantation or the induction model of endometriosis. Studies of women undergoing peritoneal dialysis and laparoscopy suggest that 76 to 90 percent have retrograde menstruation, a prevalence much higher than that of endometriosis[5,6]. This suggests that other factors such as the amount of retrograde flow or immunologic changes may determine a woman's susceptibility to endometriosis.

Peritoneal fluid inflammation

Macrophages are known to be the cell type found in greatest quantity in the peritoneal fluid[7]. The number of these cells and other leukocytes varies throughout the menstrual cycle, being greater in the follicular phase, immediately after menses. Infertile women with endometriosis appear to possess a greater number of peritoneal macrophages as compared with normal fertile women[8,9]. These cells have all the characteristics of tissue-differentiated mononuclear phagocytes and the stimulus responsible for these cyclic changes is probably retrograde menstruation. There is evidence to suggest that peritoneal macrophages from women with endometriosis possess accentuated activation characteristics resulting in enhanced phagocytic activity and secretion of several soluble substances, e.g. proteolytic enzymes, cytokines, prostaglandins, growth factors, etc.[10]. Complement components C3 and C4, mediators of host responses to inflammation, have also been reported to be increased in the peritoneal fluids of patients with endometriosis. In addition to complement components, an increase in prostaglandin levels has been reported by some but not by all investigators. What role these secretory products may play in the pathogenesis of endometriosis is not yet known. They have been indirectly implicated as adversely affecting fertility and/or enhancing the maintenance and proliferation of endometriotic implants[11]. Paradoxically, the extent of endometrial implants has been inversely correlated with peritoneal inflammation, as assessed by total number of peritoneal fluid polymorphonuclear leukocytes.

The findings summarized above are compelling evidence suggesting that the peritoneal fluid in women with endometriosis is proinflammatory. While this fact is now widely accepted, investigators have remained divided on whether these changes precede the disease or follow endometriosis as a consequence, as both macrophages and granulocytes may be chemotactically attracted to the peritoneal cavity in response to the disease. We have recently identified the presence of two proinflammatory chemoattractant cytokines for monocyte/macrophages (monocyte chemoattractant protein-l [MCP-l]) and for granulocytes (interleukin-8 [IL-8]) in the peritoneal fluid. Not only are concentrations of both IL-8 and MCP-1 elevated in the peritoneal fluid of women with endometriosis compared to that from those without endometriosis, but the levels correlate with the severity of the disease[12,13]. In the peritoneal cavity, several tissues can account for the increased levels of IL-8 and MCP-1. Besides mesothelial cells that form the majority of the cells, peritoneal macrophages and endometrial cells themselves are potential sources of these chemoattractant cytokines[14–17]. Thus, one possibility for the pathogenesis of endometriosis is the arrangement of the aforementioned factors into a complex but unrelated scheme (Figure 1). In this scheme retrograde menstruation is a requirement and each step may be influenced by estrogen. While it is unlikely that this represents the sole path for genesis of the disease, it does appear to be consistent with a substantial volume of investigational data.

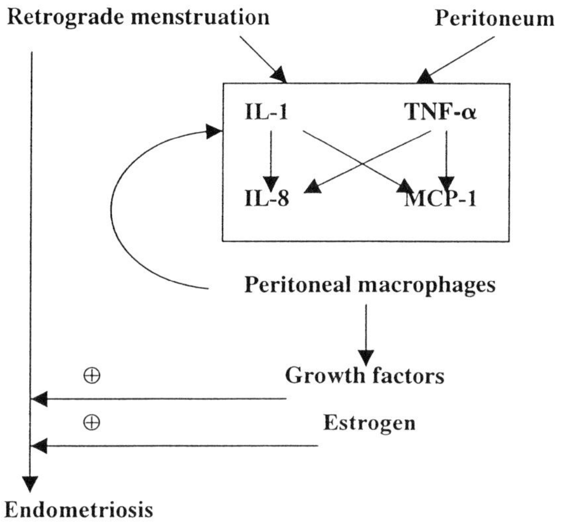

Figure 1 Role of inflammatory cytokines in the pathogenesis of endometriosis

The role of growth factors and cytokines

Several studies have documented that the increased macrophage activation in endometriosis is accompanied by their production of growth factors, that include but is not limited to fibroblast growth factor (FGF), platelet-derived growth factor (PDGF), epidermal growth factor (EGF), transforming growth factor-β (TGF-β). These growth factors have been shown to stimulate the proliferation of endometrial stromal cells *in vitro*, and it has been speculated that they may enhance the implantation of endometrial cells[18]. Many investigators have shown that viable endometrial cells can be cultured from the peritoneal fluid of virtually all normally ovulating women with patent Fallopian tubes. Thus the secretion of growth factors can be of importance in the maintenance of ectopic endometrium. In addition, EGF receptors have been demonstrated in both eutopic and ectopic endometrium. Finally, macrophage-derived growth factor (MDGF) enhances endometrial stromal cell proliferation, with maximal stimulation of growth when MDGF and estrogen are both present in the culture medium[19]. Recently, we have shown that IL-8 induces proliferation of endometrial cells and thus may play a role in the pathogenesis of endometriosis[20]. Such data suggest that a combination of factors, including the hormonal milieu and the number and secretory capacity of cells residing in the peritoneal cavity, might be required to sustain the growth of ectopic endometrium and thus induce clinical endometriosis.

CONCLUSIONS

Despite intense interest in endometriosis, there are many gaps in our understanding of its pathogenesis. But there is substantial evidence that immunologic factors play a role in the pathogenesis of endometriosis and endometriosis-associated reproductive failure. It has been established that the overwhelming majority of women regurgitate menstrual debris into the peritoneal cavity, but only a few develop endometriosis.

The initiation of endometriosis may be a function of the quantity of refluxed endometrium that is viable. Furthermore, the environment of the peritoneal cavity may play a decisive role in the development of endometriosis. Activated peritoneal macrophages and their secreted growth factors and cytokines will induce proliferation of the endometrial implants. Furthermore, these factors are also secreted by endometrium and peritoneum, suggesting an inflammatory pathogenetic cascade with multiple locations from which primary dysfunction might result in the disease endometriosis.

References

1. Meyer R. Uber den staude der frage der adenomyosites adenomyoma in allgemeinen und adenomyonetitis sarcomastosa. *Zentralblatt fur Gynakologia* 1919;36:745
2. Sampson JA. Peritoneal endometriosis due to the menstrual dissemination of endometrial tissue into the peritoncal cavity. *Am J Obstet Gynecol* 1927;14:422–69
3. Olive DL, Schwartz LB. Endometriosis. *N Engl J Med* 1993;328:1759–69
4. Merrill JA. Endometrial induction of endometriosis across Millipore filters. *Am J Obstet Gynecol* 1966;94:780–90
5. Blumenkrantz JM, Gallagher N, Bashore RA, *et al.* Retrograde menstruation in women undergoing chronic peritoneal dialysis. *Obstet Gynecol* 1981;57:667–70
6. Bartosik D, Jacobs SL, Kelly LJ. Endometrial tissue in peritoneal fluid. *Fertil Steril* 1986;46:796–800
7. Haney AF, Muscato JJ, Weinberg JB. Peritoneal fluid cell populations in infertility patients. *Fertil Steril* 1981;35:696–8
8. Halme J, Becker S, Hammond MG, *et al.* Pelvic macrophages in normal and infertile women: the role of patent tubes. *Am J Obstet Gynecol* 1982;142: 890–5
9. Dunselman GA, Hendrix MG, Bouckaert PX, *et al.* Functional aspects of peritoneal macrophages in endometriosis of women. *J Reprod Fertil* 1988;82:707–10
10. Halme J, White C, Kauma S, *et al.* Peritoneal macrophages from patients with endometriosis release growth factor activity *in vitro*. *J Clin Endocrinol Metab* 1988;66:1044–9
11. Orlicky DJ, Silio M, Williams C, *et al.* Regulation of inositol phosphate levels by prostaglandins in cultured endometrial cells. *J Cell Physiol* 1986; 128:105–12
12. Arici A, Tazuke SI, Attar E, *et al.* Interleukin-8 concentration in peritoneal fluid of patients with endometriosis and modulation of interleukin-8 expression in human mesothelial cells. *Mol Hum Reprod* 1996;2:40–5
13. Arici A, Oral E, Attar E, *et al.* Monocyte chemotactic protein-1 concentration in peritoneal fluid in patients with endometriosis and its modulation in human mesothelial cells. *Fertil Steril* 1997;67:1065–72
14. Arici A, Head JR, MacDonald PC, *et al.* Regulation of interleukin-8 gene expression in human endometrial cells in culture. *Mol Cell Endocrinol* 1993;94:195–204
15. Arici A, MacDonald PC, Casey ML. Regulation of monocyte chemotactic protein-1 gene expression in human endometrial cells in culture. *Mol Cell Endocrinol* 1995;107:189–97
16. Arici A, Seli E, Senturk LM, *et al.* Interleukin-8 in the human endometrium. *J Clin Endocrinol Metab* 1998;83
17. Arici A, Oral E, Bukulmez O, *et al.* The effect of endometriosis on implantation: results from the Yale University *in vitro* fertilization and embryo transfer program. *Fertil Steril* 1996;65:603–7
18. Hammond MG, Oh ST, Anners J, *et al.* The effect of growth factors on the proliferation of human endometrial stromal cells in culture. *Am J Obstet Gynecol* 1993;168:1131–6
19. Olive DL, Montoya I, Riehl RM, *et al.* Macrophage-conditioned media enhance endometrial stromal cell proliferation *in vitro*. *Am J Obstet Gynecol* 1991;164:953–8

20 Arici A, Seli E, Zeyneloglu HB, *et al.* Interleukin-8 induces proliferation of endometrial stromal cells: a potential autocrine growth factor. *J Clin Endocrinol Metab* 1998;83:1201–5

Endometriosis: a systemic disorder associated with immunological dysfunction

2

W.P. Dmowski and D.P. Braun

INTRODUCTION

Since the beginning of the 1980s numerous studies have been published demonstrating alterations in immune function in monkeys as well as in women with endometriosis. Some of these reported changes in humoral, others in cell mediated immunity. However, in spite of the extensive research it is still not clear whether changes in immune function precede the development of endometriosis and are causative or contributory to the pathogenesis of the disease. Alternatively, immune changes may develop as a result of endometriosis, and are simply an epiphenomenon. In support of the former concept are reports indicating that Rhesus monkeys exposed to a whole body single dose proton radiation or treated with polychlorinated biphenyls (PCBs) or dioxin, develop an advanced and aggressive form of endometriosis at least twice as frequently as unexposed controls, following a latent period of approximately 7 to 10 years[1,2,3]. Both radiation and organochlorides such as PCBs or dioxin are known to exert an adverse effect on the immune system, and it has been postulated that it is the immunosuppression that contributes to the development of the disease.

The investigators who have studied immune function in endometriosis, and who consider immune changes associated with this disease more than epiphenomena, are divided in their interpretation of the data. Some propose that humoral changes are the main hallmark of the disease, and suggest that endometriosis is a form of an autoimmune disorder[4]. Others postulate that changes in cell mediated immunity are a primary mechanism leading to the development of this disease[5]. Our group subscribes to the latter concept, which will be the basis for this presentation.

DEFECTIVE CELL MEDIATED IMMUNITY

The initial studies in rhesus monkeys and in women with endometriosis reported in 1981 and 1984 suggested that peripheral blood lymphocytes are able to recognize autologous endometrial antigens and cells, and respond with increased proliferation and cytotoxic destruction of these cells[6,7]. This effect was decreased in subjects with endometriosis. We proposed then the hypothesis that defective cell mediated immunity and abnormal immune system response to misplaced endometrial cells lead to the ectopic survival of these cells and endometriosis. Fundamental to this hypothesis were observations that endometrial cells are transported through the Fallopian tubes and can be identified in the peritoneal cavity of all menstruating females.

Our initial studies were subsequently confirmed by Oosterlynck *et al.*[8] `and by other investigators who attributed decreased cell mediated immunity in endometriosis to the decrease in NK cell cytotoxicity. These investigators reported functional alterations and a decreased differentiation of NK-cells in endometriosis and the presence of factors inhibiting NK-cell function in the sera and peritoneal fluids of affected women. Oosterlynck *et al.*[9] attributed the decrease in NK cytotoxicity to TGFβ which is increased in the peritoneal fluid in endometriosis and is produced by PBM/PM, while Vercellini *et al.*[10] proposed that decreased NK function is secondary to the decreased β-endorphin secretion by PBM. According to Oosterlynck *et al.*[11] *in vitro* treatment with IL-2 restored NK-cell cytotoxicity.

In addition to the functional changes in CTL and NK cells, circulating PBM also appear to be functionally different in endometriosis. They produce higher levels of reactive oxygen metabolites indicating an increase in their activational status, as we demonstrated using chemiluminescence, and they secrete higher levels of TNFα, IL-6 and IL-8 than PBM of healthy women[12,13]. However, the immune cells most extensively studied in endometriosis are peritoneal macrophages (PM). They are increased in number, size and activational status, and release higher levels of C3, C4, TNFα, IL-l, IL-lra, IL-6, IL-8, IL-10, fibronectin, prostaglandins $F_{2\alpha}$ and E_2, lysozomal enzymes, and growth factors such as TGFβ, EGF, MDGF and PDGF. PM from women with endometriosis also demonstrate increased expression of BCL-2 which indicates decreased apoptosis and increased PM survival[14].

ABNORMAL ENDOMETRIAL RESPONSE

Further studies of the immune and ectopic, as well as eutopic endometrial cells and their interactions, have revealed alterations in the endometrial cells in endometriosis and suggested that it is the ectopic endometrium that escapes immune detection and destruction. Endometrial cells in the ectopic locations produce a variety of immunosuppressive factors as demonstrated by Wang *et al.* in 1987[15] and subsequently Hirata *et al.* in 1994[16] and Somigliana *et al.* in 1996[17]. Furthermore, the decrease in the lymphocyte proliferation in response to autologous endometrial cells which we demonstrated in 1981[6] may also be a reflection of abnormal endometrial function, rather than the immune cell activity as recently suggested by Helvacioglu *et al*[18]. Endometrial stromal cells in advanced endometriosis may escape immunosurveillance through increased shedding of ICAM-l adhesion molecules, as suggested by Somigliana *et al*[19]. Endometrial cells also demonstrate a decreased expression of E-cadherins, an invasion suppressing molecule, which may be a mechanism to increase their invasive properties[20]. We have also recently reported a decrease in the cytolysis of ectopic as compared to eutopic endometrial cells by the PBM/PM[21].

Alterations in the endometrial-immune cell interactions may be related to the differences in antigenic/immunogenic properties of the endometrium in endometriosis. Over the years, numerous investigators have reported the presence of unique endometrial antigens of different molecular weights in the endometriotic endometrium, and absence of these antigens in the endometrium of healthy women. These antigens seem to stimulate the immune system to produce abnormal autoantibodies, the presence of which has been reported extensively in women with endometriosis. It may be relevant that increased expression of HLA-DR and upregulation of MHC class l molecules in the ectopic endometrial cells have also been reported[22,23]. Lessey *et al.*[24] and others reported aberrant expression of integrins in the endometrium of women with endometriosis, and Isaacson *et al.*[25], estradiol-independent C3 and C4 secretion. Furthermore, endometrium in endometriosis secretes a variety of proteins, qualitatively and quantitatively different than normal endometrium[26,27].

Moreover, the endometrium in ectopic locations seems to acquire a certain growth autonomy. The expression of estradiol and progesterone receptors in the ectopic endometrium is increased with loss of cyclic variability, resulting in increased ectopic endometrial cell proliferation without characteristic cyclicity[28,29]. The C-19 aromatase which converts androgens to estrogens and is absent in the normal endometrium is present in eutopic and ectopic endometrial cells of women with endometriosis and is upregulated by PGE_2[30,31]. The growth factors such as EGF, IGF-1, IGF-2, HGF and their corresponding receptors are expressed abnormally in the ectopic endometrial cells and there is aberrant secretion of IL-6, IL-6ra and other growth regulatory cytokines[32–36].

Other studies suggest that the endometrial cells in endometriosis not only modify the immune response, but also seem to subvert that response to their advantage. Several investigators have demonstrated that endometriotic cells produce chemotactic substances for macrophages and lymphocytes, and secrete higher levels of complement factors which are chemotactic for lymphocytes and macrophages[37,38]. This results in a higher number of stromal lymphocytes in endometriosis[39]. We have reported that both eutopic and ectopic endometrial cells in endometriosis respond with increased proliferation in co-culture with PBM or to PBM/PM secretions or TNFα[40–42]. In contrast, eutopic endometrial cells from healthy women decrease proliferation in response to PBM/PM, their secretions or TNFα.

CLINICAL CHANGES

Endometriotic lesions in the peritoneal cavity have a characteristic appearance. However, even more characteristic are peritoneal changes surrounding these lesions. Peritoneal defects, 'peritoneal windows' and adhesions, as well as increased congestion of the peritoneum and dilatation of the peritoneal vessels, have long been recognized as the 'tell-tale' signs of endometriosis in the absence of endometriotic lesions[43]. These 'tell-tale' signs of endometriosis seem to develop as the result of the peritoneal-endometrial-immune cell interactions at the molecular level. In endometriosis, peritoneal mesothelial cells abnormally express ICAM-1 and VCAM-l adhesion molecules, which are further upregulated by TNFα[44,45]. The endometriotic cells in turn abnormally express cadherins, integrins and ICAM-l molecules[46]. Ectopic endometrial cells and PM produce TGFβ and IL-lra, and PM high levels of TNFα[47,48]. Peritoneal macrophages in endometriosis release high levels of fibronectin, and fibronectin receptors are abnormally expressed on endometriotic cells[49]. Mesothelial cells and PM secrete IL-8 which is upregulated by IL-1 and TNFα, and increased levels of VEGF are produced by PM[50]. Interactions between the cells and molecules described above lead to peritoneal congestion, angiogenesis and adhesion development.

The characteristic chronic pelvic pain symptoms of endometriosis have long been attributed to abnormal prostaglandin production, although abnormal prostaglandin levels have been difficult to demonstrate. Nevertheless, these symptoms improve during treatment with prostaglandin synthetase inhibitors. Abnormal prostaglandin production has been demonstrated in both eutopic and ectopic endometrial cells in endometriosis, but the concentration of prostaglandins in the peritoneal fluid appears to be variable and dependent on a multitude of factors. Interestingly, however, Karck *et al.*[51] have demonstrated that PM in endometriosis produce higher levels of PGE_2 and $PGF_{2\alpha}$. It is possible that the same applies to the circulating PBM.

Both PM and PBM in endometriosis produce higher levels of TNFα, IL-6, IL-8, and perhaps other cytokines. It is quite likely that the generalized symptoms of aches and pains, general malaise, low grade fever, nausea, vomiting and diarrhea, frequently experienced by women with endometriosis, and in the past referred to as somatizations of the disease, are caused by abnormal cytokine and prostaglandin secretion, not only by the endometrial, but also by the immune cells.

The peritoneal fluid in endometriosis contains a variety of substances produced by the ectopic endometrial cells as well as the immune cells, and is known to adversely affect several steps in the reproductive function. Increased sperm phagocytosis, abnormal sperm survival, defective ovum capture by the fimbriae of the Fallopian tubes, abnormal fertilization, and embryotoxic effects of the peritoneal fluid in endometriosis, have all been reported. It is generally agreed that these effects play a role in the decreased reproductive performance associated with endometriosis. Abnormal autoantibodies to endometrial cells, as well as to a variety of cell derived antigens, are present in the circulation, peritoneal, follicular, and other body fluids in endometriosis. The presence of such autoantibodies has been associated with infertility, embryo implantation failure, and increased frequency of spontaneous abortions.

CELL CYCLE–CELL DEATH EVENTS

We have reported recently that programmed cell death or spontaneous apoptosis in the eutopic endometrium is lower in endometriosis than in healthy controls[52]. Furthermore, in women with endometriosis, spontaneous apoptosis is lower in matched ectopic than eutopic endometria. These changes overshadow cycle related variability and confirm prior results by Watanabe *et al.*[53] indicating persistent expression of BCL-2 in the ectopic endometrium during the menstrual cycle.

It is well known that in healthy women there is an increase in endometrial cell apoptosis at the end of the cycle[54]. It is quite likely that PBM/PM, PBM/PM secretions or TNFα suppress endometrial cell proliferation and signal apoptosis in the healthy endometrium[54]. In endometriosis, it appears that PBM/PM, their secretions and TNFα stimulate endometrial cell proliferation rather than apoptosis. Furthermore, PM are less effective than PBM in both eutopic and ectopic endometrial cell lysis, and ectopic endometrial cells are more resistant than eutopic to both PBM and PM mediated cell lysis[21].

TNFα is a major secretory product of PBM and PM, and its secretion is significantly upregulated in endometriosis. It has been demonstrated previously that TNFα, after binding to a cell membrane receptor, activates the sphingomyelin pathway leading to the hydrolysis of sphingomyelin by sphingomyelinase and the generation of ceramide[55]. Ceramide, a second messenger, can activate, in the same cells, either proliferation/inflammation or apoptosis pathways. Considering a divergent effect of TNFα on the endometrial cells in women with and without endometriosis, one can speculate that in endometriosis activation of the proliferation/inflammation pathway allows survival of the misplaced endometrial cells, while in normal women activation of the apoptosis pathway leads to endometrial cell death regardless of their location.

CONCLUSION/SPECULATION

The data reviewed above indicate profound changes in the immune and endometrial cell functions in endometriosis and dysregulated immune-endometrial cell communications. It is possible that dysregulated immune-endometrial cell communications and abnormal signal transduction in the sphingomyelin and other cell cycle/cell death pathways of the endometrial cells may be the cause of endometriosis.

References

1. Wood DH, Yochmowitz MG, Salmon YL, *et al.* Proton irradiation and endometriosis. *Aviat Space Environ Med* 1983;54:718–24

2. Campbell JS, Wong J, Tryphonas L, *et al.* Is simian endometriosis an effect of immunotoxicity? Proceedings of Forty-Eighth Annual Meeting,

The Ontario Association of Pathologists, London, Ontario, October 1985. *Abstract # 12, Health Protection Branch, Health & Welfare Canada,* Tunney's Pasture, Ottawa, Ontario, Canada

3. Rier SE, Martin DC, Bowman RE, *et al.* Endometriosis in rhesus monkeys (*Macaca mulatta*) following chronic exposure to 2,3,7,8-Tetrachlorodibenzo-p-dioxin. *Fundam Appl Toxicol* 1993;21:433–41
4. Gleicher N, El-Roeiy A, Confino E, *et al.* Abnormal autoantibodies in endometriosis: is endometriosis an autoimmune disease? *Obstet Gynecol* 1987;70:115–22
5. Dmowski WP, Gebel H, Braun DP. The role of cell mediated immunity in pathogenesis of endometriosis. *Acta Obstet Gynecol Scand* 1994; 73:7–14
6. Dmowski WP, Steele RW, Baker GF. Deficient cellular immunity in endometriosis. *Am J Obstet Gynecol* 1981;141: 377–83
7. Steele RW, Dmowski WP, Marmer DJ. Immunologic aspects of human endometriosis. *Am J Reprod Immunol* 1984;6:33–6
8. Oosterlynck DJ, Cornillie FJ, Waer M, *et al.* Women with endometriosis show a defect in natural killer activity resulting in a decreased cytotoxicity to autologous endometrium. *Fertil Steril* 1991;56:45–51
9. Oosterlynck DJ, Meuleman C, Waer M, *et al.* Transforming growth factor-β activity is increased in peritoneal fluid from women with endometriosis. *Obstet Gynecol* 1994;83:287–92
10. Vercellini P, Sacerdote P, Panerai AE, *et al.* Mononuclear cell β-endorphin concentration in women with and without endometriosis. *Obstet Gynecol* 1992;79:743–6
11. Oosterlynck DJ, Lacquet FA, Waer M, *et al.* Lymphokine-activated killer activity in women with endometriosis. *Gynecol Obstet Invest* 1994; 37:185–90
12. Zeller JM, Henig I, Radwanska E, *et al.* Enhancement of human monocyte and peritoneal macrophage chemiluminescence activities in women with endometriosis. *Am J Reprod Immunol Microbiol* 1987;13:78–82
13. Braun D, Gebel H, House R, *et al.* Spontaneous and induced synthesis of cytokines by peripheral blood monocytes in patients with endometriosis. *Fertil Steril* 1996;65:1125–9
14. McLaren J, Prentice A, Charnock-Jones DS, *et al.* Immunolocalization of the apoptosis regulating proteins Bcl-2 and Bax in human endometrium and isolated peritoneal fluid macrophages in endometriosis. *Hum Reprod* 1997;12:146–52
15. Wang HS, Kanasaki H, Yoshida M, *et al.* Suppression of lymphoctye reactivity *in vitro* by supernatants of explants of human endometriosis. *Am J Obstet Gynecol* 1987;157:956–63
16. Hirata J, Kikuchi Y, Imaizumi E, *et al.* Endometriotic tissues produce immuno-suppressive factors. *Gynecol Obstet Invest* 1994;37:43–7
17. Somigliana E, Vigano P, Gaffuri B, *et al.* Modulation of NK cell function by endometrial secretory factors: potential role in endometriosis. *Am J Reprod Immunol* 1996;36:295–300
18. Helvacioglu A, Aksel S, Peterson RDA. Endometriosis and autologous lymphocyte activation by endometrial cells. Are lymphocytes or endometrial cell defects responsible? *J Reprod Med* 1997;42:71–5
19. Somigliana E, Vigano P, Gaffuri B, *et al.* Human endometrial stromal cells as a source of soluble intercellular adhesion molecule (ICAM) molecules. *Hum Reprod* 1996;11:1190–4
20. Gaetje R, Kotzian S, Herrmann G, *et al.* Nonmalignant epithelial cells, potentially invasive in human endometriosis, lack the tumor suppressor molecule E-cadherin. *Am J Pathol* 1997;150:461–7
21. Braun DP, Gebel H, Rana N, *et al.* Cytolysis of eutopic and ectopic endometrial cells by peripheral blood monocytes and peritoneal macrophages in women with endometriosis. *Fertil Steril* 1998;69:1103–8
22. Ota H, Igarashi S. Expression of major histocompatibility complex class II antigen in endometriotic tissue in patients with endometriosis and adenomyosis. *Fertil Steril* 1993; 60:834–8
23. Semino C, Semino A, Pietra G, *et al.* Role of major histocompatibility complex class I expression and natural killer-like T cells in the genetic control of endometriosis. *Fertil Steril* 1995;64:909–16
24. Lessey BA, Castelbaum AJ, Sawin SW, *et al.* Aberrant integrin expression in the endometrium of women with endometriosis. *J Clin Endocrinol Metab* 1994;79:643–9
25. Isaacson KB, Galman M, Coutifaris C, *et al.* Endometrial synthesis and secretion of complement component-3 by patients with and without ednometriosis. *Fertil Steril* 1990;53:836–41
26. Sharpe KL, Zimmer RL, Griffin WT, *et al.* Polypeptides synthesized and released by human endometriosis differ from those of the uterine endometrium in cell and tissue explant culture. *Fertil Steril* 1993;60:839–51
27. Nothnick WB, Currey TE Jr, Muse KN, *et al.* Detection of a unique 32-kDa protein in the peritoneal fluid of women with endometriosis. *Fertil Steril* 1994;61:288–93
28. Nisolle M, Casanas-Roux F, Donnez J. Immunohistochemical analysis of proliferative activity and steroid receptor expression in peritoneal and ovarian endometriosis. *Fertil Steril* 1997;68:912–19
29. Fujishita A, Nakane PK, Koji T, *et al.* Expression of estrogen and progesterone receptors in

endometrium and peritoneal endometriosis: an immunohistochemical and *in situ* hybridization study. *Fertil Steril* 1997;67:856–64
30. Noble LS, Simpson ER, Johns A, *et al.* Aromatase expression in endometriosis. *J Clin Endocrinol Metab* 1996;81:174–9
31. Noble LS, Takayama K, Zeitoun KM, *et al.* Prostaglandin E_2 stimulates aromatase expression in endometriosis-derived stromal cells. *J Clin Endocrinol Metab* 1997;82:600–6
32. Sbracia M, Zupi E, Alo P, *et al.* Differential expression of IGF-I and IGF-II in eutopic and ectopic endometria of women with endometriosis and in women without endometriosis. *Am J Reprod Immunol* 1997;37:326–9
33. Sugawara J, Fukaya T, Murakami T, *et al.* Increased secretion of hepatocyte growth factor by eutopic endometrial stromal cells in women with endometriosis. *Fertil Steril* 1997;68:468–72
34. Tseng JF, Ryan IP, Milam TD, *et al.* Interleukin-6 secretion *in vitro* is up-regulated in ectopic and eutopic endometrial stromal cells from women with endometriosis. *J Clin Endocrinol Metab* 1996;81:1118–22
35. Akoum AA, Lemay A, Paradis I, *et al.* Secretion of interleukin-6 by human endometriotic cells and regulation by proinflammatory cytokines and sex steroids. *Hum Reprod* 1996;11:2269–75
36. Harada T, Yoshioka H, Yoshida S, *et al.* Increased interleukin-6 levels in peritoneal fluid of infertile patients with active endometriosis. *Am J Obstet Gynecol* 1997;176:593–7
37. Akoum A, Lemay A, Brunet C, *et al.* Cytokine-induced secretion of monocyte chemotactic protein-l by human endometriotic cells in culture. *Am J Obstet Gynecol* 1995;172:594–600
38. Akoum A, Lemay A, McColl S, *et al.* Elevated concentration and biologic activity of monocyte chemotactic protein-l in the peritoneal fluid of patients with endometriosis. *Fertil Steril* 1996;66:17–23
39. Jones RK, Bulmer JN, Searle RF. Immunohistochemical characterization of stromal leukocytes in ovarian endometriosis: comparison of eutopic and ectopic endometrium with normal endometrium. *Fertil Steril* 1996;66:81–9
40. Braun DP, Muriana A, Gebel H, *et al.* Monocyte-mediated enhancement of endometrial cell proliferation in women with endometriosis. *Fertil Steril* 1994;61:78–84
41. Braun DP, Dmowski WP. Proliferative response of eutopic endometrial cells (EC) to tumor necrosis factor-α (TNFα) in women with endometriosis (endo). Abstract presented at IFFS'98, 16th World Congress on Fertility and Sterility and 54th Annual Meeting of the American Society for Reproductive Medicine, October 1998
42. Braun DP, Dmowski WP. Eutopic and ectopic endometrial cell proliferation in endometriosis. Abstract presented at VIth World Congress on Endometriosis, Quebec, June 1998
43. Dmowski WP. Pitfalls in clinical, laparoscopic and histologic diagnosis of endometriosis. *Acta Obstet Gynecol Scand* 1984;Suppl 123:61–6
44. Jonjic N, Peri G, Bernasconi S, *et al.* Expression of adhesion molecules and chemotactic cytokines in cultured mesothelial cells. *J Exp Med* 1992; 176:1165–74
45. Zhang R, Wild RA, Ojago JM. Effect of tumor necrosis factor-α on adhesion of human endometrial stromal cells to peritoneal mesothelial cells: an *in vitro* system. *Fertil Steril* 1993;59:1196–201
46. Ota H, Igarashi S, Tanaka T. Expression of γδ T cells and adhesion molecules in endometriotic tissues in patients with endometriosis and adenomyosis. *Am J Reprod Immunol* 1996;35:477–82
47. Ignotz RA, Heino J, Massague J. Regulation of cell adhesion receptors by transforming growth factor-beta. Regulation of vitronectin receptor and LFA–l. *Biol Chem* 1989;264:389–92
48. Rana N, Braun D, House R, *et al.* Basal and stimulated secretion of cytokines by peritoneal macrophages in women with endometriosis. *Fertil Steril* 1996;65:925–30
49. Beliard A, Donnez J, Nisolle M, *et al.* Localization of laminin, fibronectin, E-cadherin, and integrins in endometrium and endometriosis. *Fertil Steril* 1997;67:266–72
50. McLaren J, Prentice A, Charnock-Jones D-S, *et al.* Vascular endothelial growth factor is produced by peritoneal fluid macrophages in endometriosis and is regulated by ovarian steroids. *JCI* 1996;98:482–9
51. Karck U, Reister F, Schafer W, *et al.* PGE_2 and $PGF_{2\alpha}$ release of human peritoneal macrophages in endometriosis. *Prostaglandins* 1996;51:49–60
52. Gebel H, Braun DP, Tambur A, *et al.* Spontaneous apoptosis of endometrial tissue is impaired in women with endometriosis. *Fertil Steril* 1998;69:1042–7
53. Watanabe H, Kanzaki H, Narukawa S, *et al.* Bcl-2 and Fas expression in eutopic and ectopic human endometrium during the menstrual cycle in relation to endometrial cell apoptosis. *Am J Obstet Gynecol* 1997;176:360–8
54. Tabibzadeh S. The signals and molecular pathways involved in human menstruation, a unique process of tissue destruction and remodelling. *Mol Hum Reprod* 1996;2:77–92
55. Pena LA, Fuks Z, Kolesnick R. Stress-induced apoptosis and the sphingomyelin pathway. *Biochem Pharmacol* 1997;52:2–7

Endometriosis and adenomyosis: a unifying hypothesis

3

J.J. Brosens and I. Brosens

Endometriosis is currently defined as the presence of endometrial-like tissue outside the uterine cavity. This definition is based on Sampson's discovery in 1921 that endometrial-like tissue in hemorrhagic (chocolate) cysts of the ovary showed evidence of menstrual shedding[1]. Sex steroid hormone-dependent bleeding is a specific activity of endometrial tissue. Before Sampson the disease was defined as the presence of adenomyotic nodules which typically occurred in the posterior fornix of the vagina[2]. These lesions were characterized by smooth muscle cell hyperplasia, glands and scanty stroma. It has been assumed that endometriosis and adenomyosis are two different diseases with a different pathogenesis and clinicopathological characteristics. In this chapter we will discuss the pathogenetic and clinicopathological aspects which support the unifying thesis that endometriosis and adenomyosis both represent the disruption of sex steroid hormone-dependent differentiation processes in the paramesonephric duct.

SEX STEROID HORMONE RESPONSIVENESS OF ENDOMETRIUM

Estrogen primed endometrial cells differentiate during the luteal phase of the menstrual cycle in response to progesterone. The responsiveness to sex steroids of both the glandular and stromal cell compartments is maximal in the superficial endometrial layer and gradually decreases towards the basalis. Such polarization of the endometrium is thought to be effected by cytokine release from CD3-positive T-lymphocyte aggregates in the endometrio-myometrial junction[3–6]. The phenotype of the basal layer is characterized by low proliferative activity with high human leukocyte antigen (HLA–DR) and integrin expression in glandular epithelial cells. The stromal cell compartment of the basal layer is characterized by a poor decidualization response in the late luteal phase. Studies *in vitro* have shown that immune cell cytokines such as interferon-γ (INF-γ), interleukin-1 (IL-1) and tumor necrosis factor-α (TNF-α) induce HLA–DR expression in glandular eptihelial cells and inhibit their proliferation consistent with the phenotype of the basalis. The expression of decidua related genes, such as prolactin, in endometrial stromal cells *in vitro* is also inhibited by IL-1 and TNF-α, illustrating further the ability of pro-inflammatory cytokines to modulate endometrial differentiation[7,8]. Some genes are expressed in the superficial but not basal endometrial layer. For instance, expression of interstitial collagenase (matrix metalloproteinase-1, MMP-1), a proteinase that controls lysis of the interstitial matrix, is limited to endometrial stromal cells of the functional layer during the late secretory phase, immediately prior to menstruation[9–11]. Differential zonal expression of genes such as MMP-1 explains why only the superficial endometrial layer is shed during menstruation.

SEX STEROID RESPONSIVENESS OF MYOMETRIUM

Zonal polarization is not limited to the endometrium. Human non-gravid myometrium also differentiates in response to ovarian sex steroids into a subendometrial layer or junctional zone and an outer myometrial layer[12,13]. Compared to the outer myometrial layer the junctional zone myocytes are characterized by higher cellular density and lower cytoplasmatic-nuclear ratio[14]. These structural differences allow *in vivo* visualization of the myometrial zonal anatomy by T2-weighted MR imaging. The human myometrium is also functionally polarized. Videovaginosonography studies have shown that propagated myometrial contractions in the non-pregnant uterus originate only from the junctional zone and that the frequency and orientation of these contraction waves are dependent on the phase of the menstrual cycle[15–17]. The mechanism underlying zonal myometrial differentiation is not known but growing evidence suggests that ovarian hormone action may be mediated through cytokines and uterotonins locally released by the basal endometrial layer and endometrio-myometrial T-lymphocytes[18].

EUTOPIC ENDOMETRIUM AND JUNCTIONAL ZONE IN ENDOMETRIOSIS AND ADENOMYOSIS

Marked biochemical disturbances characterize eutopic endometrium of endometriosis and adenomyosis compared to the endometrium from disease-free controls. The most striking differences are the expression of aromatase activity[19,20] and upregulation of IL-6 in eutopic stromal cells[21] and the failure of β3-integrin expression in eutopic glandular cells during the luteal phase of the cycle[22,23]. In addition, overexpression of HLA–DR on glandular epithelium cells[24], increased numbers of macrophages and neutrophils[25], and expression of C_3 complement components in endometrium of diseased women[26] are indicative of an abnormal local eutopic immune cell response. Locally-produced pro-inflammatory factors such as IL-1α, IL-1β, TNF-α and INF-γ, which are also elevated in the peritoneal fluid of patients with endometriosis, are implicated in such disturbance of endometrial function. These cytokines regulate the expression of IL-6[27,28], aromatase activity[29], and chemotactic cytokines such as monocyte chemotactic peptide-1 (MPC-1)[30] and RANTES[31], in eutopic and ectopic endometrial stromal cells. Elevated IL-6 and local estrogen biosynthesis by endometrial stromal cells can amplify the local immune response. Interleukin-6, a multifunctional cytokine, has been shown to act as a mitogenic factor for lymphocytes, can induce differentiation of both B cells and cytotoxic T cells, and is necessary for the production of IgG[32,33]. T-lymphocytes contain ER, which by binding to a classical estrogen response element (ERE) in the INF-γ promoter can increase INF-γ expression in response to locally produced estrogens[34].

Disruption of the specific micro-environment in the basal endometrial layer may explain the junctional zone dysfunction associated with pelvic endometriosis and subfertility[35–37]. A recent study found marked hyperperistalsis during the early and mid-follicular phase and dysperistalsis during the late follicular phase in women with endometriosis. Hysterosalpingoscintigraphy studies indicated that the hyperperistalsis was associated with a marked increase in the transport of inert particles from the vaginal depot to the peritoneal cavity while the peri-ovulatory dysperistalsis resulted in a significant decrease of uterine transport capacity in comparison with healthy controls[36].

On the other hand, irregular thickening of the junctional zone has been associated with adenomyosis[38–40]. Pathologically this has been shown to represent smooth muscle hyperplasia characterized by closely packed smooth muscle fibers that are poorly orientated and less vascular than the smooth muscle of the normal inner myometrium[39]. It is now apparent that extensive hyperplasia of the inner myometrial layer can exist with minimal or no penetration of endometrial glands and stroma into the myometrium. For instance, Reinhold[41] found that only if the junctional zone width is 12 mm or greater

Table 1 Sex steroid hormone (SSH) differentiation of ectopic endometrium

	Ovary/peritoneum	*Myometrium/rectovaginal septum*
Morphology	Surface epithelium, stroma, glands	Smooth muscle, stroma, glands
Microenvironment	Inflammation, macrophages	T-lymphocytes
Endometrial-like tissue	Superficial layer	Basal-junctional zone layer
Endometrial activity	SSH-dependent bleeding	SSH-dependent smooth muscle cell hyperplasia
Clinical presentation	Endometriosis	Adenomyosis

does it become predictive of the presence of endometrial islets at 2.5 mm or deeper below the endometrio-myometrial junction. In addition, endometrial infiltration of the myometrium is commonly patchy and focal while the myoproliferative changes often affect the entire inner myometrium as demonstrated by diffuse thickening on MR imaging. Whether pelvic endometriosis is associated with biochemical changes in inner myometrial smooth muscle cells remains to be determined.

ECTOPIC ENDOMETRIUM IN ENDOMETRIOSIS

Aberrant gene expression in eutopic endometrial cells and junctional zone dysfunction in women suffering from endometriosis indicate that endometriosis may be the consequence of the disruption of sex steroid-dependent differentiation processes in the paramesonephric or Müllerian duct. This 'aberrant' gene expression may not only predispose endometrial cells to colonize sites which allow implantation and development but also modulate the local immune response and result in the expression of endometrial-like activity. As is the case in eutopic endometrium, the topography and local micro-environment of the ectopic implant will determine if its endometrial-like activity resembles that of the eutopic superficial endometrium, with cyclic bleeding and cyst formation, or basal layer, characterized predominantly by smooth muscle hyperplasia and formation of nodular lesions (Table 1).

Sex steroid-dependent bleeding

In the cystic lesions the endometrial implant is composed of surface epithelium and stroma with or without glands. The mucosal vessels in non-fibrotic cysts bleed cyclically in response to ovarian sex steroids, similarly to the terminal spiral arteries in the upper functional layer of the uterus. Cyclic bleeding is seen in red, vesicular lesions of the peritoneum and in ovarian endometriomas. These lesions, but not black peritoneal lesions or deep nodular implants, have been shown to express MMP-1 mRNA[42]. In eutopic endometrium, MMP-1 expression is restricted to the superficial stromal cell compartment in the perimenstrual period[9–11]. This confined temporal expression is thought to be mediated through potent inhibition of MMP-1 gene transcription by estradiol and progesterone[10,43]. In ectopic implants focal expression of MMP-1 messenger RNA can be detected irrespective of the phase of the menstrual cycle[42]. This observation further indicates that although ectopic implants express estrogen and progesterone receptors, the biological activity of these steroid hormone receptors on gene transcription is impaired. The process of tissue remodeling involves proliferation, angiogenesis and hemorrhage and can result in fibrosis and healing (white lesions) or adhesions and pseudocyst formation (endometriomas) depending on the topography of the implant.

Adenomyotic lesion

The nodular type of lesion consists of marked fibromuscular tissue with some glands and stroma and the presence of T-lymphocyte aggregates. These lymphoid aggregates are characteristically found in the endometrio-myometrial junction. Nodular lesions are typically found in the posterior fornix. In ontogenetic terms the posterior fornix is derived from the lower uterine part of the paramesonephric duct and at a higher level than the anterior fornix[44]. Both fornices become hollow by the 20th postovulatory week. Light microscopy of transverse sections of the body of the foetal uterus reveals that by 14 weeks' gestation two layers of mesenchymal cells can be recognized. The outer, subserosal layer consists of elongated cells and is more cellular than the inner layer. Ultrastructurally, the mesenchymal cells of the uterus do not display characteristics of smooth muscle cells until 16 to 18 weeks of gestation. The cells in the outer layer then resemble immature smooth muscle cells. At 26 weeks the thickness of the outer layer increases markedly and by 31 weeks bundles of almost mature smooth muscle cells are present. These microscopical observations resulted in the hypothesis that mesenchymal cells of the outer layer differentiate into immature myofibroblasts and subsequently mature myocytes while those of the inner layer are the precursors of endometrial stromal cells in the adult uterus[45]. An alternative explanation, first proposed in 1898 by Werth and Grusdew[46], is that subserosal mesenchymal cells give rise to the outer myometrium while cells from the inner mesenchymal layer are the progenitors of both endometrial stromal cells and inner myometrial smooth muscle cells[46,47]. As the posterior fornix is derived from these uterine mesenchymal cells it is no surprise that lesions here resemble uterine adenomyosis. If our view is correct then rectovaginal endometriosis is not endometriosis of the rectovaginal septum but cervico-vaginal adenomyosis. This may explain the consistent involvement of the posterior fornix or cervix, but not rectal wall in these lesions. Although the molecular basis of smooth muscle hyperplasia in nodular endometriosis and adenomyosis is unknown, it is likely that the role of endometrial and immune cell interactions on smooth muscle cell differentiation will become an important area of research.

CONCLUSIONS

Endometriosis and adenomyosis represent disruptions of sex steroid hormone-dependent differentiation processes in the paramesonephric duct. It affects all compartments. The phenotypical appearance of the ectopic lesion is dependent upon topography and reflects modulations by local immune cell factors of steroid hormone-dependent gene expression in the target cells.

References

1. Sampson JA. Perforating hemorrhagic (chocolate) cysts of the ovary. *Arch Surg* 1921; 3:245–323
2. Cullen TS. The distribution of adenomyoma containing uterine mucosa. *Arch Surg* 1920;1: 215–83
3. Stewart CJR, Farquharson MA, Foulis AK. The distribution and possible function of gamma interferon-immunoreactive cells in normal endometrium and myometrium. *Virchows Archiv A Pathol Anat* 1992;420:419–24
4. Tabibzadeh SS, Geber MA, Satyaswaroop PG. Induction of HLA-DR antigen expression in human endometrial epithelial cells *in vitro* by recombinant gamma-interferon. *Am J Pathol* 1986;125:656–63

5. Tabibzadeh S. Patterns of expression of integrin molecules in human endometrium throughout the menstrual cycle. *Hum Reprod* 1992;7:876–82
6. Tabibzadeh S, Sun XZ, Kong QF, *et al.* Induction of a polarized micro-environment by human T cells and interferon-gamma in three-dimensional spheroids cultures of human endometrial epithelial cells. *Hum Reprod* 1993;7:182–93
7. Kariya M, Kanzaki H, Takakura K, *et al.* Interleukin-1 inhibits *in vitro* decidualization of human endometrial stromal cells. *J Clin Endocrinol Metab* 1992;73:1170–4
8. Jikihara H, Handwerger S. Tumor necrosis factor-α inhibits the synthesis and release of human decidual prolactin. *Endocrinology* 1994;134: 353–7
9. Hampton AL, Salamonsen LA. Expression of messenger ribonucleic acid encoding matrix metalloproteinases and their tissue inhibitors is related to menstruation. *J Endocrinol* 1994;141: R1–R3
10. Marbaix E, Kokorine I, Henriet P, *et al.* The expression of interstitial collagenase in human endometrium is controlled by progesterone and by oestradiol and is related to menstruation. *Biochem J* 1995;305:1027–30
11. Kokorine I, Marbaix E, Henriet P, *et al.* Focal cellular origin and regulation of interstitial collagenase (matrix matalloproteinase-1) are related to menstrual breakdown in the human endometrium. *J Cell Sci* 1996;109:2151–60
12. Demas BE, Hricak H, Jaffe RB. Uterine MR imaging: effects of hormonal stimulation. *Radiology* 1985;159:123–6
13. Andreyko JL, Blumenfeld Z, Marshall LA, *et al.* Use of an agonistic analog of GnRH (NAFARELIN) to treat leiomyomata: assessment by magnetic resonance imaging. *Am J Obstet Gynecol* 1988;158:903–10
14. Scoutt LM, Flynn SD, Luthringer DJ, *et al.* Junctional zone of the uterus: correlation of MRI and histologic examination of hysterectomy specimen. *Radiology* 1991;179:403–7
15. de Vries K, Lyons EA, Ballard G, *et al.* Contractions of the inner third of the myometrium. *Am J Obstet Gynecol* 1990;162:679–82
16. Lyons EA, Taylor PJ, Zheng XH, *et al.* Characterization of subendometrial myometrial contractions throughout the menstrual cycle in normal fertile women. *Fertil Steril* 1991;55:771–4
17. Kunz G, Beil D, Deininger H, *et al.* The dynamics of rapid sperm transport through the female genital tract: evidence from vaginal sonography of uterineperistalsis and hysterosalpingo-scintography. *Hum Reprod* 1996;11:627–32
18. Brosens J, Brosens I. Adenomyosis. In Cameron I, Fraser I, Smith S, eds. *Clinical disorders of the menstrual cycle and endometrium.* Oxford University Press, 1998: in press
19. Noble LS, Simpson ER, Johns A, *et al.* Aromatase expression in endometriosis. *J Clin Endocrinol Metab* 1996;81:174–9
20. Noble LS, Takayama K, Zeitoun KM, *et al.* Prostaglandin E_2 stimulates aromatase expression in endometriosis-derived stromal cells. *J Clin Endocrinol Metab* 1997;82: 600–6
21. Tseng JF, Ryan IP, Milam TD, *et al.* Interleukin-6 secretion *in vitro* is upregulated in ectopic and eutopic endometrial stromal cells from women with endometriosis. *J Clin Endocrinol Metab* 1996;81:1118–22
22. Lessey BA, Castlebaum AJ, Souvin SJ, *et al.* Aberrant integrin expression in the endometrium of women with endometriosis. *J Clin Endocrinol Metab* 1994;79:643–9
23. Ota H, Tanaka T. Integrin adhesion molecules in the endometrial glandular epithelium in patients with endometriosis or adenomyosis. *J Obstet Gynaecol Res* 1997;23:485–91
24. Ota H, Igarashi S. Expression of major histocompatibility complex class II antigen in endometriotic tissue in patients with endometriosis and adenomyosis. *Fertil Steril* 1993; 60:834–84
25. Leiva MC, Hasty LA, Lyttle CR. Inflammatory changes of the endometrium in patients with minimal-to-moderate endometriosis. *Fertil Steril* 1994;62:967–72
26. Isaacson KB, Galman M, Coutifaris C, *et al.* Endometrial synthesis and secretion of complement component-3 by patients with and without endometriosis. *Fertil Steril* 1990;53: 836–40
27. Akoum A, Lemay A, Paradis I, *et al.* Secretion of interleukin-6 by human endometriotic cells and regulation by proinflammatory cytokines and sex steroids. *Hum Reprod* 1996;11:2269–75
28. Rier SH, Zarmakoupis PN, HuX, *et al.* Dysregulation of interleukin-6 responses in ectopic endometrial stromal cells: correlation with decreased soluble receptor levels in peritoneal fluid of women with endometriosis. *J Clin Endocrinol Metab* 1995;80:1431–7
29. Simpson ER, Michael MD, Agarwal VR, *et al.* Expression of the CYP19 (aromatase) gene: an unusual case of alternative promoter usage. *FASEB J* 1997;11:29–36
30. Akoum A, Lemay A, Brunet C, *et al.* Cytokine-induced secretion of monocyte chemotactic protein-1 by human endometriotic cells in culture. *Am J Obstet Gynecol* 1995; 172:594–600
31. Hornung D, Ryan IP, Chao VP, *et al.* Immunolocalization and regulation of the chemokine RANTES in human endometrial and endometriosis tissues and cells. *J Clin Endocrinol Metab* 1997;82:1621–8
32. Le J, Vilcek J. Interleukin-6: a multifunctional cytokine regulating immune reactions and acute

phase protein response. *Lab Invest* 1989;61: 588–602
33. Houssiau F, Coulie P, van Snick J. Distinct role of IL-1 and IL-6 in human T-cell activation. *J Immunol* 1989;143:2520–4
34. Fox HS, Bond BL, Parslow TG. Estrogen regulates the INF-γ promoter. *J Immunol* 1991;146:4362–7
35. Salamanca A, Beltrán E. Subendometrial contractility in menstrual phase visualized by transvaginal sonography in patients with endometriosis. *Fertil Steril* 1995;64:193–5
36. Leyendecker G, Kunz G, Wildt L, *et al.* Uterine hyperperistalsis and dysperistalsis as dysfunctions of the mechanism of rapid sperm transport in patient with endometriosis and infertility. *Hum Reprod* 1996;11:1542–51
37. Ijland MM, Evers JLH, Dunselman GAJ, *et al.* Relation between endometrial wavelike activity and fecundability in spontaneous cycles. *Fertil Steril* 1997;67:492–6
38. Mark AS, Hricak H, LeRoy WH, *et al.* Adenomyosis and leiomyoma: differential diagnosis by means of magnetic resonance imaging. *Radiology* 1987;163:527–9
39. Togashi K, Ozasa H, Konishi I, *et al.* Enlarged uterus: differentiation between adenomyosis and leiomyoma with MRI. *Radiology* 1989;171:531–4
40. deSouza NM, Brosens JJ, Schwieso JE, *et al.* The potential value of magnetic resonance imaging in infertility. *J Radiol* 1995;50:75–9
41. Reinhold C, McCarthy S, Bret PM, *et al.* Diffuse adenomyosis – comparison of endovaginal US and MR-imaging with histopathologic correlation. *Radiology* 1996;199:151–8
42. Kokorine I, Nisolle M, Donnez J, *et al.* Expression of interstitial collagenase (matrix metalloproteinase-1) is related to the activity of human endometriotic lesions. *Fertil Steril* 1997;68: 246–51
43. Singer CF, Marbaix E, Kokorine I, *et al.* Paracrine stimulation of interstitial collagenase (MMP-1) in the human endometrium by interleukin-1 alpha and its dual block by ovarian steroids. *Proc Natl Acad Sci USA* 1997;94:10341–5
44. O'Rahilly R. Prenatal human development. In Wynn RM, ed. *Biology of the uterus.* New York: Plenum Press, 1977:748
45. Konishi I, Fujii S, Okamura H, *et al.* Development of smooth muscle in the human fetal uterus: an ultrastructural study. *J Anat* 1984;139:239–52
46. Werth R, Grusdew H. Untersuchungen uber die Entwicklung und Morphologie der menschlichen Uterusmuskulatur. *Arch Gynaekol* 1898;55:127
47. Daels J. Uterine contractility patterns of the outer and inner zones of the myometrium. *J Obstet Gynecol* 1974;44:315–16

Endometriosis is an organ-dependent disease. Peritoneal endometriosis, ovarian endometriosis and adenomyotic nodules of the rectovaginal septum are three different entities

4

J. Donnez and M. Nisolle

Several theories relating to the pathogenesis of endometriosis have been proposed since its first detailed description by von Rokitansky in 1860[1]. The most widely accepted theory, the transplantation theory, was proposed by Sampson in 1927, who observed that endometrial cells regurgitated through the Fallopian tubes during menstruation[2].

Three essential conditions must be met in order to consider retrograde menstruation as the explanation for the pathogenesis of pelvic endometriosis[3]. Firstly, endometrial cells must enter the peritoneal cavity through the Fallopian tubes. Secondly, cells within the menstrual debris must be viable and able to be transplanted onto pelvic structures. Thirdly, the anatomical distribution of endometriosis in the pelvic cavity must be correlated with the principles of transplantation for exfoliated cells.

Numerous studies have demonstrated that reflux of endometrial cells in the peritoneal cavity during menstruation is a common and physiological condition in women with patent tubes[4,5]. The viability of endometrial cells was demonstrated by culture of the menstrual effluent or the peritoneal fluid[6,7]. Experimental studies also proved that endometriosis could be induced by exposure of the pelvis to increased amounts of menstrual discharge[8,9]. Implantation of endometrial tissue also induced endometriosis in rabbits[10,11]. The second prerequisite for the transplantation theory implies that cells must not only be viable but also retain the capacity to adhere and proliferate. A large number of adhesive proteins and proteoglycans have been biochemically determined during the last decade. In our group[4,5] it was demonstrated that laminin and fibronectin are two major adhesion glycoproteins that play a key role in, respectively, anchoring epithelial cells to basement membranes and stromal cells to the interstitial matrix[12,13]. Integrins are cell surface glycoproteins which act as receptors for extracellular matrix proteins. The expression of some of them has been described in normal endometrium, where they are important in the interactions between glandular and stromal elements[12,14,15]. The first description of these glycoproteins in endometriotic tissue was given by Beliard *et al* in 1992[16]. The attachment of endometrial tissue fragments to the peritoneum could be explained by the detection of such cell adhesion molecules. Bridges *et al.*[17] described cyclical changes in integrin expression but no difference was observed when comparing endometrial and endometriotic samples. Beliard *et al.*[13] did not find any difference in the expression of laminin and fibronectin in the two tissues. However, in their study, the expression of integrins was found to be present around the endometriotic glands when compared to the endometrium. Such a difference in the expression of fibronectin receptors between the endometrium and endometriosis was not found by the study of Bridges *et al.*[17] and Van der Linden *et al*.[18]. After the adherence of the endometriotic cells to the basement membrane (peritoneum), a local degradation of the extracellular matrix is required. Recently, Marbaix *et al.*[19,20] demonstrated that the marked decline in progesterone concentration at the end of the menstrual cycle would initiate the synthesis and activation of matrix metallo-proteinases (MMP), thereby causing extracellular matrix (ECM) breakdown, tissue collapse and menstruation. The presence of collagenases was thus proved during the menstrual period, and their probable presence in the peritoneal fluid, together with regurgitated endometrial cells, could be one of the elements in the local degradation of the peritoneal extracellular matrix. Recently, Kororine *et al*.[21] detected the presence of MMP in red peritoneal lesions and in ovarian endometriomas independently of the menstrual cycle, suggesting that such lesions could present a shedding independently of the decline in progesterone concentration. This hypothesis was bolstered by the detection of amino-terminal propeptide of type III procollagen in peritoneal fluid, which is a sign of an increase in the metabolism of the extracellular matrix[22].

Recently, *in vitro* studies demonstrated that the invasion index of endometriotic cells was similar to that of bladder metastatic cells lines, suggesting that the invasiveness of endometriotic cells may contribute to the pathogenesis of endometriosis[23].

The anatomical distribution of endometriosis in the pelvic cavity was described by Jenkins *et al.*[24] and correlated to the principles of transplantation for exfoliated cells.

These data suggest that any exposure of the pelvic peritoneum to menstrual reflux would result in an increased risk of endometriosis. As retrograde menstruation can be considered as a physiological occurrence in menstruating women with patent tubes[4], how can we explain the finding that not all such women have endometriosis at laparoscopy ?

To explain the discrepancy between the occurrence of regurgitation and endometriosis, one must consider the volume of regurgitated menstrual debris: it may be determined by anatomic-mechanical predispositions. Ayers and Friedenstab[25] showed uterotubal junction hypotonia in endometriosis patients, compared with (infertile) controls. Their findings seem to be corroborated by Bartosik *et al.*[26], who found more endometrial cells in the abdominal cavity during flushing of the tubes in endometriosis patients. Recently, Salamanca & Beltran[27] demonstrated that in women with endometriosis, the propagation direction of the subendometrial myometrial contractive wave in the menstrual phase showed a predominant retrograde pattern, whereas the control group showed a normal antegrade pattern.

Short cycle lengths and long durations of menstruation with heavy flow[21,22], and therefore an increased exposure to retrograde menstruation, have been reported as risk factors for endometriosis[28]. Moreover, there is a high prevalence of endometriosis in girls with congenital menstrual outflow tract obstruction[29,30]. But even if volume is one important factor, there is no doubt that the other etiological factors such as hereditary contribution and immunologic deficiency[31,32] also account for implantation.

In 1991 Oosterlinck *et al.*[33] reported defective NK cell activity in endometriosis patients, also resulting in decreased cellular immunity. This could suggest that in endometriosis patients, macrophages may not have sufficient capacity to clean the pelvic cavity of regurgitated debris[34]. Recently, Rana *et al.*[35] reported a significantly higher basal or stimulated *in vitro* macrophage production of TNFα, IL-8 and IL-10 in the peritoneal fluid of endometriosis patients. TNFα and IL-8 are proinflammatory cytokines, being involved in the angiogenic process[36]. Moreover, TNFα could facilitate the *in vitro* adherence process of stromal cells to the mesothelium[37].

The role of traumatism of the mesothelium was suggested by Van der Linden *et al.*[38], who cultured endometrial cells on amniotic membranes. Adherence of endometrial cells on the epithelial surface of the amniotic membranes was never observed when it was intact. They suggested that an intact epithelium could be an important defense mechanism in preventing initial adhesion of retrogradely-shed endometrial fragments to peritoneum.

The coelomic metaplasia hypothesis proposed by Meyer[39] states that the original coelomic membrane undergoes metaplasia forming typical endometrial glands and stroma.

The coelomic metaplasia theory is supported by the description of cases of endometriosis in which retrograde menstruation does not occur and cannot be explained by Sampson's theory[2]. Endometriosis was described in the prostatic utricle of men with prostatic carcinoma undergoing high-dose estrogen therapy[40,41], and in patients with Rokitansky–Kuster–Hauser syndrome[42] where there is no endometrium capable of being a source of endometriotic cells. The origin of pelvic endometriosis by metaplasia from the pelvic peritoneum is consistent with the supposed Müllerian potentiality of this tissue, which has been referred to as a secondary Müllerian system[43]. Lauchlan first used the term 'secondary Müllerian system' to refer to all Müllerian-type epithelium (including endometriotic lesions) located outside the cavities of the original Müllerian ducts. Moreover, common epithelial tumors of the ovary are considered to be derived from the surface epithelium (coelomic epithelium or mesothelium) covering the ovary and from the underlying stroma[44]. Considering the metaplastic potential of the ovarian surface epithelium, ovarian endometriosis could also be explained by the metaplasia theory[45–47]. In spite of the histological reports of Fujii[45,46] and Nakamura *et al.*[47] which demonstrated the transformation of ovarian surface epithelium into other tissues (ciliated cells, endometrial-type epithelium), the metaplasia theory has not been widely supported until now, the transplantation theory of Sampson[2] being the most widely accepted.

In the pelvis, three different forms of endometriosis must be considered: (1) peritoneal endometriosis; (2) ovarian endometriosis; and (3) endometriosis of the rectovaginal septum[48].

Peritoneal endometriosis

According to our morphological data and morphometric evaluation of the stromal vascularization[49,51], there is an obvious similarity between proliferative eutopic endometrium and red peritoneal lesions. Morphologically, red peritoneal lesions are systematically located on the peritoneal surface and characterized by numerous proliferative glands with a columnar or pseudostratified epithelium, as observed in proliferative eutopic endometrium. Hyperplasia areas, characterized by an increase in the number of endometrial glands in relation to the stroma, were observed in 12% of red lesions[50,51]. In such cases, the distinction between peritoneal lesions and eutopic endometrium was very difficult for the pathologist. The glandular proliferative status of red lesions is similar to that observed in eutopic endometrium, revealing a similar degree of activity. Indeed, the glandular proliferation index, immunohistochemically evaluated with the monoclonal antibody Ki-67, was similar in eutopic endometrium and red lesions during the proliferative phase[50,51]. The stromal vascularization measured by the capillaries/stroma surface area was similar in eutopic endometrium and red lesions[49]. An increase in the stromal vascularization was observed during the secretory phase in both tissues, corroborating the morphological characteristics which have been described by several authors in eutopic endometrium[52,53]. The gradual increase in the arborization and coiling of spiral arteries during the preovulatory phase is amplified in the postovulatory period.

When compared with eutopic endometrium[54], the presence of a lower expression of cytokeratin in the epithelium of peritoneal endometriosis could be interpreted as a lower degree of differentiation or as a delay in the differentiation. Indeed, in hyperplastic endometrial lesions, the loss of vimentin expression and the absence of secretory changes give rise to suspicion regarding their benign process[55]. It has also been interpreted as a low degree of cell differentiation. The loss of vimentin in eutopic endometrium during the secretory phase could be responsible for the cell disorganization associated with an ischemic process and could play a role in menstruation and implantation[56]. It may also reflect a change in glandular function[54]. A similar decrease throughout the cycle was observed in eutopic endometrium as well as in ectopic peritoneal endometrium.

The significantly lower vimentin expression in the epithelium of red lesions led us to suggest that it can be related to a trend toward hyperplasia.

Our morphological and morphometric data allow us to suggest that eutopic endometrium and red peritoneal lesions are similar tissues, red lesions being recently implanted regurgitated endometrial cells[50,51]. These data constitute an argument in favor of the transplantation theory for peritoneal endometriosis.

Following endometrial tissue transplantation, the factors that regulate the attachment phase and thereafter initiate ectopic growth are not known. We demonstrated that red lesions are consistently located on the surface of the peritoneum, which histologically consists of a thin layer of loose connective tissue covered with a layer of mesothelium. There is a rich supply of subperitoneal blood vessels and lymphatics[57]. We recently observed in red flame-like lesions, biopsied together with the normal peritoneum surrounding them, that between the stroma which had recently implanted onto the peritoneal surface and the peritoneal and subperitoneal layers, an extensive vascular network was obviously present in fresh lesions, demonstrating the importance of angiogenesis in the early stages of development after implantation[50,51]. In our opinion, vascularization of endometriotic implants is probably one of the most important factors of growth and invasion of other tissue by endometrial glands[49,58]. The 3-dimensional representation of the vascular network located at the junction between the red lesions and the peritoneum revealed to us the main role of angiogenesis[50,51]. The high stromal vascularization suggests an angiogenesis induced by recent implantation[59] via growth factors or cytokine secreted in the stroma. Hypervascularization permits further implantation in the subperitoneal fatty tissue[58].

Once implantation has occurred, possibly facilitated by the NK defect according to the hypothesis of Oosterlinck[33], the further growth of the lesions will depend on the formation of new capillaries. Soluble substances involved in angiogenesis have been detected in the peritoneal fluid of women with endometriosis[60]. It seems reasonable to infer that the angiogenic factors, present in the peritoneal fluid of 58.3% of women with endometriosis, will facilitate the growth of the endometriotic implants. These angiogenic factors could be produced by peritoneal macrophages, retrogradely-menstruated endometrial cells, and/or the ectopic endometriotic lesions themselves[60].

The hypothesis that endometriotic implants secrete cytokines that recruit and activate peritoneal macrophages has been proposed[61]. Macrophage chemotactic activity is present in the peritoneal fluid of women with endometriosis. Khorram *et al.*[61] demonstrated the presence of cytokines at higher concen-trations in the peritoneal fluid of women with endometriosis than in normal controls. Activated peritoneal macrophages could be an important source of peritoneal fluid IL-8. Recently, Ryan *et al.*[62] pointed out a significant correlation between peritoneal fluid IL-8 concentration and the stage of endometriosis, and suggested that IL-8 is an important angiogenic factor that contributes to the pathogenesis of endometriosis by promoting the neovascularization and proliferation of ectopic endometrial implants. Further studies are needed to find a relation between high PF IL-8 concentrations and the presence of red peritoneal lesions.

Immunohistochemical studies have demonstrated the presence of angiogenic factors in eutopic and ectopic endometrium[62]. In 1993 Ferriani *et al.*[63] detected fibroblast growth factor immunoreactivity in normal and endometriotic tissue, suggesting its role in the proliferation and angiogenesis of normal and ectopic human endometrium.

Red flame-like lesions and glandular excrescences are thus probably the first stage of early implantation of endometrial glands and stroma[50,51]. Their significantly higher stromal vascularization and epithelial mitotic index are responsible for the invasion of ectopic sites by glands and stroma. Thereafter, detachment of glands from viable red endometrial implants, explained by the presence of matrix metallo-proteinases (MMP)[21], could initiate their implantation in other peritoneal sites, as in a metastatic process. Indeed, preliminary data from our group[21] reveal the presence of MMP in the stroma of red lesions throughout the menstrual cycle (although in eutopic endometrium, MMP are detected only during the marked decline in progesterone). After this partial shedding, the remaining red lesion always regrows constantly until the next shedding, but menstrual shedding finally induces an inflammatory reaction, provoking a scarification process which encloses the implant. The enclosed implant becomes a 'black' lesion because of the presence of intraluminal debris. This scarification process is probably responsible for the reduction in vascularization, as proved by the significant decrease in the capillaries/stroma relative surface area[49]. In some cases, the inflammatory process and subsequent fibrosis totally devascularize the endometriotic foci, and white plaques of old collagen are all that remain of the ectopic implant[50,51]. White opacification and yellow-brown lesions are latent stages of endometriosis[49]. They are probably nonactive lesions which could be quiescent for a long time.

In agreement with Brosens[64], we regard red lesions as early endometriosis and black lesions as advanced endometriosis[49,65]. White lesions are believed to be healed endometriosis or quiescent or latent lesions[49].

This hypothesis corroborates the clinical studies of Redwine[66] and Goldstein *et al.*[67] that red lesions precede the others, and that with time their presence decreases, being replaced by black and ultimately white lesions. Red petechial lesions were found in adolescents[67]. The shedding and implantation of endometrial cells is a process that occurs during the initial phase of reproductive life. The fact that this period is characterized by anovulatory cycles is in accordance with the hypothesis that anovulation, with a low progesterone concentration in the peritoneal fluid, is the favored time for the implantation of endometriosis[68] (Figure 2).

In our study, black lesions rarely demonstrated typical progestational changes, although some authors have reported that 70% of foci with a cycle pattern underwent changes that were considered synchronous (± 3 days) with the eutopic endometrium[50,51,69]. This probably is owing to the fact that, in some cells (but < 20%), some basal vacuoles can be observed. Nevertheless, this sign cannot be interpreted as a typical secretory change because it has to be revealed in > 50% of the epithelial cells to be considered a secretory change and because basal vacuoles can also be observed in anovulatory cycles or in the absence of progesterone[52,70]. The comparison of the steroid receptor content of endometriosis with eutopic endometrium and their cyclic changes is a subject of controversy. This discrepancy between the results of the different studies may be due to the different assay methods used. In particular, biochemical assays which require a tissue homogenate obscure the heterogeneity of receptor content between glands and stroma, and between endometriotic implants and non-endometrial tissue[71]. It could also be explained by the selection of the endometriotic implants; indeed in most studies, both peritoneal and ovarian lesion data were mixed up. Metzger[72] found that ER and PR content of endometriotic implants correlated well with the receptor content of the corresponding endometrium, although only 13% of endometrial implants were found histologically synchronous with the corresponding intrauterine endometrium. The discrepancy between the apparent lack of histological response and the apparently appropriate steroid receptor regulation suggests that histological transformation is influenced by factors other than steroid receptor regulation.

In our quantitative immunohistochemical study, cyclic changes were noted in eutopic endometrium as well as in black lesions[73]. Indeed, the ER content of glandular epithelium and stroma decreased significantly during the secretory phase in the same way in both ectopic and eutopic endometrium. The ER content was, however, lower in the glandular epithelium of black lesions than in eutopic endometrium. The PR content and its cyclic changes were similar in both endometrium and endometriosis, except in the glandular epithelium during the late secretory phase where a persistently high PR content was observed in black lesions[50,51].

The ectopic foci are more or less autonomous, not governed by the normal control mechanisms governing the uterine endometrial glands and stroma. The exact reason why a number of implants or cells do not respond to hormonal therapy is not known, but at least four hypotheses have been proposed: (1) the drug does not gain access to the endometriotic foci because fibrosis surrounding the foci prevents access locally; (2) endometriotic cells may have their own genetic programming, while endocrine influence appears to be only secondary and dependent on the degree of differentiation of the individual cell; (3) fewer estrogen receptors are present in peritoneal ectopic endometrium when compared to eutopic endometrium; (4) the different regulatory mechanisms of endometriotic steroid receptors may result in deficient endocrine dependency because the receptors, although present, are biologically inactive. In our opinion, the persistence of PR in both the epithelium and stroma of endometriotic lesions may explain the inadequacy of medical theory, and may be the reason why peritoneal endometriosis can quickly recur after cessation of medical therapy[74].

In peritoneal endometriosis, after GnRH agonist administration, we recently demonstrated a low rate of mitosis and a poor stromal vascularization[75]. Our hypothesis is that under GnRH agonist, lesions are in latent stages. They are probably non-active lesions which could be quiescent as long as estrogen secretion is suppressed. But the fact that residual areas of active endometriosis are present in 78% of cases explains the quick recurrence observed after cessation of therapy.

Ovarian endometriosis

The pathogenesis of typical ovarian endometriosis is a source of controversy. The original paper by Sampson[76] on this condition reported that perforation of the so-called chocolate cyst led to spillage of adhesions and the spread of peritoneal endometriosis. The findings of Hughesdon[77] contradicted Sampson's hypothesis and suggested that adhesions are not the consequence but the cause of endometrioma formation. He demonstrated by serial section of ovaries containing an endometrioma that 90% of typical endometriomas are formed by invagination of the cortex following the accumulation of menstrual debris from bleeding of endometrial implants, which are located on the ovarian surface and adherent to the peritoneum. The site of perforation, as described by Sampson[76], could represent the stigma of invagination. The observations of Brosens *et al.*[78], based on ovarioscopy and *in situ* biopsies, were in agreement with the hypothesis of Hughesdon[77]. In 93% of typical endometriomas, the pseudocyst is formed by an accumulation of menstrual debris from the shedding and bleeding of active implants located by ovarioscopy[78] at the site of inversion, resulting in a progressive invagination of the ovarian cortex. Other authors[79] have suggested that large endometriomas may develop as a result of the secondary involvement of functional ovarian cysts in the process of endometriosis. Donnez and Nisolle[58,80] recently published a different hypothesis on the development of ovarian endometriosis. Coelomic metaplasia of invaginated epithelial inclusions could be responsible for this pathogenesis. This hypothesis, based on the metaplastic potential of the pelvic mesothelium, is already a widely accepted theory on the pathogenesis of common epithelial ovarian tumors[44].

According to our classification[81], there are three different types of ovarian endometriosis: (1) superficial hemorrhagic lesions; (2) hemorrhagic cysts (endometriomas); and (3) deep-infiltrating ovarian endometriosis. The presence of active foci deeply infiltrating the ovarian cortex led us to suggest that different pathogeneses must be considered as such a development from epithelial inclusions in the ovary.

Although recent papers and debates[78,79] have tried to classify endometriomas, considerable uncertainty still exists. We believe that ovarian endometriosis is caused by metaplasia of the invaginated coelomic epithelium. Our arguments are the following[50,51]: (1) In our series, we found 12% of endometriomas not fixed to the broad ligament and Hughesdon's theory cannot explain the formation of the endometrioma in these cases. (2) It was not unusual to find multilocular endometriomas, which cannot be explained by the theory of adhesions and bleeding of active superficial implants adherent to the peritoneum. (3) The epithelium covering the ovary, which is the mesothelium, can invaginate in the ovarian cortex. Invaginations of the mesothelial layer covering the ovarian tissue were described by Motta *et al.*[82] in animal and fetal ovaries, and were also visualized in human adult ovaries. Indeed, in our serial sections of the ovary, it is common to see mesothelial inclusions. Under the influence of so far unknown growth factors, these inclusions could be transformed into intra-ovarian endometriosis by metaplasia. (4) The fact that primordial follicles were found surrounding the endometriotic cyst is also in agreement with our hypothesis[80]. When the mesothelium invaginates deep in the ovary, the follicles located at the invagination site are pushed concomitantly with the mesothelium. (5) Our main argument the presence of epithelial invaginations in continuum with endometrial tissue, proving the metaplasia theory[50,51,80]. (6) Another major argument is the demonstration, in our study[50,51,80], of the capacity of the endometrioma wall to invaginate secondarily into the ovarian cortex. Such secondary invaginations were observed in 33% of our cases and represent the so-called deep-ovarian endometriosis which is in fact just an extension of the endometrioma wall. (7) Arguments can also be found in the literature. Endometriomas have been described in patients suffering from the Rokitansky–Kuster–Hauser syndrome characterized by the absence of a uterus, and, therefore, without retrograde menstruation[42]. Common epithelial tumors of the ovary are considered to be derived from the surface epithelium covering the ovary and from the underlying stroma[44].

Our theory is thus different from the theory of Hughesdon[77] and Brosens[78], who consider that the pathogenesis of the typical ovarian endometrioma has now been clarified as a process originating from a free superficial implant which is in contact with the ovarian surface and is sealed off by adhesions, the menstrual shedding and bleeding of this small implant resulting in a progressive invagination of the ovarian cortex and the formation of the pseudocyst.

In our opinion, the endometrioma must be considered as an invagination, but not as the result of the bleeding of a superficial implant. Indeed, metaplasia of the coelomic epithelium invaginated into the ovarian cortex was proved and explains the endometrioma formation[80]. In fact, the 'deep-infiltrating ovarian endometriosis' described by our group[81] is only the consequence of invagination of endometriotic tissue into the ovary and is probably responsible for the recurrence of ovarian endometriosis after cyst excision or vaporization[50,51,81,82,83].

Adenomyotic nodules

Another form of the disease is 'deep-infiltrating endometriosis of the rectovaginal septum'. Sampson, in 1922[84], defined cul-de-sac obliteration as 'extensive adhesions in the cul-de-sac, obliterating its lower portion and uniting the cervix or the lower portion of the uterus to the rectum; with adenoma of the endometrial type invading the cervical and the uterine tissue and probably also (but to a lesser degree) the anterior wall of the rectum'.

The endometriotic nodule of the rectovaginal septum was considered by Koninckx and Martin[85] as the consequence of deep-infiltrating endometriosis, and these authors described three subtypes of deep endometriosis according to the depth of infiltration. The rectovaginal septum endometriotic nodule was considered the deepest form of endometriosis and a result of the natural evolution of peritoneal endometriosis in some women. For us, the nodule of the rectovaginal septum is an entity different from peritoneal endometriosis and has another pathogenesis and we strongly suggest that it corresponds to an adenomyotic nodule originating from Müllerian remnants by metaplasia[48,50,51,86,87].

Deep vaginal endometriosis associated with pelvic endometriosis can take the form of nodular or polyploid masses, involving the posterior vaginal fornix[85,86]. The differential diagnosis of vaginal endometriosis, particularly of the superficial type, includes vaginal adenosis of the tuboendometrial variety, but the latter lacks endometrial stroma and the characteristic inflammatory response of endometriosis[88]. In the uterus corpus, adenomyosis is a common condition characterized pathologically by the presence of endometrial glands and stroma within the myometrium. Adenomyosis exhibits a varied functional response to ovarian hormones. Proliferative glands and stroma are generally observed in the first half of the menstrual cycle. Adenomyosis may not respond to physiologic levels of progesterone, and secretory changes are frequently absent or incomplete during the second half of the menstrual cycle. Similar histological observations (no case showed cellular differentiation in phase with eutopic endometrium) can be made at the level of the 'endometriotic' rectovaginal nodule which is, like an adenomyoma, a circumscribed nodular aggregate of smooth muscle, endometrial glands and usually endometrial stroma[48,87]. This lesion originates from the rectovaginal septum tissue and consists essentially of smooth muscle with active glandular epithelium and scanty stroma. The invasion of the smooth muscle by very active glandular epithelium without stroma proves that the stroma is not mandatory for invasion and that the nodule is different from peritoneal endometriosis, in which epithelial glands are systematically surrounded by endometrial-type stroma[50,51]. The very similar histological descriptions to uterine adeno-myosis have led us to suggest, like Brosens[64], that the so-called endometriotic nodule of the rectovaginal septum is, in fact, just like an adenomyoma or an adenomyotic nodule. Nevertheless, the coexpression of vimentin and cytokeratin indicates a close relationship with their mesodermal Müllerian origin[50,51,87]. The significantly lower vimentin expression in the epithelium of nodules[119], when compared to black lesions and eutopic endometrium, has led us to suggest, as we have for red peritoneal lesions, that a low expression of vimentin can be related to a trend towards hyperplasia[54,55,87]. Indeed, very often, the invasion of glandular cells without stroma in the smooth muscle of nodules was clearly seen.

In two recent studies[48,87], we described the differences observed between peritoneal and nodular lesions and we suggested that the nodule is not the consequence of deep-infiltrating endometriosis, as has been

Table 1 Classification of peritoneal endometriosis (typical and subtle) according to its macroscopic appearance

	Macroscopy	*Microscopy*
Black	Puckered black lesions	Endometrial glands and typical stroma with hemosiderin. Intraluminal debris
Red	Red flame-like lesions (vesicular)	Numerous active endometrial glands surrounded by stroma
	Glandular excrescences (vesicular)	Numerous active endometrial glands surrounded by stroma
	Areas of petechial peritoneum, areas of hypervascularization	Numerous red blood cells and rare endometrial glands
White	White opacification of the peritoneum	Occasional retroperitoneal glandular structures and scanty stroma
	Yellow-brown peritoneal patches	Hemosiderin deposits among the stromal cells
	Subovarian adhesions	Connective tissue with sparse endometrial glands
	Circular peritoneal defects	Scarring associated with rare glandular structures

suggested by Koninckx & Martin[85]. These authors suggest that the 'endometriotic' nodule is the consequence of deep infiltration by an active disease and that three types of 'deep-infiltrating endometriosis' can be distinguished according to the depth of infiltration.

Smooth muscle proliferation and fibrosis, consistently observed, are responsible for the nodular aspect of endometriosis located in the rectovaginal septum. The clinical diagnosis is only made when smooth muscle proliferation is sufficient to be felt by vaginal examination. At least two hypotheses could explain this smooth muscle proliferation: (1) endometriotic foci involving smooth muscle are typically associated with a striking proliferation of the smooth muscle, creating an adeno-myomatous appearance similar to that of adenomyosis in the endometrium[89]; (2) the endometriotic stroma may exhibit smooth muscle metaplasia, as has been demonstrated within the wall of ovarian endometriotic cysts[90].

We believe that the first hypothesis is the more accurate. Indeed, the presence of smooth muscle in the organ affected by endometriosis is the condition for smooth muscle proliferation. When endometriotic glands affect the rectovaginal septum, which contains smooth muscle, smooth muscle proliferation can take place and the nodule thus develops. Hyperplasia of the smooth muscle present in the septum provokes perivisceritis at radiography, owing to the inflammatory process and secondary retraction of the rectal serosa. The absence of evolution of the 'rectal lesion' after removal of the nodule supports our hypothesis concerning its pure rectovaginal septum origin[48,86].

The variations of estrogen receptors and progesterone receptors in the nodules throughout the cycle suggest that they are probably not regulated by steroids. In our study, the very low glandular epithelium and stroma estrogen receptor content during the follicular phase can explain the absence of any secretory change in the glandular epithelium nodule[50,87]. In a recent study[91], it was suggested that a low estrogen receptor level was the key factor in explaining the out-of-phase endometrium despite normal progesterone levels, but the reduction in progesterone receptors also could cause resistance to progesterone action and result in inadequate secretory transformation. The absence of response to progesterone levels suggests that the different regulatory mechanisms of endometriotic steroid receptors result in deficient endocrine dependency or that the receptors are present but biologically inactive[92,93]. The low mitotic activity, another low steroid receptor consequence, observed in this pathology can account for the relatively slow evolution of the adenomyoma[86,94].

The very low vimentin immunoreactivity and the absence of any decrease throughout the cycle in the glandular epithelium of nodules account for the low degree of differentiation and the unresponsiveness to endogenic hormonal variations. Nevertheless, the coexpression of vimentin and cytokeratin indicates a close relationship with their mesodermal Müllerian origin.

CONCLUSION

Peritoneal endometriosis is probably caused by the implantation of regurgitated menstrual cells. Rectovaginal endometriosis is, in fact, an adenomyotic lesion and can develop from Müllerian remnants. In conclusion, peritoneal endometriosis, ovarian endometriosis and rectovaginal adenomyotic nodules must be considered as three separate entities with different pathogeneses.

References

1. von Rokintansky C. Ueber Uterusdrusen-Neubildung in Uterus and Ovarialsarcomen. *Zkk Gesellsch d Aerzte zu Wien* 1860; 37:577
2. Sampson JA. Peritoneal endometriosis due to menstrual dissemination of endometrial tissue into the peritoneal cavity. *Am J Obstet Gynecol* 1927; 14:422–69
3. Donnez J, Nisolle M, Casanas-Roux F, *et al.* Endometriosis: pathogenesis and pathophysiology. In: *Endometriosis.* Shaw RW (ed).Carnforth, UK: Parthenon Publishing 1990:11–29
4. Halme J, Hammond MG, Hulka JF, *et al.* Retrograde menstruation in healthy women and in patients with endometriosis. *Obstet Gynecol* 1984;64:151–4
5. Liu DTY, Hitchcock A. Endometriosis: its association with retrograde menstruation, dysmenorrhea and tubal pathology. *Br J Obstet Gynaecol* 1986; 93:859–62
6. Keettel WC, Stein RJ. The viability of the cast-off menstrual endometrium. *Am J Obstet Gynecol* 1951; 61:440–2
7. Kruitwagen RF, Poels LG, Willemsen WN, *et al.* Endometrial epithelial cells in peritoneal fluid during the early follicular phase. *Fertil Steril* 1991 (a); 55:297–303
8. Te Linde RW, Scott RB. Experimental endometriosis. *Am J Obstet Gynecol* 1950;60:1147–73
9. Scott RB, Te Linde RW, Wharton LR Jr. Further studies on experimental endometriosis. *Am J Obstet Gynecol* 1953;66:1082–103
10. Schenken RS, Asch RH, Williams RF, *et al.* Etiology of infertility in monkeys with endometriosis: luteinized unruptured follicles, luteal phase defects, pelvic adhesions, and spontaneous abortions. *Fertil Steril* 1984 (a); 41:122–30
11. Donnez J, Wayembergh M, Casanas-Roux F, *et al.* Effect on ovulation of surgically induced endometriosis in rabbits. *Gynecol Obstet Invest* 1987 (b); 24:131–7
12. Foidart JM, Beliard A, Donnez J. Endometriosis and invasion. In Brosens I, Donnez J, eds. *Current Status of Endometriosis Research and Management.* Carnforth, UK: Parthenon Publishing 1993:35–39
13. Beliard A, Donnez J, Nisolle M, *et al.* Expression of laminin, fibronectin and integrins in endometrium and endometriosis. *Fertil Steril* 1997; 67:266–72
14. Lessey BA, Damjanovich L, Coutifaris C, *et al.* Integrin adhesion molecules in the human endometrium. Correlation with the normal and abnormal menstrual cycle. *J Clin Invest* 1992; 90:188–95
15. Tabibzadeh S, Sun XZ. Cytokine expression in human endometrium throughout the menstrual cycle. *Hum Reprod* 1992;7:1214–21
16. Beliard A, Donnez J, Foidart JM. Laminin and fibronectin expression in endometriotic tissue. In *Proceedings of IIIrd World Congress on Endometriosis,* Brussels, 1992 (Abstract)
17. Bridges JE, Prentice A, Roche W, *et al.* Expression

of integrin adhesion molecules in endometrium and endometriosis. *Br J Obstet Gynecol* 1994; 101:696–700

18. Van der Linden PJ, De Goeij AF, Dunselman GA, *et al.* Expression of cadherins and integrins in human endometrium throughout the menstrual cycle. *Fertil Steril* 1995 (b); 63:1210–16
19. Marbaix E, Kokorine I, Henriet P, *et al.* The expression of interstitial collagenase in human endometrium is controlled by progesterone and by estradiol and is related to menstruation. *Biochem J* 1995;305:1027–30
20. Marbaix E, Kokorine I, Donnez J, *et al.* Regulation and restricted expression of interstitial collagenase suggest a pivotal role in the initiation of menstruation. *Hum Reprod* 1996;11 (Suppl 2):134–43
21. Kokorine I, Nisolle M, Donnez J, Eeckhout Y, Courtoy PJ, Marbaix E. Expression of interstitial collagenase (matrix metalloproteinase-1) is related to the activity of human endometriotic lesions. *Fertil Steril* 1997;68:246–51
22. Spuijbroek MD, Dunselman GA, Menheere PP, Evers JL. Early endometriosis invades the extracellular matrix. *Fertil Steril* 1992;58:929–33
23. Gaetje R, Kotzian S, Hermann G, *et al.* Invasiveness of endometriotic cells *in vitro. Lancet* 1995 ; 346:1463–4
24. Jenkins S, Olive DL, Haney AF. Endometriosis: pathogenetic implications of the anatomic distribution. *Obstet Gynecol* 1986;67:335–8
25. Ayers JW, Friedenstab AP. Utero-tubal hypotonia associated with pelvic endometriosis. *Proc 41st Am Fertil Soc* 1985; 131 (abstract)
26. Bartosik D, Jacobs SL, Kelly LJ. Endometrial tissue in peritoneal fluid. *Fertil Steril* 1986;46:796–800
27. Salamanca A, Beltran E. Subendometrial contractility in menstrual phase visualized by transvaginal sonography in patients with endometriosis. *Fertil Steril* 1995;64:193–5
28. Cramer DW, Wilson E, Stillman RJ, *et al.* The relation of endometriosis to menstrual characteristics, smoking, and exercise. *J Am Med Assoc* 1986; 255:1904–8
29. Sanfilippo JS, Wakim NG, Schikler KN, *et al.* Endometriosis in association with uterine anomaly. *Am J Obstet Gynecol* 1986;154:39–43
30. Olive DL , Henderson DY. Endometriosis and Müllerian anomalies. *Obstet Gynecol* 1987; 69:412–15
31. Simpson JL, Elias S, Malinak LR, *et al.* Heritable aspects of endometriosis. I. Genetic studies. *Am J Obstet Gynecol* 1980;137:327–31
32. Steele RW, Dmowski WP, Marmer DJ. Immunologic aspects of human endometriosis. *Am J Reprod Immunol* 1984;6:33–6
33. Oosterlinck D, Cornillie FJ, Waer M, *et al.* Women with endometriosis show a defect in natural killer cell activity resulting in a decreased cytotoxicity to autologous endometrium. *Fertil Steril* 1991; 56:45–51
34. Dunselmann GA, Hendricx MG, Bouckaert PX, *et al.* Functional aspects of peritoneal macrophages in endometriosis of women. *J Reprod Fertil* 1988; 82:707–10
35. Rana N, Braun DP, House R, *et al.* Basal and stimulated secretion of cytokines by peritoneal macrophages in women with endometriosis. *Fertil Steril* 1996;65:925–30
36. Koch AE, Polverini PJ, Kunkel SL, *et al.* Interleukin 8 as a macrophage derived mediator of angiogenesis. *Science* 1992;258:1798–801
37. Zhang R, Wild R, Ojago J. Effect of tumor necrosis factor-α on adhesion of human endometrial cells to peritoneal mesothelial cells: an in vitro system. *Fertil Steril* 1993;59:1196–201
38. Van der Linden PJ, de Goeij AF, Dunselman GA, *et al.* Endometrial cell adhesion in an in vitro model using intact amniotic membranes. *Fertil Steril* 1996;65:76–80
39. Meyer R. Ueber den Stand der Frage der Adenomyositis und Adenomyome in Algemeinen und Insbesondere ueber Adenomyositis seroepithelialis und Adenomyometritis sacromatosa. *Zbl Gynaekol* 1919;43:745–50
40. Melicow MM, Pachter MR. Endometrial carcinoma of the prostatic utricle (uterus masculinus). *Cancer* 1967;20:1715–22
41. Schrodt GR, Alcorn MD, Ibanez J. Endometriosis of the male urinary system: a case report. *J Urol* 1980;124:722–3
42. Rosenfeld D L, Lecher BD. Endometriosis in a patient with Rokitansky-Kuster-Hauser syndrome. *Am J Obstet Gynecol* 1981;139;105
43. Lauchlan SC. The secondary Müllerian system. *Obstet Gynecol Surv* 1972;27:133–46
44. Serov SF, Scully RE, Sobin LH. Histological Typing of Ovarian Tumors. In: *International Histological Classification of Tumors.* No9. Geneva, World Health Organization, 1973:17–21
45. Fujii S. Secondary Müllerian system and endometriosis. *Am J Obstet Gynecol* 1991;162:219–25
46. Fujii S. Metaplasia: secondary Müllerian system and endometriosis. In Brosens IA, Donnez J, eds. *Current Status of Endometriosis Research and Management*, Carnforth, UK: Parthenon Publishing 1993:19–34
47. Nakamura M, Katabuchi H, Tohya TR, *et al.* Scanning electron microscopic and immunohistochemical studies of pelvic endometriosis. *Hum Reprod* 1993;8:2218–26
48. Donnez J, Nisolle M, Casanas-Roux F, *et al.* Stereometric evaluation of peritoneal endometriosis and endometriotic nodules of the rectovaginal septum. *Hum Reprod* 1995;11:224–8
49. Nisolle M, Casanas-Roux F, Anaf V, *et al.* Morphometric study of the stromal vascularization in peritoneal endometriosis. *Fertil Steril* 1993;59:681–4

50. Nisolle M. Peritoneal, ovarian and rectovaginal endometriosis are three distinct entities. Thèse d'Agrégation de l'Enseignement Supérieur, Université Catholique de Louvain 1996
51. Nisolle M, Donnez J, eds. *Peritoneal Ovarian and Rectovaginal Endometriosis: The Identification of Three Separate Diseases.* Carnforth: Parthenon Publishing, 1996
52. Ferenczy A. Anatomy and histology of the uterine corpus. In Kurman RJ, ed. *Blaustein's Pathology of the Female Genital Tract.* New York: Springer-Verlag, 1987:257–91
53. Peek M, Landgren BM, Johannisson E. The endometrial capillaries during the normal menstrual cycle: a morphometric study. *Hum Reprod* 1992;7:906–11
54. Nisolle M, Casanas-Roux F, Donnez J. Coexpression of cytokeratin and vimentin in eutopic endometrium and endometriosis throughout the menstrual cycle: evaluation by a computerized method. *Fertil Steril* 1995;64:69–75
55. Nakopoulou L, Minaretzia D, Tsionou C, *et al.* Value of immunohistochemical demonstration of several epithelial markers in hyperplasia and neoplastic endometrium. *Gynecol Oncol* 1990; 37:346–53
56. Norwitz ER, Fernandez-Shaw S, Barlow DH, *et al.* Expression of intermediate filament in endometrial glands changes with the onset of pregnancy and in endometriosis. *Hum Reprod* 1991;6:1470–3
57. Bloom W, Fawcett DN. *A Textbook of Histology.* Philadelphia, WB Saunders, 1978:186–7
58. Donnez J, Nisolle M. L'endométriose péritonéale, le kyste endométriotique ovarien et le nodule de la lame rectovaginale sont trois pathologies différentes – Editorial. *Références Gynécol Obstétr* 1995;3:121–3
59. Smith SK. Vascular endothelial growth factor and the endometrium. *Hum Reprod* 1996;11(2 Suppl):56–61
60. Oosterlynck DJ, Meuleman C, Sobis H, *et al.* Angiogenic activity of peritoneal fluid from women with endometriosis. *Fertil Steril* 1993; 59:778–82
61. Khorram O, Taylor RN, Ryan IP, *et al.* Peritoneal fluid concentrations of the cytokine RANTES correlate with the severity of endometriosis. *Am J Obstet Gynecol* 1993;169:1545–9
62. Ryan IP, Tseng JF, Schriock ED, *et al.* Interleukin-8 concentrations are elevated in peritoneal fluid of women with endometriosis. *Fertil Steril* 1995; 63:929–32
63. Ferriani RA, Charnok-Jones DS, Prentice A, *et al.* Immunohistochemical localization of acidic and basic fibroblast growth factors in normal human endometrium and endometriosis and the detection of their mRNA by polymerase chain reaction. *Hum Reprod* 1993;8:11–16
64. Brosens IA. Is mild endometriosis a disease? Is mild endometriosis a progressive disease? *Hum Reprod* 1994;9:2209–11
65. Donnez J, Casanas-Roux F, Nisolle M. Peritoneal endometriosis: new histological aspects. In Brosens I, Donnez J, eds. *Current State of Endometriosis Research and Management.* Carnforth, UK: Parthenon Publishing, 1993:75–87
66. Redwine DB. Age-related evolution in color appearance of endometriosis. *Fertil Steril* 1987; 48:1062–3
67. Goldstein MP, de Cholnoky C, Emans SJ, *et al.* Laparoscopy in the diagnosis and management of pelvic pain in adolescents. *J Reprod Med* 1980; 44:251–8
68. Brosens IA, Koninckx PR, Corveleyn PA. A study of plasma progesterone, oestradiol-17 beta, prolactin and LH levels and of the luteal phase appearance of the ovaries in patients with endometriosis and infertility. *Br J Obstet Gynaecol* 1978;85:246–50
69. Bergqvist A, Ljunberg O, Myhre E. Human endometrium and endometriotic tissue obtained simultaneously: a comparative histologic study. *Int J Gynecol Pathol* 1984;3:135–45
70. Mazur T, Kurman RJ. Normal endometrium and infertility evaluation. In *Diagnosis of endometrial biopsies and curettings. A practical approach.* New York: Springer-Verlag, 1995:7–32
71. Bergqvist A, Ferno M. Estrogen and progesterone receptors in endometriotic tissue and endometrium: comparison of different cycle phases and ages. *Hum Reprod* 1993;8:2211–7
72. Metzger DA. Cyclic changes in endometriosis implants. In Brosens IA, Donnez J, eds. *The Current Status of Endometriosis. Research and Management.* Carnforth, UK: Parthenon Publishing, 1993;89
73. Nisolle M, Casanas-Roux F, Wyns Ch, *et al.* Immunohistochemical analysis of estrogen and progesterone receptors in endometrium and peritoneal endometriosis: a new quantitative method. *Fertil Steril* 1994;62:751–9
74. Evers JL. The second-look laparoscopy for evaluation of the result of medical treatment of endometriosis should not be performed during ovarian suppression. *Fertil Steril* 1987;47:502–4
75. Nisolle M, Casanas-Roux F, Donnez J. Histological study of ovarian endometriosis after hormonal therapy. *Fertil Steril* 1988;49:423–6
76. Sampson JA. Perforating hemorrhagic (chocolate) cysts of the ovary; their importance and especially their relation to pelvic adenomas of endometrial type (adenomyoma of the uterus *Arch Surg* 1921;3:245–323
77. Hughesdon PE. The structure of endometrial cysts of the ovary. *J Obstet Gynaecol Br Emp* 1957; 44:69–84
78. Brosens J, Puttemans P, Deprest J, Rombauts L.

The endoscopic localization of endometrial implants in the ovarian chocolate cyst. *Fertil Steril* 1994; 61:1034–8
79. Nezhat F, Nezhat C, Allan CJ, *et al.* A clinical and histological classification of endometriomas: implications for a mechanism of pathogenesis. *J Reprod Med* 1992;37:771–6
80. Donnez J, Nisolle M, Gillet N, *et al.* Large ovarian endometriomas. *Hum Reprod* 1996;11:641–6
81. Donnez J, Nisolle M, Casanas-Roux F. Classification and endoscopic treatment of ovarian endometriosis. In Popkin E, ed. *Woman's Health Today*. Carnforth, UK: Parthenon Publishing, 1994
82. Motta PM, Van Blerkom J, Mekabe S. Changes in the surface morphology of ovarian germinal epithelium during the reproductive live and in some pathological conditions. *Submicr Cytol* 1992; 99:664–7
83. Donnez J, Nisolle M, Casanas-Roux F, *et al.* Endometriosis: rationale for surgery. In Brosens I, Donnez J, eds. *Current Status of Endometriosis. Research and Management*. Carnforth, UK: Parthenon Publishing, 1993:385–95
84. Sampson JA. Intestinal adenomas of endometrial type. *Arch Surg* 1922;5:21
85. Koninckx PR, Martin D. Deep endometriosis: a consequence of infiltration or retraction or possible adenomyosis externa? *Fertil Steril* 1992; 58:924–8
86. Donnez J, Nisolle M, Casanas-Roux F, *et al.* Rectovaginal septum, endometriosis or adenomyosis: laparoscopic management in a series of 231 patients. *Hum Reprod* 1995;2:630–5
87. Donnez J, Nisolle M, Smoes P, *et al.* Peritoneal endometriosis and 'endometriotic' nodules of the rectovaginal septum are two different entities. *Fertil Steril* 1996; 66:362–8
88. Zaloudek C, Norris HJ. Mesenchymal tumors of the uterus. In Kurman R, ed. *Blaustein's pathology of the female genital tract*. Springer-Verlag 1987: 373
89. Scully RE. Smooth-muscle differentiation in genital tract disorders (Editorial). *Arch Pathol Lab Med* 1981;105:505–7
90. Scully RE. Tumors of the ovary and maldeveloped gonads. *Atlas of Tumor Pathology*. Washington DC: Armed Forces Institute of Pathology, series 2, fascicle 16, 1979:153–4
91. Hirama Y, Ochiai K. Estrogen and progesterone receptors of the out-of-phase endometrium in female infertile patients. *Fertil Steril* 1995;63: 984–8
92. Laatikainen T, Andersson B, Karkkainen J, *et al.* Progestin receptor levels in endometriomas with delayed or incomplete changes. *Obstet Gynecol* 1983;62:592–5
93. Spirtos NY, Yurewicz EC, Moghissi KS, *et al.* Pseudocorpus luteum insufficiency: a study of cytosol progesterone receptors in human endometrium. *Obstet Gynecol* 1985;65:535–40
94. Donnez J, Nisolle M, Smets M, *et al.* Recto-vaginal septum adenomyotic nodule: a distinct entity. A series of 500 cases. *Br J Obstet Gynaecol* 1997;104: 1014–18

Endometriosis is not a disease but an epiphenomenon

5

J.L.H. Evers and G.A.J. Dunselman

INTRODUCTION

In The Netherlands, people believe that babies are brought by storks; tradition calls for a mock stork, carrying a mock baby in its bill, to be placed in front of every house where a baby has recently been born. However, the stork population in The Netherlands is dwindling, as is the number of babies being born each year. This is causing the authorities great concern: it has even been suggested that to counteract the aging of society we need to provide better opportunities for storks to nest! In reproductive medicine, we also apparently are great supporters of popular beliefs. How else can our eagerness to ligate the internal spermatic veins of every oligospermic man with a varicocele be explained? Ample scientific evidence exists from prospective randomized controlled studies that varicocelectomy will not improve pregnancy rates in couples with oligospermic male partners. Yet, thousands of subfertile men are subjected to this procedure annually. And we prescribe cough mixtures for cervical mucus problems. So what about treating endometriosis in subfertile women? Does it help to make a woman hypo-estrogenic for six months? Does it help to laser all visible spots in her abdominal cavity? What is the evidence? Is there any evidence? Is it valid?

MORTALITY AND DENTURES, FERTILITY AND ENDOMETRIOSIS

In developed society, mortality in people with dentures is higher than in people without. This does not mean, however, that dentures kill. It only reflects the increased average age in people needing dentures. Having dentures is an epiphenomenon. (An epiphenomenon [Gr. epi-, and Gr. phainomenon] is a phenomenon that occurs with and seems to result from another.) So, what about fertility in patients with endometriosis? There are many ways to address causality. For example, Wheeler & Malinak[1] have looked at Koch's postulates and have concluded that, with regard to endometriosis-associated subfertility, there is no sound scientific evidence from experiments in humans for the putative relationship; that there is no strong association, if any, between endometriosis and subfertility, except for the severe cases with adhesions and endometriomas; that the association is not consistent from study to study; that the temporal relationship is not correct; that there does not exist a dose–response relationship; that the association is not specific, and that the situation in subfertile endometriosis patients does not show a clear analogy to proved causal relations in other fields of medicine. They only could confirm that the association between endometriosis and decreased fertility may make some epidemiological and biological sense[1], so they necessarily had to conclude that, only two of nine tests of causality being positive, there was insufficient scientific evidence for endometriosis and subfertility to be causally related.

In this chapter we wish to focus on three main issues: (1) is endometriosis more frequent in subfertile women? (2) Do endometriosis patients have a lower fecundity? and (3) Does treatment improve pregnancy rates?

Is endometriosis more frequent in subfertile women?

The prevalence of endometriosis varies from 1–5% in retrospective chart reviews of patients at the time of tubal ligation to 21–72% in unexplained subfertility patients in whom extensive attention was also paid to finding the smallest amounts of endometriosis, sometimes including blind biopsies in patients without visible lesions (Table 1). Balasch and co-workers[2], for example, found histologic evidence of endometriosis in blind biopsies from normal-appearing peritoneum in five of 47 endometriosis patients (11%) and in three of 50 non-endometriosis patients (6%). This confirmed earlier findings by Nisolle and co-workers[3], who also found 6% positive biopsies in non-endometriosis patients. These investigators only took one biopsy per patient. This means that, if they had taken > 16 biopsies per patient, and if sufficient sections had been studied, then all women would have had endometriosis. If endometriosis occurs in all women it is not the condition *per se* which establishes subfertility (if at all) in those patients in whom the lesions are large enough to become visible to the laparoscoped eye.

Table 1 Prevalence of endometriosis. Data taken from reference 15

	Prevalence (%)
Sterilization patients	1–5
Sterilization plus extra attention	10–18
Chronic pelvic pain	9–47
Unexplained subfertility	21–72
Reversal of sterilization	18

Table 2 Spontaneous pregnancy rate in patients with unexplained subfertility. Data taken from reference 4

	Number of patients	*Pregnancy rate*	*95% confidence interval*
Unexplained subfertility	2026	33%	31–35%
Endometriosis	290	28%	23–33%

Do endometriosis patients have a lower fecundity?

The best way to study the putative effect of endometriosis on fertility would be to document the spontaneous pregnancy rate in women with endometriosis but without infertility factors, and to compare it to the spontaneous pregnancy rate in women without endometriosis and without subfertility factors (i.e.'normal' women), all other – known and unknown – factors being kept equal. This for obvious reasons will never be done. Second best, but far worse, is to study the spontaneous occurrence of pregnancies in subfertility patients with endometriosis only, i.e. with no other fertility impairing factors, and to compare it to the spontaneous pregnancy rate in patients of the same age with unexplained subfertility of the same duration. The latter method can be found in Taylor & Collins's review[4] from 1993, in which they collected data from 20 studies (2026 couples) and found a (crude) spontaneous pregnancy rate of 33% (Table 2). The spontaneous pregnancy rate in the non-treated controls of the only (six) randomized controlled studies (RCTs) on endometriosis treatment published so far was 28% (Table 2), and did not differ significantly from that in the unexplained subfertility review[4].

Another way to look at endometriosis and fertility would be to study the results of artificial insemination with donor semen in women with azoospermic husbands. Three studies[5–7] have been published so far (Table 3), documenting pregnancies in 38 out of 59 cases (64%), compared to 46 out of 91 (51%) controls (i.e women without laparoscopic evidence of endometriosis).

Van Rozendaal and co-workers[8] studied the problem directly and found no significant differences in cumulative pregnancy rates

Table 3 Artificial insemination by donor (AID) in endometriosis patients

	Patients	*Pregnancies*	*CPR 12 months*	*95% CI*
Portuondo *et al.*[5]	31 cases	19	61%	42–78%
Jansen[6]	7 cases	2	29%	4–71%
	91 controls	46	51%	40–61%
Rodriquez-Escudero *et al.*[7]	21 cases	17	81%	58–95%

between rAFS-1 endometriosis patients and patients with unexplained subfertility. Also in this way a causal relationship between endometriosis and fertility impairment can not be established.

Does treatment improve pregnancy rates?

Five RCTs[9–13], leading to seven publications, on medical treatment of minimal and mild endometriosis and one on surgical treatment have been published so far (Table 4). The odds ratio for medical treatment to result in pregnancy within 12 months was not in favor of a positive effect (0.9; 95% confidence interval 0.5–1.5). The OR for surgical treatment was 2.0 (95% CI 1.2–3.3). Surgical treatment consisted of excision or ablation of lesions and lysis of adhesions, whereas in controls no removal of lesions and no lysis of adhesions was performed. This study has been criticized because the patients were informed about the procedure having been performed, which as such might have affected pregnancy rates, but it remains the single largest RCT on endometriosis performed to date, and it provides evidence that surgical treatment of minimal and mild endometriosis improves the pregnancy chances of a given patient, although not to the level one would expect in patients like these (Table 5), and definitely

Table 4 Odds ratios (ORs) in six randomized controlled studies (RCTs) of medical and surgical treatment of minimal and mild endometriosis

	Cases		*Controls*			
	Number	*Number pregnant*	*Number*	*Number pregnant*	*OR*	*95% CI*
Medical treatment						
Bayer *et al.*[9]	37	13	36	17	0.6	0.2–1.7
Fedele *et al.*[10]	35	17	36	17	1.1	0.4–3.0
Thomas & Cooke[11]	20	5	17	4	1.1	0.2–6.7
Telimaa[12]	18	6	14	6	0.7	0.1–3.6
Overton *et al.*[13]	32	15	18	7	1.4	0.4–5.4
Common OR					**0.9**	**0.5–1.5**
Surgical treatment						
Marcoux *et al.*[14]	172	50	169	29	2.0	1.2–3.3
Common OR					**2.0**	**1.2–3.3**

not to those of unaffected women. Whether electrocoagulation of the peritoneum, or of the lesions or lysis of adhesions causes the modest increase in fertility remains to be elucidated.

In conclusion, there is insufficient evidence to support the contention that endometriosis *per se* causes subfertility.

Table 5 36 weeks spontaneous pregnancy rates in Marcoux *et al*.s' study[14]

	Patients	*Pregnancy rate*	*95% CI*
Surgery	172	29%	22–36%
No surgery	169	17%	12–24%

References

1. Wheeler JM, Malinak LR. Does mild endometriosis cause infertility? *Seminars Reprod Endocrinol* 1988;6:239–51
2. Balasch J, Creus M, Fabregues F, *et al*. Visible and non-visible endometriosis at laparoscopy in fertile and infertile women and in patients with chronic pelvic pain: a prospective study. *Hum Reprod* 1996;11:387–91
3. Nisolle M, Paidaveine B, Bourdon A, *et al*. Histologic study of peritoneal endometriosis in infertile women. *Fertil Steril* 1990;53:984–8
4. Taylor PJ, Collins JA. *Unexplained Infertility*. Oxford: Oxford Medical Publications, 1992
5. Portuondo JA, Echanojauregui AD, Herran C, *et al*. Early conception in patients with untreated mild endometriosis. *Fertil Steril* 1983;39:22–5
6. Jansen RPS. Minimal endometriosis and reduced fecundability: prospective evidence from an artificial insemination by donor program. *Fertil Steril* 1986;46:141–3
7. Rodriguez-Escudero FJ, Neyro JL, Corcostegui B, *et al*. Does minimal endometriosis reduce fecundity? *Fertil Steril* 1988;50:522–4
8. Van Rozendaal M, Dunselman GAJ, Evers JLH. Selecting the proper control group in trials of rAFS-1 endometriosis associated subfertility. *Hum Reprod* 1994;9:161–2
9. Bayer SR, Seibel MM, Saffan DS, *et al*. Efficacy of danazol treatment for minimal endometriosis in infertile women. *J Reprod Med* 1988;33:179–83
10. Fedele L, Parazzinni F, Radici E, *et al*. Buserelin acetate versus expectant management in the treatment of infertility associated with minimal or mild endometriosis: a randomized clinical trial. *Am J Obstet Gynecol* 1992;166:1345–50
11. Thomas EJ, Cooke ID. Impact of gestrinone on the course of asymptomatic endometriosis. *Br Med J* 1987; 294:272–4
12. Telimaa S. Danazol and medroxyprogesterone acetate inefficacious in the treatment of infertility in endometriosis. *Fertil Steril* 1988; 50:872–5
13. Overton CE, Lindsay PC, Johal B, *et al*. A randomized, double-blind, placebo-controlled study of luteal phase dydrogesterone in women with minimal and mild endometriosis. *Fertil Steril* 1994;62:701–7
14. Marcoux S, Maheux R, Berube S, the Canadian Collaborative Group on Endometriosis. Laparoscopic surgery in infertile women with minimal or mild endometriosis. *N Engl J Med* 1997;337:217–22
15. Dunselman GAJ. *Endometriosis, clinical and experimental aspects*. Thesis Maastricht University, Maastricht, 1988

Epidemiologic issues in the study of endometriosis

6

B. Eskenazi and M. Warner

The purpose of this paper is to review the challenges which confront epidemiologists in determining the frequency of endometriosis in the general population and to review the factors which have been associated with a woman's risk for developing endometriosis. A relatively new hypothesis about a possible causal agent will be discussed.

The frequency of endometriosis in the population depends on its definition and the population studied[1]. For example, in some epidemiologic investigations, endometriosis is defined by visualization and in other studies only by biopsy confirmation. In addition, frequency of endometriosis will vary by the population studied, e.g. clinic-based population or the general population. Also, among clinic-based populations, the prevalence of endometriosis may vary by the reason for presentation.

To illustrate this point, data were accumulated from multiple papers and examined, by indication for surgery, for the prevalence of endometriosis (see Table 1)[1–47]. For example, approximately a quarter of women presenting with pelvic pain will have endometriosis on laparoscopy compared to 20% of those presenting with infertility and 4% of those undergoing tubal sterilization.

The fact that 4% of women undergoing tubal sterilization have endometriosis illustrates the problem in including only symptomatic women in determining the prevalence of the disease in the general population. Clearly, pain is subjective and not all those who experience pain seek treatment and are diagnosed. Using infertility patients to estimate prevalence of disease can also lead to biased estimates since fertility may be untested and, thus, is not known for all women of reproductive age in the population. Estimating population prevalence from women undergoing laparoscopy because of pelvic pain or infertility will probably overestimate the prevalence in the general population. In contrast, estimating population prevalence from a sample of women undergoing tubal ligation is likely to underestimate prevalence in the general population because these women are presumably asymptomatic and fertile[1]. There are a number of population based studies in

Table 1 Prevalence of endometriosis during laparoscopy by indication for surgery

	Total N	*n with endometriosis*	*%*	*Range in %*	*% with minimal/ mild disease*	*Range in %*
Pelvic pain*	2400	588	24.5	4.5–82	70	61–100
Infertility†	14 371	2812	19.6	2.1–78	66	16–95
Tubal Sterilization‡	10 634	433	4.1	0.7–43	92	20–100

Adapted from Eskenazi & Warner[1]. Data from: *, 2–15; †, 2–5, 7–9, 11, 16–38; ‡, 10, 11, 22, 36, 39–47

Table 2 Estimates of incidence of endometriosis by Houston *et al.*[52]

	Number with endometriosis	*Age-specific incidence 100 000 person years*			
Histologically confirmed	171	108.8			
Surgically visualized	81		160.4		
Clinically probable	121			237.4	
Clinically possible	15				246.9
Total	388				

the scientific literature. 'Population' prevalence of endometriosis has been estimated from hospitalized women[48], by report of prior laparoscopy-confirmed diagnosis of endometriosis among women attending family planning clinics[49] and by report of prior diagnoses in population samples of women such as that conducted by the National Health Interview Survey[50] and by Moen and Schei in Norway[51]. All of these studies are likely to lead to a biased estimate of prevalence in that disease cannot be diagnosed in women who have not been examined, undergone laparoscopy/laparotomy, or reported symptoms[1].

Only one study, by Houston *et al.*[52], truly attempted a population-based study. Houston *et al.*[52] examined the medical records of in-patient and out-patient visits of all 15 to 49-year-old female residents in Rochester, Minnesota, between 1970 and 1979. Using census data for the denominator, they estimated the incidence (number of new cases diagnosed during this period of time). They defined cases in four ways from most definite to least definite: histologically confirmed, surgically visualized, clinically probable based on pain and a positive pelvic examination, and clinically possible based on only a positive exam. If all cases are summed (see Table 2), the age-specific incidence per 100 000 person years is 246.9. There were also 131 cases which were lost because of unreviewed medical records.

Prevalence of disease is equal to the incidence multiplied by the average duration of disease. If we assume that the average age of diagnosis of endometriosis is the mid 20s and the disease is present until the end of the reproductive years, approximately age 50, then the average duration may be around 25 years. In this case, the prevalence of endometriosis in the general population should be around 6%, i.e. 246.9 per 100 000 person years multiplied by 25 years. If those 131 cases which Houston *et al.*[52] were not able to review were included, the prevalence could rise to approximately 8%.

Most studies designed to identify risk factors for endometriosis are case-control studies. Of almost 100 studies reviewed, we have identified only a handful which include a laparoscopy-confirmed case group, clear criteria for selection of controls, and have adjusted for potential confounders[21,45,53–62].

In these case-control studies, risk factors which have been found to be associated with an increased risk for endometriosis include older age[45], older age at marriage or first regular intercourse[58], higher social class[53], low alcohol use ($\leq$ 1 drink/week)[55], high caffeine use[54], and being taller[21,63]. In addition, cases compared to controls are more likely to have used tampons for > 14 years, to have longer menstrual flow ($\geq$ 6 days), heavier flow[56], and shorter or longer than average cycle length[21,45]. Endometriosis cases compared to controls are more likely to have used oral contraceptives (OC) in the past[59,60]. Cases are less likely than controls to exercise[21], to smoke (during adolescence)[21,56], to currently or recently have used OCs or intrauterine

Table 3 Endocrine disruptors and endometriosis in humans

Authors	*Study design*	*Size*	*Measured exposure*	*Results*
Mayani *et al.*[65] Israel	laparoscopy case-control	44 cases 35 controls	Dioxin	% positive for TCDD cases 18% controls 3%
Lebel *et al.*[66] Quebec	laparoscopy case-control	86 cases 70 controls	PCBs Chlorinated pesticides	no relationship
Boyd *et al.* (unpublished) Pennsylvania	laparsocopy case-control	15 cases 15 controls	Dioxin Furan PCBs	no relationship
Eskenazi *et al.*[67] Italy	cohort	750 women	TCDD	to be completed 1999

devices[45], to be parous or gravid[51,61,62], and to have irregular cycles[61,62]. Not all the above risk factors have been consistent across all studies. If there are differences across studies in the referral patterns, indication for surgery, or differences in diagnostic criteria (e.g. biopsy, visualization, etc.), it is not surprising that the risk factors identified would be different, since case definition would differ.

Furthermore, it is difficult to infer causal relationships from case-control studies, because it is often difficult to know the temporal relationship between the risk factor and endometriosis. For example, exercise rates may be lower in cases than controls, not because those who exercise are less likely to develop disease, but because women with endometriosis experience pelvic discomfort and, therefore, are less likely to exercise; that is, the risk factor was the 'effect of' rather than the 'cause of' the disease.

A potentially interesting 'risk factor' has been reported in recent years. Tetrachlorodibenzo-*p*-dioxin (TCDD), a ubiquitous chemical in the environment, has been associated with endometriosis in a study of Rhesus monkeys[64]. TCDD, or dioxin, is a by-product of various chemical reactions including chlorine bleaching of paper and combustion processes. It is one of a class of chemicals thought to be an endocrine disruptor and it may also have immunologic effects. The study by Rier *et al.*[64] found that both the incidence of endometriosis and the severity of the disease were related to TCDD exposure in Rhesus monkeys.

As shown in Table 3, four case-control studies have been conducted in humans to explore the association between endocrine disruptors, in particular dioxin, and endometriosis[65, 66]. The cases and controls were drawn from very low exposed populations in Israel[65], in Quebec[66] and in Pennsylvania (Boyd *et al.*, unpublished data). All these studies are fairly small. The studies by Boyd *et al.* and Lebel *et al.*[66] revealed no differences between cases and controls in serum levels of dioxin or dioxin-like chemicals. However, Mayani *et al.*[65] reported that 8 out of 44 cases (18%) had blood samples positive for dioxin compared to 1 out of 35 (3%) of controls (OR = 7.6; 95% CI = 0.9,170). Also, among the Stage III and IV (r-AFS) cases, 25% (5 of 20 women) were positive for dioxin, whereas among Stage I and II cases 12.5% (3 of 24 women) were positive for dioxin.

We are currently studying the frequency of endometriosis in a heavily-exposed population. If an association between TCDD and endometriosis is found in a heavily-exposed population, then it would be important to determine if there is a threshold for that effect or a sub-population which may be particularly susceptible. There are a number of heavily-exposed female populations, but only one with large numbers of women with well-documented exposure levels. This population in Seveso, Italy, a town about 14 kilometers north of Milan, was exposed to high levels of TCDD as a result of an explosion which took place at a chemical plant on 10 July, 1976. This population has been exposed to the highest levels of TCDD known in humans, exposure was to relatively pure TCDD, and individual TCDD exposure could be measured from the blood which was collected and stored between 1976 and 1980.

One disadvantage of studying endometriosis in an exposed cohort is that laparoscopy can only be offered when it is medically indicated and, therefore, disease may not be diagnosed. Our approach is similar to that proposed by Houston *et al.*[52]. We have developed a probability scale for diagnosis. All women in our study were interviewed, had a pelvic examination and vaginal ultrasound, and completed a menstrual diary. Using standardized criteria for diagnosis and for offering laparoscopy, we diagnosed a woman as definitely having or not having endometriosis if she had laparoscopy; women with positive ultrasounds with suspected endometriomas were considered 'highly probable' for disease; women with signs on pelvic examination and clear symptoms were considered 'probable' for disease; women with symptoms *or* signs were considered 'possible' for disease; and women with neither signs nor symptoms were considered 'unlikely' for disease. Data collection has been completed and data analysis is underway.

In conclusion, there are few well-designed case-control studies, there is little consistency in diagnostic criteria for endometriosis, and only one study to date has attempted to estimate true 'population' frequency. There are a number of important areas for future epidemiologic research in endometriosis. The development of an agreed-upon definition and criteria for endometriosis would allow for greater comparison across studies. If a non-invasive biomarker of endometriosis which is both sensitive and specific could be identified, then epidemiologists can help to validate these biomarkers, cohort studies could be more readily conducted, 'population' frequency could be better estimated, the natural history of the disease from menarche to menopause could be investigated, and risk factors which precede rather than follow the onset of disease could be identified. The relationship of endometriosis and endocrine disruptors needs to be understood, given the chronic low level exposure in industrialized populations and, thus, the potential for large and growing impact. Identifying a relationship with endocrine disruptors may provide clues to the pathophysiology of endometriosis.

ACKNOWLEDGEMENTS

We would like to acknowledge the technical support of Rosemary Castorina, MPH and Valerie Taylor. This research was supported by Grant Nos. R824761-01 from the Environmental Protection Agency, R01 ES07171-01 from the National Institutes of Health, and EA-M1977 from the Endometriosis Association.

References

1. Eskenazi B, Warner M. Epidemiology of endometriosis. *Obstet Gynecol Clin North Am* 1997;24:235–58
2. Ajossa S, Mais V, Guerriero S, *et al.* The prevalence of endometriosis in premenopausal women undergoing gynecological surgery. *Clin Exp Obstet Gynecol* 1994;21:195–7
3. Blunt A. The place of laparoscopy in "normal" gynaecological practice. *Aust NZ J Obstet Gynaecol* 1972;12:194–7
4. Cornillie FJ, Oosterlynck D, Lauweryns JM, *et al.* Deeply infiltrating pelvic endometriosis: histology and clinical significance. *Fertil Steril* 1990;53:978–83
5. Duignan NM, Jordan JA, Coughlan BM, *et al.* One thousand consecutive cases of diagnostic

laparoscopy. *J Obstet Gynaecol Br Commonwealth* 1972;79:1016–24

6. Goldstein DP, deCholnoky C, Emans SJ, *et al.* Laparoscopy in diagnosis and management of pelvic pain in adolescents. *J Reprod Med* 1980; 24:251–6
7. Gruppo Italiano per lo Studio dell'Endometriosi. Prevalence and anatomical distribution of endometriosis in women with selected gynaecological conditions: results from a multi-centric Italian study. *Hum Reprod* 1994;9:1158–62
8. Hasson HM. Incidence of endometriosis in diagnostic laparoscopy. *J Reprod Med* 1976;16: 135–8
9. Kleppinger RK. One thousand laparoscopies at a community hospital. *J Reprod Med* 1974;13: 13–20
10. Kresch AJ, Seifer DB, Sachs LB, *et al.* Laparoscopy in 100 women with chronic pelvic pain. *Obstet Gynecol* 1984;64:672–4
11. Mahmood TA, Templeton A. Prevalence and genesis of endometriosis. *Hum Reprod* 1991;6: 544–9
12. Mathias SD, Kuppermann M, Liberman RF, *et al.* Chronic pelvic pain: prevalence, health-related quality of life, and economic correlates. *Obstet Gynecol* 1996;87:321–7
13. Pent D. Laparoscopy: its role in private practice. *Am J Obstet Gynecol* 1972;113:459–68
14. Vercellini P, Fedele L, Arcaini L, *et al.* Laparoscopy in the diagnosis of chronic pelvic pain in adolescent women. *J Reprod Med* 1989; 34:827–30
15. Vercellini P, Fedele L, Molteni P, *et al.* Laparoscopy in the diagnosis of gynecologic chronic pelvic pain. *Int J Gynaecol Obstet* 1990;32:261–5
16. Arumugam K, Templeton AA. Endometriosis and race. *Aust NZ J Obstet Gynaecol* 1992;32:164–5
17. Beral V, Rolfs R, Joesoef MR, *et al.* Primary infertility: characteristics of women in North America according to pathological findings. *J Epidemiol* 1994;48:576–9
18. Berger MJ, Alper MM. Intractable primary infertility in women exposed to diethylstilbestrol *in utero*. *J Reprod Med* 1986;31:231–5
19. Brincat M, Galea R, Buhagiar A. Polycystic ovaries and endometriosis: a possible connection. *Br J Obstet Gynaecol* 1994;101:346–8
20. Chang YS, Lee JY, Moon SY. Diagnostic laparoscopy in gynecologic disorders. *Asia Oceania J Obstet Gynaecol* 1987;13:29–34
21. Cramer DW, Wilson E, Stillman RJ, *et al.* The relation of endometriosis to menstrual characteristics, smoking, and exercise. *J Am Med Assoc* 1986;255:1904–8
22. Drake TS, Grunert GM. The unsuspected pelvic factor in the infertility investigation. *Fertil Steril* 1980;34:27–31
23. Dunphy BC, Kay R, Barratt CLR, *et al.* Female age, the length of involuntary infertility prior to investigation and fertility outcome. *Hum Reprod* 1989;4:527–30
24. El-Yahia AW. Laparoscopic evaluation of apparently normal infertile women. *Aust NZ J Obstet Gynaecol* 1994;34:440–2
25. Fedele L, Bianchi S, Di Nola G, *et al.* Endometriosis and nonobstructive Müllerian anomolies. *Obstet Gynecol* 1992;79:515–17
26. Federici D, Conti E, Costantini W, *et al.* Endometriosis and infertility: our experience over five years. *Hum Reprod* 1988;3:109–11
27. Filer RB, Wu CH. Coitus during menses: its effect on endometriosis and pelvic inflammatory disease. *J Reprod Med* 1989;34:887–90
28. Forman RG, Robinson JN, Mehta Z, *et al.* Patient history as a simple predictor of pelvic pathology in subfertile women. *Hum Reprod* 1993;8:53–5
29. Liston WA, Bradford WP, Downie J, *et al.* Laparoscopy in a general gynecologic unit. *Am J Obstet Gynecol* 1972;113:672–7
30. Mahmood TA, Templeton A. The relationship between endometriosis and semen analysis: a review of 490 consecutive laparoscopies. *Hum Reprod* 1989;4:782–5
31. Matorras R, Rodriguez F, Pijoan JI, *et al.* Are there any clinical signs and symptoms that are related to endometriosis in infertile women? *Am J Obstet Gynecol* 1996;174:620–3
32. Moeloek FA, Affandi B, Samil RS. Peritoneal factors in infertile women in Jakarta, Indonesia. *J Reprod Med* 1984;29:603–8
33. Musich JR, Behrman SJ. Infertility laparoscopy in perspective: review of five hundred cases. *Am J Obstet Gynecol* 1982;143:293–303
34. Sarram M, Rezazadeh A. Endometriosis in diagnostic laparoscopy in Isfahan, Iran. *Int Fed Gynaecol Obstet* 1986;24:117–19
35. Singh KB, Patel YC, Wortsman J. Coexistence of polycystic ovary syndrome and pelvic endometriosis. *Obstet Gynecol* 1989;74:650–2
36. Strathy JH, Molgaard CA, Coulam CB, *et al.* Endometriosis and infertility: a laparoscopic study of endometriosis among fertile and infertile women. *Fertil Steril* 1982;38:667–72
37. Waller KG, Lindsay P, Curtis P, *et al.* The prevalence of endometriosis in women with infertile partners. *Eur J Obstet Gynecol Reprod Biol* 1993;48:135–9
38. Woodworth SH, Singh M, Yussman MA, *et al.* A prospective study on the association between red hair color and endometriosis in infertile patients. *Fertil Steril* 1995;64:651–2
39. Dodge ST, Pumphrey RS, Miyazawa K. Peritoneal endometriosis in women requesting reversal of sterilization. *Fertil Steril* 1986;45:774–7
40. Kirshon B, Poindexter AN, Fast J. Endometriosis in multiparous women. *J Reprod Med* 1989;34: 215–17

41. Liu DTY, Hitchcock A. Endometriosis: its association with retrograde menstruation, dysmenorrhoea and tubal pathology. *Br J Obstet Gynaecol* 1986;93:859–62
42. Moen MH. Endometriosis in women at interval sterilization. *Acta Obstet Gynecol Scand* 1987;66: 451–4
43. Moen MH. Is a long period without childbirth a risk factor for developing endometriosis? *Hum Reprod* 1991;6:1404–7
44. Moen MH, Muus KM. Endometriosis in pregnant and non-pregnant women at tubal sterilization. *Hum Reprod* 1991;6:699–702
45. Sangi-Haghpeykar H, Poindexter AN. Epidemiology of endometriosis among parous women. *Obstet Gynecol* 1995;85:983–92
46. Trimbos JB, Trimbos-Kemper GCM, Peters AAW, *et al.* Finding in 200 consecutive asymptomatic women, having a laparoscopic sterilization. *Arch Gynecol Obstet* 1990;247:121–4
47. Wheeler JM. Epidemiology of endometriosis-associated infertility. *J Reprod Med* 1989;34:41–6
48. National Center for Health Statistics – McCarthy E. *Inpatient Utilization of Short-Stay Hospitals by Diagnosis: United States, 1980.* Hyattsville, MD: National Center for Health Statistics, 1982
49. Vessey MP, Villard-Mackintosh L, Painter R. Epidemiology of endometriosis in women attending family planning clinics. *Br Med J* 1993;306:182–4
50. Kjerulff KH, Erickson BA, Langenberg PW. Chronic gynecological conditions reported by US women: findings from the National Health Information Survey, 1984 to 1992. *Am J Public Health* 1996;86:195–9
51. Moen MH, Schei B. Epidemiology of endometriosis in a Norwegian county. *Acta Obstet Gynecol Scand* 1997;76:559–62
52. Houston DE, Noller KL, Melton LJ, *et al.* Incidence of pelvic endometriosis in Rochester, Minnesota, 1970–1979. *Am J Epidemiol* 1987;125: 959–69
53. Obermeyer CM, Armenian HK, Azoury R. Endometriosis in Lebanon. *Am J Epidemiol* 1986; 124:762–7
54. Grodstein F, Goldman MB, Ryan L, *et al.* Relation of female infertility to consumption of caffeinated beverages. *Am J Epidemiol* 1993;137:1353–60
55. Grodstein F, Goldman MB, Cramer DW. Infertility in women and moderate alcohol use. *Am J Public Health* 1994;84:1429–32
56. Darrow SL, Vena JE, Batt RE, *et al.* Menstrual cycle characteristics and the risk of endometriosis. *Epidemiol* 1993;4:135–41
57. McCann SE, Freudenheim JL, Darrow SL, *et al.* Endometriosis and body fat distribution. *Obstet Gynecol* 1993;82:545–9
58. Darrow SL, Selman S, Batt RE, *et al.* Sexual activity, contraception, and reproductive factors in predicting endometriosis. *Am J Epidemiol* 1994;140:500–9
59. Parazzini F, Ferraroni M. Epidemiology of endometriosis. *Br Med J* 1993;306:930–1
60. Parazzini F, Ferraroni M, Bocciolone L, *et al.* Contraceptive methods and risk of pelvic endometriosis. *Contraception* 1994;94:47–55
61. Parazzini F, Ferraroni M, Fedele L, *et al.* Pelvic endometriosis: reproductive and menstrual risk factors at different stages in Lombardy, northern Italy. *J Epidemiol Community Health* 1995;49:61–4
62. Candiani GB, Danesino V, Gastaldi A, *et al.* Reproductive and menstrual factors and risk of peritoneal and ovarian endometriosis. *Fertil Steril* 1991;56:230–4
63. Laufer MR, Goitein L, Bush M, *et al.* Prevalence of endometriosis in adolescent girls with chronic pelvic pain not responding to conventional therapy. *J Pediatr Adolesc Gynecol* 1997;10:199–202
64. Rier S, Martin D, Bowman R, *et al.* Endometriosis in Rhesus monkeys (*Macaca mulatta*) following chronic exposure to 2,3,7,8-tetrachlorodibenzo-p-dioxin. *Fund Appl Toxicol* 1993;21:433–41
65. Mayani A, Barel S, Soback S, *et al.* Dioxin concentrations in women with endometriosis. *Hum Reprod* 1997;12:373–5
66. Lebel G, Dodin S, Ayotte P, *et al.* Organochlorine exposure and the risk of endometriosis. *Fertil Steril* 1998;69:221–8
67. Eskenazi B, Mocarelli P, Warner M, *et al.* Seveso Women's Health Study: a study of the effects of TCDD on reproductive health. *Chemosphere* 1999, in press

Endometriosis in adolescence: epidemiology, investigation and diagnosis

7

M.R. Laufer

INTRODUCTION

Adolescents frequently complain of dysmenorrhea and pelvic pain. Traditionally, non-steroidal anti-inflammatory drugs (NSAIDs) and oral contraceptive pills (OCPs) are the first line of treatment; however, many adolescents continue to describe pelvic pain despite these medications. For these young women, it is important to include endometriosis in the differential diagnosis. Endometriosis in adult women is commonly associated with cyclic pelvic pain; however the symptoms in adolescents may include acyclic and cyclic pain. Treatment of endometriosis usually combines surgery and hormonal therapy. It is estimated that 4 to 17% of postmenarchal females have some degree of endometriosis[1]. Although in the past it was assumed that endometriosis presented only after many years of men-struation, numerous series have shown rates of endometriosis at 50–70% of adolescents undergoing laparoscopy for pelvic pain who did not control it with OCPs and NSAIDs[2,3,4].

With education of young women, pediatricians, nurse practitioners, family practitioners, gynecologists, and pediatric surgeons we may be able to decrease the length of time from the onset of symptoms to presentation, and from the time of presentation to diagnosis. In addition, with early diagnosis of endometriosis it may be possible to decrease the long-term effects of the disease (pain, masses and infertility), and thus improve the quality of life of young women who are affected.

THE ORIGIN OF ENDOMETRIOSIS

It is important to note that some patients may have a genetic predisposition towards developing endometriosis. This is suggested by the observation that 6.9% of first degree female relatives of patients with endometriosis are affected, as compared to 1% or less of controls[5].

The source of endometrial tissue outside the uterus is still debated, but there are four widely supported theories which have been formulated to explain the origin of endometriosis. In a classic 1927 article, Sampson suggested that retrograde menstruation through the Fallopian tubes results in seeding the pelvis with endometrial tissue[6]. This theory is supported by the observation that endometriosis occurs most commonly in the dependent portion of the pelvis. Furthermore, obstructive anomalies of the female genital tract that enhance retrograde flow have been associated with endometriosis in the adolescent population[7–9]. Schiffren and colleagues identified six adolescents with Müllerian anomalies associated with endometriosis, the youngest being a 12-year-old with vaginal atresia and bicornuate uterus leading to a hematocolpos[8]. Furthermore, repair of this type of obstructive anomaly has been associated with resolution of endometriosis[9].

In the second theory seeking to explain the origin of endometriosis, Meyer proposed that metaplastic cells transform into endometrial cells[10]. The third theory suggests endometriosis metastasizes through lymphatic and vascular channels[11]. This would explain the finding of endometriosis in tissue remote from the pelvis such as the lung, brain, and skin. The most recent theory suggests that a deficiency in cellular immunity allows the ectopic endometrial tissue to proliferate[12].

All these theories help explain some aspects of endometriosis, but no single theory explains all cases of endometriosis, especially when relating to adolescents. One very challenging scenario is that of post-pubertal/ pre-menarcheal endometriosis. Most probably the cause of endometriosis is multifactorial, and all proposed mechanisms may contribute to the etiology of this disease process.

DIAGNOSIS OF ENDOMETRIOSIS

Evaluation of pelvic pain

In adult women endometriosis is suspected when a patient presents with chronic pelvic pain, dysmenorrhea, dyspareunia, a pelvic mass, or infertility. In adults the pain of endometriosis is most often cyclic pain, but in the adolescent population pelvic pain is most often acyclic and cyclic[4]. In addition, bowel and bladder symptoms may be common in adolescents found to have endometriosis[4].

Initial evaluation of an adolescent with pelvic pain should include a thorough history. A pain diary documenting frequency and character of pain will help the adolescent and her caregiver to determine whether pain is cyclic, or whether it is related to bowel or bladder function. Complaints of difficulty participating in normal activities, missing school or avoiding extracurricular activities secondary to pain suggest that medical intervention is appropriate. A family history of endometriosis is correlated with a higher likelihood of endometriosis in the patient[5]. A history of sexual abuse or physical abuse may also be associated with chronic pelvic pain[13], but should not preclude further evaluation.

The gynecological examination is very important. For an adolescent who is not sexually active, a rectal-abdominal exam may be better tolerated than a vaginal-abdominal exam. Common findings in the setting of endo-metriosis include cul-de-sac tenderness and nodularity[14]. Cultures for gonorrhea and chlamydia should be performed and a stool hemoccult may also be helpful.

Laboratory studies should include a pregnancy test. A CBC (complete blood count) and erythrocyte sedimentation rate will rule out an inflammatory process. Urinalysis and urine culture help identify a urinary tract source of pain. In patients with a known diagnosis of endometriosis, CA-125 may be used to follow the progress of disease, but this assay is not a useful screening test owing to its high rate of false positives[15]. We prefer to rely on reporting of symptoms to follow endometriosis, and do not use CA-125 in clinical management.

Ultrasound evaluation of the pelvis is the most helpful radiological study in the setting of pelvic pain. In adults endometriomas may often be identified on ultrasound; however, endometriomas are rarely seen in adolescents. Ultrasound can identify other causes of pelvic pain such as ovarian cysts, torsion, tumors, genital tract anomalies and appendicitis. CT scan with contrast may help rule out appendicitis in cases of acute pain, but is otherwise not helpful. MRI is an excellent but expensive modality for evaluation of genital tract anomalies.

Empiric treatment

The differential diagnosis of chronic pelvic pain is wide ranging[16]. When the evaluation of pain suggests a non-acute gynecological source such as primary dysmenorrhea, endometriosis or adhesions, a trial of non-steroidal anti-inflammatory agents (NSAIDs) is recommended. The patient should begin the medication before the expected onset of severe pain if possible. A low-dose oral contraceptive may also improve symptoms of dysmenorrhea by suppressing hormonal stimulation associated with ovulation, and decreasing menstrual flow.

In cases where disabling pain persists laparoscopy to rule-out endometriosis is essential. We have found that 69% of adolescents with pelvic pain not responding to a trial of NSAIDs and OCPs were found to have cyclic endometriosis[4].

Laparoscopy

In the adolescent population it is especially important to achieve a good cosmetic result with laparoscopy. To minimize visible scarring, the laparoscope trocar can be placed through a vertical umbilical incision. Additional operative ports should be placed symmetrically 1 to 2 cm above the pubic symphysis so that the pubic hair will grow over the incision site(s).

Endometriotic implants have variable morphology which has been described in the revised American Society of Reproductive Medicine classification of endometriosis[17]. Only one series has objectively compared lesions in adolescents to those found in adults[18]. This series suggests red-flame lesions are more common in adolescents with endometriosis than in adult patients. Powder-burn lesions are less common in adolescents, which is consistent with the presumption that these lesions represent older, more advanced implants. Peritoneal Alan–Masters windows between the uterosacral ligaments are also common in adolescents. Care must be taken to identify subtle lesions of endometriosis which often appear as clear shiny peritoneal vesicles. Visualization of lesions through a liquid distention medium may facilitate identification of clear vesicular lesions[19]. If no evidence of endometriosis is identified, a cul-de-sac biopsy to rule out microscopic disease should be performed as endometriosis may be identified without visualization on laparoscopy. Although one study suggests a low prevalence of microscopic endometriosis[14], another report shows a significant rate of microscopic endometriosis in adults[20]. Recent experience at the Children's Hospital in Boston, MA, suggests a significant amount (3%) of microscopic endometriosis in adolescents with a visually normal pelvis[4].

At the time of laparoscopy, endometriosis should be staged according to the revised ASRM classification of endometriosis[17] in order to facilitate follow-up and comparison if future surgery is performed. Interestingly, although most adolescents present with Stage I–II disease, in one reported series of 36 adolescents with endometriosis, 31% had stage IV disease[18]. When counseling patients post-operatively, it is important to remember that the severity of symptoms has not been found to correlate with the extent or location of endometriosis[21].

TREATMENT OF LAPAROSCOPICALLY PROVEN ENDOMETRIOSIS

Laparoscopic treatment

Operative laparoscopy provides the means towards ablation or resection of endometriosis in the least invasive and most cost-effective fashion. Removal of endometriosis may be performed with electrocautery, endocoagulation or laser[22]. We favor the use of CO_2 laser. Regardless of the technique, care must be taken to avoid damage to the ureters, major vessels, bowel and bladder. Resection of adhesions is easily performed with electrocautery and scissors. As noted previously, endometriomas are rare in adolescents; however, large ovarian cysts should be removed, taking care to preserve ovarian tissue.

Medical management of endometriosis

Adolescent patients with disabling endometriosis confirmed by laparoscopy should receive medical treatment for their disease. The choice of treatment depends on the severity of the patient's symptoms, the extent of disease and compliance. Although numerous options have been described for the treatment of endometriosis[23], at the Children's Hospital in Boston, MA, continuous oral contraceptives or gonadotropin-releasing hormone agonists are usually first line therapy. We offer either therapy to women over age 16, and only continuous oral contraceptives to women less than 16 years old for concern of the effects of the GnRH agonist on the formation of normal bones and bone density.

Nonsteroidal anti-inflammatory agents

As noted earlier in this report, NSAIDs are appropriate empiric treatment for dysmenorrhea. NSAIDs are also helpful adjuvant agents for the treatment of pelvic pain associated with endometriosis.

Hormonal suppression

Clearly, not all patients with endometriosis find relief from symptoms with NSAIDs alone[24]. Hormonal suppression of endometriosis generally achieves superior pain control. By hormonally decreasing the stimulus to endometriotic tissue, regression of disease and improved pain control may be achieved.

Oral contraceptives

Continuous low-dose oral contraceptives diminish pain from endometriosis by creating a hormonal pseudopregnancy state in which endometrial implants are relatively inactive. Gynecologists and pediatricians have extensive experience with OCP administration in adolescents. OCPs are generally well tolerated, and may be safely used for at least ten years without an associated increase in mortality[25].

Gonadotropin-releasing hormone agonists

GnRH agonists may also be prescribed in the adolescent population. We generally prescribe depot leuprolide acetate 11.25 mg intramuscularly every 3 months for two doses. With this dose more than 90% of patients will become amenorrheic and hypoestrogenic[26]. Upon completion of this therapy the patient begins continuous OCPs. Nafarelin (nasal spray), one puff twice daily intranasally, is an alternative GnRH agonist; however, compliance is often unpredictable in the adolescent population. The most common complaints arising from GnRH agonists in the adolescent population include hot flashes, headaches, and difficulty sleeping. Further studies are needed to determine if GnRH-agonist with 'add-back' therapy is safe for adolescents[27].

Danazol

Danazol is a 17-alpha-ethinyltestosterone derivative which also creates an acyclic environment, and multiple studies show its efficacy in treating endometriosis to be equivalent to a variety of GnRH agonists[28–34]. Danazol has significant androgenic side-effects secondary to binding sex-hormone-binding-globulin resulting in an increase of free testosterone. For example, in a series by Buttram of 220 patients, complaints included weight gain, depression, muscle cramps, decreased breast size, flushing, oily skin and hair, acne, hirsutism, irreversible deepening of the voice, and skin rash[35]. In this particular series 7% of patients discontinued the drug because of intolerable side-effects. Compared with patients using danazol, patients using GnRH agonists report a better quality of life[36]. Given the side-effects, this medication would probably be poorly tolerated by adolescents, and is not used in our practice.

Progestins

Progestins such as medroxyprogesterone acetate will induce ameneorrhea at high doses (30–50 mg daily by mouth, or medroxyprogesterone acetate 150 mg intramuscularly every 1 to 3 months), and will improve symptoms of 80 to 100% of patients with endometriosis[37–39]. At therapeutic doses, progestins are associated with significant side-effects such as weight gain, bloating, depression and irregular bleeding. This medication also has the benefit of providing birth control.

SUMMARY POINTS

(1) Evaluation of pelvic pain in adolescents begins with history and physical examination, pain calendar, laboratory evaluation, and ultrasound.

(2) Empiric treatment of chronic pelvic pain in adolescents may include non-steroidal anti-inflammatory agents and oral contraceptive agents.

(3) A definitive diagnosis of endometriosis can only be made by laparoscopy. Forty-five to 70% of adolescents with chronic pelvic pain have endometriosis diagnosed at the time of laparoscopy.

(4) In adolescents, the laparoscopic appearance of endometriosis may be subtle, with red-flame lesions and clear shiny peritoneal vesicles.

(5) Surgical management involves diagnosis of endometriosis and ablation of lesions.

(6) Medical management of endometriosis in adolescents is achieved with hormonal suppression using continuous oral contraceptives, gonadotropin-releasing hormone agonists, or other medications.

References

1. Ranney B. Etiology, prevention and inhibition of endometriosis. *Clin Obstet Gynecol* 1980;23: 875–82
2. Emans SJ, Laufer MR, Goldstein DP. *Pediatric and Adolescent Gynecology* (4th edition), Philadelphia: Lippincott/Raven Publishing Company, 1998
3. Reese KA, Reddy S, Rock JA. Endometriosis in an adolescent population: the Emory experience. *J Pediatr Adolesc Gynecol* 1996; 9:125–8
4. Laufer MR, Goitein L, Bush M, *et al.* Prevalence of endometriosis in adolescent women with chronic pelvic pain not responding to conventional therapy. *J Pediatr Adolesc Gynecol* 1997;10:199–202
5. Simpson JL, Elias S, Malinak LR, *et al.* Heritable aspects of endometriosis. *Am J Obstet Gynecol* 1980; 137:327–31
6. Sampson JA. Peritoneal endometriosis due to the menstrual dissemination of endometrial tissue into the peritoneal cavity. *Am J Obstet Gynecol* 1927;14:422–69
7. Goldstein DP, De Cholnoky C, Leventhal JM, *et al.* New insights into the old problem of chronic pelvic pain. *J Ped Surg* 1979;14:675–80
8. Schifrin BS, Erez S, Moore JG. Teenage endometriosis. *Am J Obstet Gynecol* 1973;116:973–80
9. Sanfilippo JS, Wakim NG, Schikler KN, *et al.* Endometriosis in association with uterine anomaly. *Am J Obstet Gynecol* 1986;154:39–43
10. Meyer R. Uber entzundliche neterope epithelwucherungen im weiblichen Genetalg ebiet und uber eine bis in die Wurzel des Mesocolon ausgedehnte benigne Wucherung des Dar mepithel. *Virch Arch Pathol Anat* 1909; 195:487
11. Halban J. Hysteroadenosis metastica. *Wien Klin Wochenschr* 1924;37:1205–28
12. Dmowski W, Braun D, Gebel H. Endometriosis: genetic and immunologic aspects. *Prog Clin Biol Res* 1990;323:99–122
13. Walling MK, Reiter RC, O'Hara MW, *et al.* Abuse history and chronic pain in women: I. prevalences of sexual abuse and physical abuse. *Obstet Gynecol* 1994;84:193–9
14. Redwine DB, Yocom LB. Serial section study of visually normal pelvic peritoneum in patients with endometriosis. *Fertil Steril* 1990;54:648–51
15. Pittaway DE, Fayez JA. Use of CA–125 in the diagnosis and management of endometriosis. *Fertil Steril* 1986;46:790–5
16. Rapkin AJ, Reading AE. Chronic pelvic pain. *Curr Probl Obstet Gynecol Fertil* 1991;14:101–37
17. American Society for Reproductive Medicine. Revised American Society for Reproductive Medicine classification of endometriosis: 1966. *Fertil Steril* 1997;67:817
18. Davis GD, Thillet E, Lindemann J. Clinical characteristics of adolescent endometriosis. *J Adol Health* 1993;14:362–8
19. Laufer MR. Identification of clear vesicular lesions of atypical endometriosis: a new technique. *Fertil Steril* 1997;68:739–40
20. Nisolle M, Berliere M, Paindaveine B, *et al.* Histologic study of peritoneal endometriosis in infertile women. *Fertil Steril* 1990;53:984–8

21. Fedele L, Parazzini F, Bianchi S,*et al.* Stage and localization of pelvic endometriosis and pain. *Fertil Steril* 1990;53:155–8
22. Cook AS, Rock JA. Role of laparoscopy in the treatment of endometriosis. *Fertil Steril* 1991; 55:663–749
23. Laufer MR. Endometriosis in adolescents. *Curr Opin Ped* 1992;4:582–9
24. Ylikorkala O, Viinikka L. Prostaglandins and endometriosis. *Acta Obstet Gynecol Scand Suppl* 1983;113:105–7
25. Colditz GA. Oral contraceptive use and mortality during 12 years of follow-up: the nurses health study. *Ann Intern Med* 1994;120:821–6
26. Barbieri RL. Treatment of endometriosis with the GnRH agonists. In Barbieri RL, Friedman AJ. *Gonadotropin Releasing Hormone Analogs: Applications in Gynecology*. New York: Elsevier Science, 1991:63–7
27. Lubianca JN, Gordon CM, Laufer MR. Addback therapy for endometriosis in adolescents. *J Reprod Med* 1998;43:164–72
28. Kennedy SH, Williams IA, Brodribb J, *et al.* Comparison of nafarelin acetate and danazol in the treatment of endometriosis. *Fertil Steril* 1990;53:998–1000
29. Wheeler JM, Knittle JD, Miller JD. Depot leuprolide acetate versus danazol in the treatment of women with symptomatic endometriosis: a multicenter, double-blind randomized clinical trial. II. Assessment of safety. The Lupron Endometriosis Study Group. *Am J Obstet Gynecol* 1993;169:26–33
30. Rock JA, Truglia JA, Caplan RJ. Zoladex (goserelin acetate implant) in the treatment of endometriosis: a randomized comparison with danazol. The Zoladex Endometriosis Study Group. *Obstet Gynecol* 1993;82:198–205
31. The Nafarelin European Endometriosis Trial Group (NEET). Nafarelin for endometriosis: a large-scale, danazol-controlled trial of efficacy and safety, with 1 year follow-up. *Fertil Steril* 1992;57:514–22
32. Leuprorelin acetetate depot vs danazol in the treatent of endometriosis: results of an open multicentre trial. *Clin Therap* 1992;14A:29–36
33. Shaw RW. An open randomized comparative study of the effect of goserelin depot and danazol in the treatment of endometriosis. Zoladex edometriosis study team. *Fertil Steril* 1992;58: 265–72
34. Shaw RW. Nafarelin in the treatment of pelvic pain caused by endometriosis. *Am J Obstet Gynecol* 1990;162:574–6
35. Buttram VC, Reiter RC, Ward S. Treatment of endometriosis with danazol: report of a 6-year prospective study. *Fertil Steril* 1985;43:353–60
36. Burry KA. Nafarelin in the management of endometriosis: quality of life assessment. *Am J Obstet Gynecol* 1992;166:735–9
37. Luciano AA, Turksoy RN, Carleo J. Evaluation of oral medroxyprogesterone acetate in the treatment of endometriosis. *Obstet Gynecol* 1988;72:323–7
38. Moghissi KS, Boyce CR. Management of endometriosis with oral medroxyprogesterone actetate. *Obstet Gynecol* 1976;47:265–7
39. Vercellini P, De Giorgi O, Oldani S, *et al.* Depot medroxyprogesterone acetate versus an oral contraceptive combined with very-low-dose danazol for long-term treatment of pelvic pain associated with endometriosis. *Am J Obstet Gynecol* 1996;175:396–401

Chronic pelvic pain in UK primary care: patterns of diagnosis 8

K.T. Zondervan, P.L. Yudkin, M.P. Vessey, M.G. Dawes, D.H. Barlow and S.H. Kennedy

INTRODUCTION

Chronic pelvic pain (CPP) is commonly defined as non-malignant pain in the lower abdominal region lasting for at least six months, and excludes pain occurring only during periods (dysmenorrhea) or intercourse (dyspareunia). Though the condition can have a profound effect on the quality of life and general well-being of women, no published data exist on its epidemiology in the general UK population or in primary care [1].

Clinical experience indicates that women with CPP can often be labeled with a variety of diagnoses, including irritable bowel syndrome, pelvic inflammatory disease, and endometriosis. The aim of this study was to provide an insight into the diagnostic process involving women of reproductive age being seen in general practice with CPP for the first time, using data from the national general practice database *MediPlus®* UKPCD. Particular emphasis was given to women labeled with endometriosis.

METHODS

MediPlus®, the UK primary care database (UKPCD)

MediPlus® UKPCD is a national database containing clinical and prescribing data on approximately 1 700 000 patients from 140 general practices. It is representative of the general UK population regarding age, sex, and regional distribution, except that Scottish practices are under-represented (IMS International, personal communication). More details regarding *MediPlus®* UKPCD and quality assurance methods have been published elsewhere [2].

The data in *MediPlus®* UKPCD are recorded individually by date, providing anonymized longitudinal records of patients for the time they remain within the practice. Each item of data can be a symptom, diagnosis, type of medication, referral, or procedure. The codes used for items are selected from a comprehensive list, which includes codes from the International Classification of Diseases, ninth revision (ICD–9), Read codes [3], and other codes built in by IMS on request. The study period for our analyses was 1 January 1991 to 31 December 1995.

Definitions

Pelvic pain contact: a date at which a code is entered that suggests pelvic pain (e.g. 'lower abdominal pain', 'pelvic inflammatory disease', 'endometriosis'). Each contact could be a visit to the GP, a telephone encounter, or a repeat prescription. Contacts occurring during pregnancy, or indicating upper abdominal symptoms, were excluded.

CPP case: a woman with at least two pelvic pain contacts covering a time-period of at least six months, but with no gap between contacts of more than one year. Time of onset of CPP was defined as six months after the first CPP contact. Cases with cancer in the lower abdominal region, or a chronic inflammatory bowel disorder were excluded, as were cases with dysmenorrhea or dyspareunia codes *only*.

Incidence: The number of new CPP cases as a

proportion of the unaffected population at risk. Within the period 1991–1995, complete incidence rates could only be determined from July 1992 to December 1994, because of the definition of a CPP case previously described.

Prevalence: The number of existing CPP cases – estimated after following the accumulation of incident cases from July 1992 onwards towards a steady state[4] – as a proportion of the total population at risk. Further details on the method of incidence and prevalence calculation are given elsewhere (K.T. Zondervan, submitted for publication).

Population at risk: All women (n = 176 915) aged 18–50 in 1992 who were free of CPP before July 1992 and who were registered with their practice for the whole time-period of 1991–95.

CPP cohort: CPP cases who were incident in July 1992 to June 1993. This cohort consisted of 3357 women, who were followed up until the end of 1995 (mean follow-up 3.5 years) to investigate patterns of diagnosis and referral.

Duration of symptoms: Time between the first and the last registered pelvic pain contact of an incident CPP case.

Diagnostic label: A diagnosis relevant to CPP occurring in the follow-up of a CPP case. The term 'diagnostic label' was used to indicate that diagnoses could be suspected or confirmed. Diagnostic labels were grouped into nine categories: cystitis, irritable bowel syndrome, other gastrointestinal diagnoses (e.g. diverticular disease, diverticulitis, GIT infections), pelvic inflammatory disease, endometriosis, ovarian cysts, uterine fibroids, adhesions, and the pelvic congestion syndrome.

Statistical methods

All analyses were performed using SAS version 6.12. Differences in mean age (normally distributed) between diagnostic groups were assessed using analysis of variance, whereas differences in median duration of symptoms (not normally distributed) were assessed using the Kruskal–Wallis non-parametric test. Differences in numbers of diagnosis and referral rates between diagnostic groups were assessed using Pearson χ^2 tests.

RESULTS

The annual prevalence of CPP in primary care in women aged 18–50 was 37.2/1000 (95% confidence interval: 36.3–38.1). This rate was comparable to prevalence rates in primary care reported for other common chronic conditions, such as migraine (25/1000), asthma (37/1000), and back pain (38/1000) in women aged 16–44[5].

Duration of symptoms and patterns of diagnosis and referral were investigated in the cohort of 3357 incident CPP cases. Table 1 shows that more than a third of women continued to have symptoms for at least two years, with a median duration of 16.1 months (interquartile range: 10.1–31.8).

Frequencies of diagnostic labels ever given to women in follow-up are shown in Table 2. A quarter of all CPP cases never received a diagnostic label in their entire follow-up (this figure was 20.4% for women with symptoms lasting more than two years). Cystitis was the most common diagnostic label (31.3%), followed by irritable bowel syndrome (30.5%) and pelvic inflammatory disease (15.1%). Only 6.3% of women ever received the diagnostic label of endometriosis.

For further analyses, CPP cases were grouped into three diagnostic categories (Table 3): women with an endometriosis label (n = 210) in follow-up; women with only

Table 1 Duration of symptoms in follow-up of 3357 women

*Duration**	*Number of women* (%)
6 months – 1 year	1250 (37.2)
> 1–2 years	948 (28.2)
> 2 years	1159 (34.5)
Total	3357 (100)

*Median duration (interquartile range) = 16.1 months (10.1–31.8)

Table 2 Types of diagnostic labels in follow-up of 3357 women

Diagnostic label	*Number of women with diagnostic label (%)**
None	852 (25.4)
Cystitis	1051 (31.3)
Irritable bowel syndrome (IBS)	1025 (30.5)
Pelvic inflammatory disease (PID)	507 (15.1)
Endometriosis	210 (6.3)
Other gastrointestinal diagnoses[1]	154 (4.6)
Ovarian cysts	116 (3.5)
Uterine fibroids	110 (3.3)
Adhesions	24 (0.7)
Pelvic congestion syndrome	8 (0.2)
Total	3357 (100)

*Percentages do not add up to 100% as some women had more than one diagnosis
[1], Mainly diverticular disease, diverticulitis, and GIT infections

diagnostic labels other than endometriosis ($n = 2295$); and women without any diagnostic label ($n = 852$). The three groups were similar regarding mean age. Median duration of symptoms differed significantly between diagnostic groups ($p < 0.0001$), varying from a median of 28.6 months in the endometriosis group to 13.7 months in the group without a diagnosis. The majority of women with an endometriosis label (74.5%) had an indication of a gynecological referral or a laparoscopy before the endometriosis diagnosis was entered, providing some evidence of its validity.

Women with an endometriosis label were more likely to have received more than one diagnostic label compared to women with other diagnostic labels (Table 3). The most frequent other diagnostic labels in the 210 women with an endometriosis label were the irritable bowel syndrome (20.5%), pelvic inflammatory disease (13.8%), and cystitis (12.9%).

Fifty-three per cent of all 3357 CPP cases and 40% of those with symptoms for at least two years had no indication of any hospital referral in follow-up. Table 4 shows that women with an endometriosis label were much more likely to have had any hospital referral than women in the other groups. This indicated that diagnoses commonly suspected to be the cause of CPP – such as cystitis, irritable bowel syndrome, and pelvic inflammatory disease – were more commonly managed within primary care.

In all three diagnostic groups, women were most often referred to a gynecology department (Table 4). A small proportion of all women with CPP (6.9%) were referred to more than one specialty, the most common combination being gynecology and general surgery (3.2%).

Table 3 Characteristics of women by diagnostic label (ever) in follow-up

	Ever in follow-up:		
	Endometriosis ($n = 210$)	*Diagnoses other than endometriosis* ($n = 2295$)	*No diagnosis* ($n = 852$)
Mean age (SD)*	34.5 (7.8)	34.4 (9.0)	34.9 (9.1)
Median duration in months (interquartile range)†	28.6 (14.5–39.3)	16.5 (10.2–31.6)	13.7 (9.4–29.0)
Number of diagnostic labels†			
1	51.4%	78.0%	–
2	34.3%	19.6%	–
> 2	14.3%	2.4%	–

*Difference between groups: $p = 0.45$; †Difference between groups: $p < 0.001$

Table 4 Specialties to which women were referred by type of diagnostic label

	Ever in follow up:		
	Endometriosis (n = 210)	*Diagnosis, but no endometriosis* (n = 2295)	*No diagnosis* (n = 852)
Number (%) referred to specialty			
Any referral*	177 (84.3)	986 (43.0)	414 (48.6)
Gynecology	170 (81.0)	733 (31.9)	313 (36.7)
Gastroenterology	4 (1.9)	90 (3.9)	26 (3.1)
Urology	4 (1.9)	63 (2.7)	17 (2.0)
General surgery	18 (8.6)	151 (6.6)	81 (9.5)
General medicine	12 (5.7)	78 (3.4)	32 (3.8)

*Difference between groups: $p < 0.001$

CONCLUSIONS

CPP is a common condition in UK primary care, with consultation rates comparable to migraine, back pain, and asthma. Duration of symptoms is often long, with one-third of women continuing to have symptoms two years after their first consultation. Only a minority of women (6.3%) received the label of endometriosis in 3–4 years of follow-up after first consultation. These women had the longest duration of symptoms on the database, and were most likely to have been referred to secondary care. However, 50% of all CPP cases and a third of those with at least two years of symptoms had no indication of referral in their follow-up. These results indicate that women seen in secondary care for CPP, who may be diagnosed with endometriosis, are likely to represent only the tip of the iceberg.

ACKNOWLEDGEMENTS

We would like to thank all general practitioners who have contributed to *MediPlus*® UKPCD and thus made this study possible. Furthermore, we would like to thank Intercontinental Medical Statistics Ltd and Pharmacia & Upjohn Ltd for their help and for providing access to *MediPlus*® UKPCD. We gratefully acknowledge Dr Rosemary Painter for her help with Fortran programming.

References

1. Zondervan KT, Yudkin PL, Vessey MP, *et al.* The prevalence of chronic pelvic pain in women in the UK – a systematic review. *Br J Obstet Gynaecol* 1998;105:93–99
2. Lloyd DCEF, Harris CM, Roberts DJ. Specific therapeutic group age-sex related prescribing units (STAR-PUs): weightings for analysing general practices' prescribing in England. *Br Med J* 1995;311:991–4
3. Chisholm J. The Read clinical classification. *Br Med J* 1990;300:1092
4. Rothman KJ, Greenland SG. Measures of disease frequency. In Rothman KJ, Greenland SG, eds. *Modern Epidmiology*. Philadelphia: Lippincot-Raven, 1998:29–46
5. Office of Population Censuses & Surveys. *Morbidity Statistics from General Practice.* Fourth national study 1991–1992. London, HMSO, 1995;MB5 no 3:24–78

Histopathology of endometriosis: study of activity, angiogenesis and steroid receptor expression in peritoneal endometriosis

9

M. Nisolle, F. Casanas-Roux and J. Donnez

INTRODUCTION

Differences in activity have been noted between the different macroscopic appearances of peritoneal endometriotic lesions. Indeed, a higher stromal vascularization and increased mitotic activity have been observed in red peritoneal lesions, which can be considered as the most active[1]. In order to evaluate the proliferation index of the different types of peritoneal endometriosis, we used Ki 67 immunohistochemically[2]. This monoclonal antibody recognizes a nuclear antigen which is expressed in all stages of the cell cycle, except GO[3]. It can be widely used to assess the proliferative status of cell populations in a variety of neoplastic conditions, in non-neoplastic conditions and in normal tissue.

Vascular endothelial growth factor (VEGF), also known as vascular permeability factor, is a heparin-binding glycoprotein with potent angiogenic, endothelial cell-specific mitogenic and vascular permeability activities. Its presence has also been demonstrated in human endometrium and may be important in both physiologic and pathologic angiogenesis[4,5].

The aim of this study was to evaluate the proliferative status of the glandular epithelium and stroma of endometriotic tissue throughout the menstrual cycle and to compare the data with those obtained from eutopic endometrium. A new stereographic computer technology enabled us to evaluate estrogen receptors (ER) and progesterone receptors (PR) in both endo-metriotic tissue and eutopic endometrium[6].

We also compared the VEGF content of eutopic endometrium and black and red peritoneal lesions throughout the menstrual cycle in order to clarify the role of VEGF in the pathogenesis of endometriosis[7].

MATERIALS AND METHODS

Patients

In women undergoing laparoscopy for infertility, biopsies of both typical black lesions ($n = 27$) and red flamelike lesions ($n = 19$) were taken. All the women had regular ovulatory cycles, and none were given hormonal therapy for at least 3 months before surgery.

Measurement of proliferative activity

The proliferative status of endometriotic cells was measured by the evaluation of the percentage of Ki 67 positive-staining nuclei examined (proliferation index).

Tissue samples were fixed in formaldehyde and Ki 67 labeling was determined by immunoperoxidase techniques using the peroxidase-antiperoxidase (PAP) complex. Six micron-thick tissue sections were mounted on Superfrost Plus slides and stained according to the immunocytochemical assay (Clone MIB1, Immunotech, Marseille, France).

The number of labeled glandular and stromal nuclei per 500 cells was counted using the 40× objective of a light microscope (Zeiss, Oberkochen, Germany).

Table 1 Proliferation index (glandular and stromal) in eutopic endometrium and peritoneal endometriosis according to the phase of the menstrual cycle (% of Ki 67 positive-staining nuclei). All values are means ± SEM

	Eutopic endometrium ($n = 25$)	*Black lesions* ($n = 27$)	*Red lesions* ($n = 19$)
Glandular epithelium			
Late proliferative phase	35.7 ± 4.9‡	13.5 ± 3.5+§	25.5 ± 15.8‡
Early secretory phase	12.7 ± 6.0	6.2 ± 1.7	1.4 ± 0.6
Mid to late secretory phase	0	1.4 ± 0.7§	1.0 ± 0.8§
Stroma			
Proliferative phase	17.0 ± 3.3	1.4 ± 0.8+§	5.4 ± 1.4§
Early secretory phase	9.1 ± 3.7	2.4 ± 0.8§	4.8 ± 1.9
Mid to late secretory phase	10.1 ± 1.2	0.6 ± 0.3§	5.4 ± 1.8

+Significantly higher than the late secretory phase ($p < 0.05$); ‡significantly higher than the early and late secretory phases ($p < 0.05$); §significantly different from the percentage observed in eutopic endometrium during the corresponding phase ($p < 0.05$)

Steroid receptor expression

Immunostaining quantitative analysis was performed with a computerized microscope image processor as previously described, giving the results of the degree of intensity in terms of an optical density. The distribution of specific staining was thus evaluated according to an optical density scale[6] using the values of all the positive nuclei of a given receptor; the quantitative H-score (QH-score) was calculated as follows: QH-score = $\Sigma P i$, where i is the optical density degree: from 0 (negative nuclei) to 3 (high optical density) and P is the percentage of stained cells for each given i (from 0% to 100%). This method is a modification of the semi-quantitative H-score analysis described by McCarty *et al*[8].

The Chi-square test and the median test were used for statistical analysis. The data were analyzed by one-way analysis of variance (ANOVA).

VEGF content

Ten women without endometriosis at laparoscopy (Group I) and 43 women with endometriosis (Group II) were evaluated. Measurement of VEGF staining on tissue was based on immuno-labeling with a polyclonal antibody, which recognizes the 165, 189 and 121 amino acid splice variants of VEGF of human origin. This technique has been previously described[7].

RESULTS

Proliferative activity

Table 1 represents the proliferation index in the glandular and stromal cells of eutopic and ectopic endometrium according to the phase of the menstrual cycle.

In *eutopic endometrium*, the glandular epithelium revealed a significantly ($p < 0.01$) higher proliferation index (35.7 ± 4.9%) during the proliferative phase than during the early and mid to late secretory phases (12.7 ± 6.0% and 0% respectively). In the stroma, no significant cyclic variations were observed.

In *typical black peritoneal lesions*, the glandular proliferation index was found to be significantly higher during the late proliferative phase (13.5 ± 3.5%) than during the early secretory phase (6.2 ± 1.7%) and the mid to late secretory phase (1.4 ± 0.7%) ($p < 0.02$). In the stroma, the proliferation index was found to be higher during the late proliferative phase (1.4 ± 0.3%) and the early secretory phase (2.4 ± 0.8%) when compared

Table 2 QH-score of steroid receptors in eutopic endometrium and endometriosis throughout the cycle. All values are given as means ± SEM

	Estrogen receptor		*Progesterone receptor*	
	Glandular epithelium	*Stroma*	*Glandular epithelium*	*Stroma*
Eutopic endometrium				
Proliferative phase ($n = 9$)	234 ± 24	126 ± 25	274 ± 13	207 ± 12
Early secretory phase ($n = 10$)	156 ± 41	$8 \pm 4^{‡}$	264 ± 18	209 ± 22
Late secretory phase ($n = 7$)	0^{+}	0^{+}	0^{+}	$115 \pm 18^{+}$
Black peritoneal lesions				
Proliferative phase ($n = 8$)	$124 \pm 28^{§}$	88 ± 25	281 ± 14	215 ± 14
Early secretory phase ($n = 3$)	94 ± 94	$0^{‡}$	$73 \pm 73^{‡§}$	130 ± 130
Late secretory phase ($n = 7$)	$4 \pm 4^{‡}$	$1 \pm 1^{‡}$	$201 \pm 44^{§}$	200 ± 36
Red peritonral lesions				
Proliferative phase ($n = 4$)	216 ± 28	182 ± 33	273 ± 13	197 ± 31
Early secretory phase ($n = 4$)	158 ± 64	$113 \pm 54^{§}$	$108 \pm 71^{‡§}$	156 ± 58
Late secretory phase ($n = 8$)	$57 \pm 41^{§‡}$	$22 \pm 8^{§+}$	$14 \pm 17^{§}$	$52 \pm 11^{§+}$

$^{+}$Significantly different from the proliferative phase and the early secretory phase ($p < 0.001$); ‡significantly different from the proliferative phase ($p < 0.02$); §significantly different from the eutopic endometrium during the same phase ($p < 0.005$)

with the mid to late secretory phase (0.6 ± 0.3%) ($p < 0.05$).

In *red peritoneal lesions*, the glandular proliferation index was found to be significantly ($p < 0.05$) higher during the late proliferative phase (25.5 ± 15.8%) than during the early secretory phase (1.4 ± 0.6%) and the mid to late secretory phase (1.0 ± 0.8%). In the stroma, the proliferation index was found to be similar throughout the menstrual cycle.

Comparison between eutopic endometrium and ectopic endometrium

During the late proliferative phase, the percentages of Ki 67 positive-staining nuclei were similar in the glandular epithelium of red lesions (25.5 ± 15.8%) and in eutopic endometrium (35.7 ± 4.9%). The percentage observed in black lesions (13.5 ± 3.5%) was significantly lower ($p < 0.05$). During the late secretory phase, the eutopic glandular epithelium did not reveal Ki 67 positive-staining nuclei while the ectopic glandular epithelium did.

The stromal proliferation index was consistently lower in black endometriotic lesions than in eutopic endometrium throughout the different phases of the cycle ($p < 0.05$). In red lesions, it was significantly lower ($p < 0.05$) than in eutopic endometrium only during the late proliferative phase.

Steroid receptors

The results of the measurement of ER and PR content of eutopic and ectopic endometrium according to the QH-score are shown in Table 2.

Comparison between eutopic endometrium and ectopic endometrium

The ER content was found to be lower in the glandular epithelium of black lesions than in eutopic endometrium, but similar cyclic changes (a decrease during the secretory phase) were observed. In the stroma, the ER content and its cyclic variations were similar in eutopic endometrium and black peritoneal lesions.

A similar ER content was observed in the glandular epithelium of eutopic endo-

Table 3 Vascular endothelial growth factor (VEGF) H-score in the glandular cells of eutopic and ectopic endometrium according to the phase of the menstrual cycle. Values are means ± SD

Patients	*Cycle*	*Proliferative phase*	*Early secretory phase*	*Late secretory phase*
Women without endometriosis (Group I, n =10)				
eutopic endometrium	9.7 ± 4.3 (n = 10)	10.3 ± 0.6 (n = 3)	10.7 ± 3.0 (n = 4)	6.0 ± 6.6 (n = 3)
Women with endometriosis (Group II; n = 43)				
eutopic endometrium	10.3 ± 2.3 (n = 43)	9.9 ± 2.6 (n = 16)	10.6 ± 2.2^{+} (n = 13)	10.1 ± 1.9^{++} (n = 14)
black lesions	8.6 ± 2.7 (n = 29)	8.8 ± 1.2 (n = 8)	8.4 ± 2.7 (n = 12)	8.8 ± 3.6 (n = 9)
red lesions	11.1 ± 3.0 (n = 22)	9.8 ± 4.0 (n = 6)	12.0 ± 2.7^{+} (n = 6)	11.3 ± 2.7^{++} (n =10)

$^{+}$significantly different from the values observed in black lesions ($p < 0.04$); $^{++}$significantly different from the values observed in the eutopic endometrium of Group I ($p < 0.04$)

metrium and red peritoneal lesions during the proliferative phase. During the late secretory phase, ER were still found in the glandular epithelium of red lesions while they were systematically absent from eutopic endometrium. In the stroma, the ER content was similar during the proliferative phase but significantly higher ($p < 0.02$) in red peritoneal lesions during the late secretory phase.

The PR content was found to be similar in the glandular epithelium of eutopic endometrium and black and red peritoneal lesions during the proliferative phase.

A significantly higher ($p < 0.005$) PR content was observed in the glandular epithelium of black peritoneal lesions during the late secretory phase than that observed in eutopic endometrium where there were no PR. In the stroma, the PR content was similar in eutopic endometrium and black peritoneal lesions throughout the cycle, but differences were observed between eutopic endometrium and red peritoneal lesions.

VEGF content

Tables 3 and 4 represent the VEGF H-scores found in the glandular and stromal cells of eutopic and ectopic endometrium according to the phase of the menstrual cycle.

Comparative study of VEGF content in eutopic endometrium in patients with and without endometriosis

During the proliferative and early secretory phases, the glandular VEGF H-scores in eutopic endometrium were found to be similar in both groups. However, during the late secretory phase, the VEGF H-score was significantly higher in the eutopic endometrium of endometriosis patients than in control eutopic endometrium (10.1 ± 1.9 and 6.0 ± 6.6 respectively) ($p < 0.04$).

In the stroma, no significant differences were observed between the VEGF H-scores found in the eutopic endometrium of the two groups of patients throughout the menstrual cycle.

Comparative study of VEGF content in black and red peritoneal lesions

In the glandular epithelium, the VEGF H-score was significantly ($p < 0.004$) higher in red peritoneal lesions than in black peritoneal lesions during the early secretory phase (12.0

Table 4 Vascular endothelial growth factor (VEGF) H-score in the stromal cells of eutopic and ectopic endometrium according to the phase of the menstrual cycle. Values are means ± SD

Patients	*Cycle*	*Proliferative phase*	*Early secretory phase*	*Late secretory phase*
Women without endometriosis (Group I)				
eutopic endometrium	4.0 ± 2.6⁺ (n = 3)	5.7 ± 2.1⁺ (n = 3)	3.7 ± 2.4* (n = 4)	2.7 ± 3.8 (n = 3)
Women with endometriosis (Group II)				
eutopic endometrium	3.6 ± 2.3⁺ (n = 43)	4.0 ± 2.7 (n = 16)	3.1 ± 1.8* (n = 13)	3.3 ± 2.1 (n = 14)
black lesions	1.6 ± 1.6 (n = 27)	2.0 ± 1.7 (n = 6)	1.6 ± 1.8* (n = 12)	1.4 ± 1.3 (n = 9)
red lesions	5.1 ± 3.0⁺ (n = 24)	3.8 ± 1.6⁺ (n = 6)	7.1 ± 3.9‡ (n = 7)	4.5 ± 2.5⁺ (n =11)

*significantly different from the values observed in red lesions ($p < 0.03$); ⁺significantly different from the values observed in black lesions ($p < 0.03$); ‡significantly different from the proliferative phase ($p < 0.05$)

± 2.7 and 8.4 ± 2.7 respectively). During the late secretory phase, the VEGF H-scores in red lesions (11.3 ± 2.7) and in the eutopic endometrium (10.1 ± 1.9) of women with endometriosis (Group II) were significantly ($p < 0.04$) higher than in the eutopic endometrium of women without endometriosis (6.0 ± 6.6) (Group I).

In the stroma, the VEGF H-score was significantly ($p < 0.03$) higher in red lesions during the late secretory phase than in black lesions (4.5 ± 2.5 and 1.4 ± 1.3 respectively).

DISCUSSION

In the present study, the decrease in the proliferation index of the glandular epithelium throughout the menstrual cycle and the absence of positive-staining nuclei during the mid to late secretory phase corroborates the normal morphological changes described by several authors[9–11]. Jones *et al.* also noted the absence of cells expressing the Ki 67 antigen during the late secretory phase[12]. Our data, however, are at odds with those of Klein *et al.*[13] who reported very low percentages of Ki 67 positive-staining nuclei (proliferative phase: 5.7%; secretory phase: 3.3%), while our own results demonstrated percentages > 30% during the proliferative phase.

In the stroma, the persistence of Ki 67 positive-staining nuclei during the mid to late secretory phase is also in accordance with the results of light microscopy, which revealed a first peak of stromal mitoses around ovulation (10%) and a second peak just before menstruation[9,10].

The disappearance of PR from the essential glandular epithelium during the late secretory phase can reflect its declining functional importance during early pregnancy in cell populations, whereas the stroma, which becomes decidualized, would logically require receptors to support its further growth and development.

In black peritoneal lesions, while the proliferation index was significantly lower than in eutopic endometrium, it was nevertheless much higher than that described by Klein *et al.*, who observed only occasional cells staining positive for Ki 67 at a rate of less than 1%[13]. In contrast to eutopic endometrium, positive-staining nuclei were observed in the glandular epithelium of peritoneal endometriosis during the late secretory phase, although a significant decrease was observed in this phase. The persistence of proliferative activity confirms the results obtained by light microscopy studies which revealed the persistence of mitosis during the late secretory phase, leading us to suggest a relative hormonal unresponsiveness of this epithelium. The persistence of PR in the glandular epithelium of endometriotic lesions observed in this study reinforces this hypothesis. When the data were analyzed according to the macroscopic appearance, differences were observed. Indeed, during the proliferative phase, a higher glandular proliferation index was noted in red endometriotic lesions (25.5 ± 15.8) when compared to black lesions (13.5 ± 3.5). A high stromal proliferation index was also noted in red peritoneal lesions during the secretory phase. Interestingly, extensive stromal vascularization was observed in red peritoneal lesions[9,11]. The high proliferative activity of the stroma and the extensive vascular network of such endometriotic lesions led us to suggest that the endometriotic stroma probably plays a primordial role in the development and growth of endometriotic lesions.

All these results suggest that the hormonal regulation of endometriotic tissue is different from that of endometrium and that PR are synthesized but are not completely biologically active. Indeed, the higher proliferative activity of endometriotic lesions in the secretory and menstrual phases may be explained by the failure of PR expression levels to suppress proliferative activity in the secretory phase. The persistence of PR in both the epithelium and stroma of endometriotic lesions may explain the relative inefficacy of medical therapy, and why a recurrence of peritoneal endometriosis can be observed soon after cessation of medical therapy[14].

In eutopic endometrium, the morphological changes and the decrease in the proliferation index throughout the menstrual cycle can be explained by its hormonal control and steroid receptor content. In ectopic endometrium, however, the absence of morphological changes during the secretory phase, the persistence of mitotic activity during the mid to late secretory phase and the persistence of PR in glandular cells during the late secretory phase suggest its relative hormonal independence, or at least the existence of a different mechanism of proliferation control.

In human endometrium, Smith[5] and Shifren *et al.*[15] described cyclic changes in the distribution of VEGF and m-RNA expression throughout the cycle and Greb *et al.* suggested that VEGF expression is under steroid control, being upregulated in response to estradiol[16]. On the other hand, McLaren *et al.*[17] observed low expression of VEGF, mostly seen in macrophages distributed throughout the stroma of endometriotic lesions.

In our study, we immunohistochemically compared the VEGF content in the glandular epithelium and stroma of eutopic endometrium and endometriotic lesions, making a clear distinction between black and red peritioneal lesions[18].

In the group of patients without endometriosis, there were no significant variations in VEGF content in the eutopic glandular epithelium or stroma throughout the menstrual cycle. But differences were noted between the eutopic endometrium of women with and without endometriosis. Indeed, VEGF content was significantly higher in the eutopic glandular epithelium of endometriosis patients during the late secretory phase, suggesting that the endometrium of women with endometriosis is more likely to implant than that of women without endometriosis.

During the luteal phase, significantly higher levels of VEGF immunostaining were observed in both the glandular epithelium and stroma of red peritoneal endometriotic lesions than in black lesions, suggesting an active angiogenic process in red lesions, as active as in eutopic endometrium. On the contrary, black lesions were characterized by a poor angiogenesis. This confirms the differences in the stromal vascularization index between red and black lesions that we observed in a previous study[1]. The similar VEGF content found in red lesions and

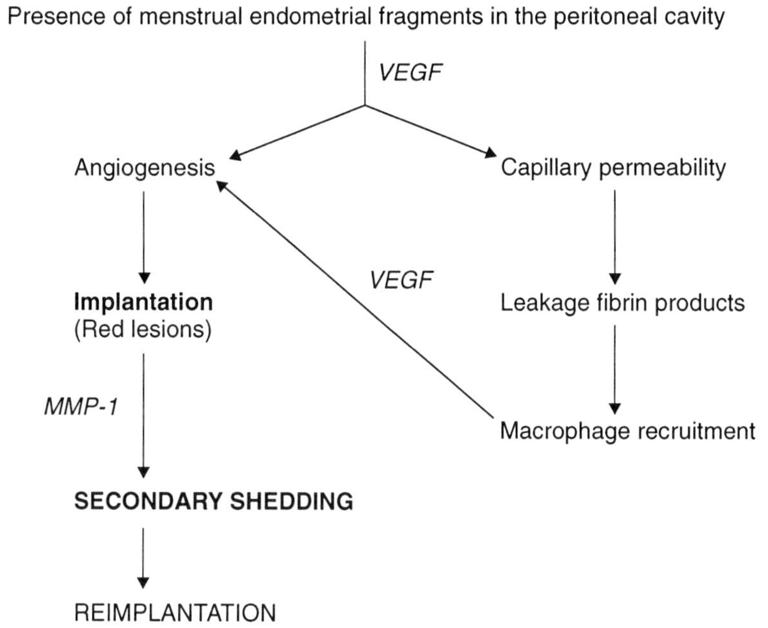

Figure 1 Hypothesis of the histogenesis of peritoneal endometriosis: the role of eutopic endometrium

eutopic glandular epithelium is another argument in favor of the transplantation theory. Red lesions must therefore be considered as the first stage of endometriosis and as freshly implanted lesions.

The fact that red lesions are characterized by high levels of VEGF and the presence of matrix metallo-proteinases (MMP-1) throughout the cycle[19] could be the key point of the transplantation theory. Indeed, under the influence of MMP-1, partial shedding of red lesions and their implantation elsewhere in the peritoneal cavity under the influence of VEGF could explain the development of peritoneal endometriosis.

From our data, we are able to suggest that the eutopic endometrium itself plays a crucial role in the histogenesis of endometriosis (Figure 1). Indeed, during retrograde menstruation, endometrial implants with a high VEGF content in glandular cells enter the peritoneal cavity. This high VEGF content found in the glandular cells of menstruating endometrium was also noted in the study by Smith[5]. The attachment phase is influenced by the presence of attachment proteins and MMP-1, as has been proved in two of our studies[19,20]. Indeed, we observed a correlation between MMP-1 expression and the activity of endo-metriotic tissue, suggesting its involvement in tissue remodeling and bleeding, and, possibly, in the secondary shedding and reimplantation of endometriotic lesions. After the attachment phase, the high VEGF levels could provoke an increase in the subperitoneal vascular network and facilitate implantation and viability. Moreover, VEGF, in addition to being angiogenic, causes increased permeability of the capillary bed, and similarly to the mechanisms involved in pathologic angiogenesis, this could suggest that in freshly implanted endometriotic lesions, the higher expression of VEGF might explain a higher permeability of the capillary bed[21]. This may lead to a leakage of fibrin products into the extracellular space which will increase the recruitment of macrophages, whose angiogenic activity is increased by the secretion of TNF-α, known to be secreted by macrophages when these cells are activated by certain large molecules, such as bacterial endotoxins of fibrin products.

The high VEGF content demonstrated in

our study has led to the hypothesis that VEGF-induced angiogenesis may be a critical aspect of the pathophysiology of this disease and suggests, as Smith already has, that anti-angiogenic therapies could be considered as a new clinical approach to this disease.

References

1. Nisolle M, Casanas-Roux F, Anaf V, *et al.* Morphometric study of the stromal vascularization in peritoneal endometriosis. *Fertil Steril* 1993;59:681–4
2. Nisolle M, Casanas-Roux F, Donnez J. Immunohistochemical analysis of proliferative activity and steroid receptor expression in peritoneal and ovarian endometriosis. *Fertil Steril* 1997; 68:912–19
3. Gerdes J, Schwab U, Lemke H, *et al.* Production of a mouse monoclonal antibody reactive with a human nuclear antigen associated with cell proliferation. *Int J Cancer* 1983;31:13–20
4. Charnock-Jones D, Sharkey A, Raffut-Williams J, *et al.* Identification and localization of alternately spliced mRNAs for vascular endothelial growth factor in human uterus and estrogen regulation in endometrial carcinoma cell lines. *Biol Reprod* 1993;48:1120–8
5. Smith SK. Vascular endothelial growth factor and the endometrium. *Hum Reprod* 1996;11:56–61
6. Nisolle M, Casanas-Roux F, Wyns Ch, *et al.* Immunohistochemical analysis of oestrogen and progesterone receptors in endometrium and peritoneal endometriosis: a new quantitative method. *Fertil Steril* 1994;4:751–9
7. Donnez J, Smoes P, Gillerot S, *et al.* Vascular endothelial growth factor (VEGF) in endometriosis. *Hum Reprod* 1998;13:1686–90
8. McCarty Jr KS, Miller LS, Cox EB, *et al.* Estrogen receptor analyses: correlation of biochemical and immunohistochemical methods using monoclonal antireceptor antibodies. *Arch Pathol Lab Med* 1985;109:716–21
9. Noyes RW, Hertig AT, Rock J. Dating the endometrial biopsy. *Fertil Steril* 1950;1:3–25
10. Johannisson E, Parker R, Landgren B, *et al.* Morphometric analysis of the human endometrium in relation to peripheral hormone levels. *Fertil Steril* 1982;38:564–71
11. Mazur T, Kurman RJ. *Diagnosis of Endometrial Biopsies and Curettings. A Practical Approach.* New York: Springer Verlag, 1995:7–32
12. Jones RK, Bulmer JN, Searle RF. Immunohistochemical characterization of proliferation, oestrogen receptor and progesterone receptor expression in endometriosis: comparison of eutopic and ectopic endometrium with normal cycling endometrium. *Hum Reprod* 1995;10: 3272–9
13. Klein N, Pergola G, Tekmal R, *et al.* Cytokine regulation of cellular proliferation in endometriosis. *Ann Acad Sci* 1994;734:322–32
14. Evers JHL. The second-look laparoscopy for evaluation of the result of medical treatment of endometriosis should not be performed during ovarian suppression. *Fertil Steril* 1987;47:502–4
15. Shifren JL, Tseng JF, Zaloudek CJ, *et al.* Ovarian steroid regulation of vascular endothelial growth factor in the human endometrium: implications for angiogenesis during the menstrual cycle and in the pathogenesis of endometriosis. *J Clin Endocrinol Metab* 1996;81:3112–18
16. Greb RR, Heikinheimo O, Williams RF, *et al.* Vascular endothelial growth factor in primate endometrium is regulated by oestrogen-receptor and progesterone-receptor ligands *in vivo. Hum Reprod* 1997;12:1280–92
17. McLaren J, Prentice A, Charnock-Jones DS, *et al.* Vascular endothelial growth factor is produced by peritoneal fluid macrophages in endometriosis and is regulated by ovarian steroids. *J Clin Invest* 1996;98:482–9
18. Nisolle M, Donnez J. Peritoneal endometriosis, ovarian endometriosis and adenomyotic nodules of the recto-vaginal septum are three different entities. *Fertil Steril* 1997;68:585–96
19. Kokorine I, Nisolle M, Donnez J, *et al.* Expression of interstitial collagenase (matrix metalloproteinase-1) is related to the activity of human endometriotic lesions. *Fertil Steril* 1997;68: 246–51
20. Beliard A, Donnez J, Nisolle M, *et al.* Localization of laminin, fibronectin, E-cadherin, and integrins in endometrium and endometriosis. *Fertil Steril* 1997;67:266–71
21. Folkman J, Shing Y. Angiogenesis. *J Biol Chem* 1992;267:10931–4

Histopathology and tissue remodeling: hormone receptors

10

A. Bergqvist

The steroid hormone receptors of interest are estrogen receptors (ER), progesterone receptors (PR) and androgen receptors (AR). Most studies have been performed on ER and PR – very few on AR. Endometriotic tissue is fairly heterogenous, which has to be kept in mind when different biochemical substances are studied. Conflicting data have been published on steroid receptor levels, mainly relating to different assay techniques. The different principles for available receptor assays focus on binding capacity, protein level or localization. Steroid receptors may be studied in tissue homogenates or tissue sections. In homogenates the receptor protein from all the cells in the sample is obtained[1]. Such techniques give a mean of the receptor level in a fairly large tissue volume and are routinely used for many clinical receptor assays, for example in breast cancer. However, steroid receptors appear heterogenously throughout different tissues, including endometrium and endometriotic tissue, which means that these techniques provide no information about the variation in receptor concentration in different areas. Moreover, the receptor concentration in epithelial cells related to stromal cells varies according to site and menstrual cycle phase, and the mean level obtained depends on the quantity of glands related to stroma. The receptors may be localized morphologically in histological sections, but that technique, however, only allows an estimation of a minor part of the tissue volume[2]. Moreover, the visual evaluation of the stained tissue sections gives, so far, only semi-quantitative information. As these two principles of receptor assays in tissue homogenates or tissue sections are completely different, the results are not well correlated to each other, but are complementary[3].

The level of steroid receptors varies to a high degree according to the levels of steroids available. The synthesis of the receptors is regulated by the steroids themselves. Estrogen induces the synthesis of both ER and PR, and progesterone has an inhibitory effect. Steroids have a rapid effect on the concentration of receptors. Endometrial cells in culture have shown a three-fold increase in receptor concentration within one day after administration of physiological doses of estrogen[4]. The effect of progesterone on human endometrial function is of short duration, because of the self-provoked downregulation of the receptor. A large dose of medroxyprogesterone acetate (MPA) was found to significantly suppress endometrial ER and PR concentrations in premenopausal women within four hours[5].

It is now known that different subtypes of steroid receptors exist as well as different isoforms of receptor mRNA. However, until very recently, only one type of ER was known, and all studies on endometriotic tissue published hitherto have looked at this form of ER. It is nowadays called ERα, since another subtype, ERβ, was described at our hospital in 1996[6]. ERβ has now been identified in different human tissues including: breast, ovarian granulosa cells, osteoblasts, nervous system and developing spermatids. Studies on ERβ in endometrium and endometriotic tissue are ongoing, but data are not yet available.

There is also a variety of estrogenic agents, including physiological estrogens (estrone and estriol), plant and environmental estrogens (genisten, conmestrol, bisphenol A,

Table 1 Publications on quantitative assays of ER and PR in endometriotic tissue

Author	*Year*	*Endometriotic samples* *n*	*Control endometrium*
Tamaya *et al.*[8]	1979	7	controls ($n = 5$)
Bergqvist *et al.*[9]	1981	20	paired ($n = 12$) and controls ($n = 30$)
Jänne *et al.*[10]	1981	47	controls ($n = 9$)
Lyndrup *et al.*[11]	1987	14	paired ($n = 14$)
Bergqvist *et al.*[12]	1993	62	paired ($n = 49$)

methoxychlor) and pharmacological agents (tamoxifen, 4-hydroxytamoxifen), known to compete effectively for estradiol binding at both receptors[7].The binding pharmacology among these agents differs, which should be taken into consideration when studying and describing the effects of estrogen, estrogen agonists/antagonists and environmental estrogens on endometrium and endometriotic tissue.

The first studies on steroid receptors in endometriotic tissue used quantitative ligand techniques, as no specific antibodies had been developed then (Table 1)[8–12]. These studies showed a lower level of both ER and PR in endometriotic tissue compared to endometrium, also in paired endometrium from the same woman. The development of specific monoclonal antibodies made quantitative enzyme immunoassays possible, which verified the results from previous ligand technique studies, although those two techniques are not directly comparable[1]. The ligand technique gives information about the level of unoccupied receptors with the capacity to bind hormone and the immunoassay gives information about the level of receptor protein, independent of whether it is biologically active or not. The ligand technique indicates that there are unbound receptors in the tissues ready to bind steroids available, transforming the hormonal message. Immunoassay requires very small tissue samples, which is attractive for studies on endometriosis. We used mainly endometriotic tissue scraped from the inside of endometriotic cysts, which means that a minimum of other cells was included. Paired samples of endometriotic tissue and endometrium from 58 women were studied using both the ligand technique and immunoassay[1]. Although the steroid receptors reside mainly in the nucleus, large quantities are found also in the cytosol, in all types of tissue studied, probably because of release from the nucleus during preparation. We found that the ER level was lower in endometriotic tissue than in endometrium, both in cytosol and the nuclear compartment. The ER level in endometrium showed a cyclic variation related to ovarian hormone cycles, being highest in the proliferative phase, but this was less obvious in endometriotic tissue. Also the level of PR was lower in endometriotic tissue than in endometrium during the follicular phase, but increased to become as high as in endometrium in the luteal phase.

Several studies localizing the receptors immunohistochemically (IHC) have been published (Table 2)[2, 13–20]. We studied 63 endometriotic samples and paired endometrium from 25 of the same women using IHC and found again lower receptor levels in endometriotic tissue than in the endometrium, but this difference was limited only to epithelial cells, not to stromal cells, and was significant only for PR[2]. There was a significant correlation between ER score in endometriotic tissue and endometrium, but not for the PR score. No significant difference was found for stromal cells. Thus expressions for a different hormonal regulation of ER and PR have been found. A consequence is that the hormonal message transferred to endometriotic cells is different to that in endometrial cells. No studies have shown any significant differences in steroid receptor levels in endometrium from women with

Table 2 Immunohistochemical studies on ER and PR in tissue sections of endometriotic tissue and endometrium

Author	*Year*	*Endometriotic samples* *n*	*Endometrial samples*
Bur *et al.*[13]	1987	19	$n = 0$
Lessey *et al.*[14]	1989	19	non-paired controls $n = 34$
Bergqvist *et al.*[2]	1993	63	paired $n = 25$
Gu *et al.*[15]	1996	15	paired $n = 15$
Donnez *et al.*[16]	1996	120	$n = 0$
Nisolle *et al.*[17]	1997	46	paired $n = 25$
Prentice *et al.*[18]	1992	25	non-paired controls $n = 25$; endometriotic controls $n = 27$
Jones *et al.*[19]	1995	30	paired $n = 30$; non-paired controls $n = 30$
Fujishita *et al.*[20]	1997	18	non-paired controls $n = 38$

endometriosis compared to control women. It is tempting to quantify the binding pattern of steroids in histological sections, but when enzyme immunoassay and IHC were compared in the same tissue samples, using the same antibodies, the correlation was low[3].

Thus the receptor concentration in epithelial cells related to the concentration in stromal cells varies according to the menstrual cycle phase, but there are also differences between different localizations. We found, when using enzyme immunoassay, that the ER level was significantly lower in ovarian endometriosis, including endometriotic cysts, compared to endometrium from the same woman[21]. No significant difference was found concerning PR. Peritoneal endometriosis did not differ from intra-uterine endometrium. IHC showed a lower score for PR in ovarian endometriosis, including endometriotic cysts, than in paired endometrium or vaginal or peritoneal endometriosis[2]. This technique did not reveal any obvious differences concerning ER. A difference in receptor concentration is also seen between different areas of the intra-uterine endometrium, illustrating that vascular and other growth regulating factors as well as different paracrine factors might influence the steroid receptor status. The clinical consequence of these differences might be that endometriotic lesions in different localizations respond differently to hormonal stimulation, endogenous as well as exogenous, and also hormonal depletion.

We have also tried to study whether steroid regulation is different in primary disease and in recurrences[21]. For clinical practical reasons it is difficult, or impossible to really know whether a lesion is primary or a recurrence in the same spot. We found that in women operated on because of clinical recurrence, the ER level in endometriotic lesions was significantly lower than in paired endometrium. No difference between endometrium and endometriotic tissue was found for PR. In endometriotic tissue the PR level was significantly higher in lesions from recurrent disease than from primary disease. No difference was found for ER.

Different factors are involved in the regulation of steroid receptors. As the estrogenic influence seems to be less pronounced in endometriotic tissue than in endometrium, other factors must be involved. It is known that steroid action in the uterus is mediated by more localized autocrine and paracrine regulatory systems of other growth regulating factors, such as epidermal growth factor (EGF), which is involved at least by having a stimulatory effect on protein synthesis, including receptor protein. EGF-R is found in endometrium and most endometriotic lesions[22]. A dramatic reduction of EGF-R in endometriotic lesions has been shown after treatment with a GnRH-agonist[23].

Only a few studies on AR have been published and all of them were on only a few samples[8,24]. Expression of AR mRNA has also been shown in endometriotic tissue[25]. The AR level does not seem to change cyclically. Although it is believed that androgens perform their endocrine effect partly by binding to other steroid receptors, AR may also play some role in the modulation of the endometrium and endometriotic tissue.

In conclusion, the levels of ER and PR are lower in endometriotic tissue than in endometrium, differ in various localizations and show a less pronounced cycle than in uterine endometrium. The reason for this is not clear, but might be dependent on influences from surrounding tissues and paracrine factors. The result might be a lower sensitivity to hormonal influence, which, in fact, is one of our great clinical dilemmas. Assays of steroid receptors as clinical routines is not meaningful, contrary to, for example, breast cancer diagnostics. However, the knowledge about steroid receptor function in endometriotic tissue helps us to understand the varying results we often obtain from hormonal treatment. Concerning hormonal replacement therapy of post-menopausal women, this knowledge has recently been taken into consideration and different schedules of intermittent hormonal treatment have been studied[26]. I am sure that this knowledge may be explored further when treatment of endometriosis is discussed.

References

1. Bergqvist A, Fernö M. Oestrogen and progesterone receptors in endometriotic tissue and endometrium: comparison of different cycle phases and ages. *Hum Reprod* 1993;8:2211–17
2. Bergqvist A, Ljungberg O, Skoog L. Immunohistochemical analysis of oestrogen and progesterone receptors in endometriotic tissue and endometrium. *Hum Reprod* 1993;8:1915–22
3. Bergqvist A, Fernö M, Skoog L. Quantitative enzyme immunoassay and semiquantitative immuno-histochemistry of oestrogen and progesterone receptors in endometriotic tissue and endometrium. *J Clin Pathol* 1997;50:496–500
4. Eckert RL, Katznellenbogen BS. Human endometrial cells in primary tissue culture: modulation of the progesterone receptor level by natural and synthetic estrogens *in vitro*. *J Clin Endocrinol Metab* 1981;52:699–708
5. Neumannova M, Kauppila A, Kivinen S, *et al.* Short-term effects of tamoxifen, medroxyprogesterone acetate, and their combination on receptor kinetics and 17β-hydroxysteroid dehydrogenase in human endometrium. *Obstet Gynecol* 1985;66:695–700
6. Kuiper GG, Gustafsson JÅ. The novel estrogen receptor-beta subtype: potential role in the cell- and promoter-specific actions of estrogens and anti-estrogens. *FEBS Letters* 1997;410:87–90
7. Petersen DN, Tkalcevic GT, Koza-Taylor PH, *et al.* Identification of estrogen receptor beta 2, a functional variant of estrogen receptor beta expressed in normal rat tissues. *Endocrinology* 1998;139:1082–92
8. Tamaya T, Motoyama T, Ohono Y, *et al.* Steroid receptor level and histology of endometriosis and adenomyosis. *Fertil Steril* 1979; 31:396–400
9. Bergqvist A, Rannevik G, Thorell JI. Estrogen and progesterone cytosol receptor concentrations in endometriotic tissue and intrauterine endometrium. *Acta Obstet Gynecol Scand Suppl* 1981; 101:53–8
10. Jänne O, Kauppila A, Kokko E, *et al.* Estrogen and progestin receptors in endometriosis lesions: comparison with endometrial tissue. *Am J Obstet Gynecol* 1981;141:562–6
11. Lyndrup J, Thorpe G, Glenthøj A, *et al.* Altered progesterone/estrogen receptor ratios in endometriosis. A comparative study of steroid receptors and morphology in endometriosis and endometrium. *Acta Obstet Gynecol Scand* 1997; 66:625–9
12. Bergqvist IA. Hormonal regulation of endometriosis and the rationales and effects of gonadotrophin-releasing hormone agonist treatment: a review. *Hum Reprod* 1995;10: 446–52
13. Bur ME, Greene GL, Press MF. Estrogen receptor localization in formalin-fixed, paraffin-embedded endometrium and endometriotic tissue. *Int J Gynecol Pathol* 1987;6:140–51
14. Lessey BA, Metzger DA, Haney AF, *et al.* Immunohistochemical analysis of estrogen and progesterone receptors in endometriosis: comparison with normal endometrium during the menstrual cycle and the effect of medical therapy. *Fertil Steril* 1989;51:409–15

15. Gu L, Zhang L, Gu F. Histologic examination and immunohistochemical analysis of estrogen and progesterone receptors of eutopic and ectopic endometrium in patients with endometriosis. *Clin J Obstet Gynecol* 1996;31:582–5
16. Donnez J, Nisolle M, Smoes P, *et al.* Peritoneal endometriosis and "endometriotic" nodules of the rectovaginal septum are two different entities. *Fertil Steril* 1996;66:362–8
17. Nisolle M, Casanas-Roux F, Donnez J. Immunohistochemical analysis of proliferative activity and steroid receptor expression in peritoneal and ovarian endometriosis. *Fertil Steril* 1997;68:912–19
18. Prentice A, Randall BJ, Weddell A, *et al.* Ovarian steroid receptor expression in endometriosis and in two potential parent epithelia: endometrium and peritoneal mesothelium. *Hum Reprod* 1992;7:1318–25
19. Jones RK, Bulmer JN, Searle RF. Immunohistochemical characterization of proliferation, oestrogen receptor and progesterone receptor expression in endometriosis: comparison of eutopic and ectopic endometrium with normal cycling endometrium. *Hum Reprod* 1995;10: 3272–9
20. Fujishita A, Nakane PK, Koij T, *et al.* Expression of estrogen and progesterone receptors in endometrium and peritoneal endometriosis: an immunohistochemical and *in situ* hybridization study. *Fertil Steril* 1997;67:856–64
21. Bergqvist A, Fernö M. Estrogen and progesterone receptors in endometriotic tissue and endometrium: comparison according to localization and recurrence. *Fertil Steril* 1993;60:63–7
22. Bergqvist A, Borg Å, Ljungberg O. Protooncogenes in endometriotic and endometrial tissue. *Ann NY Acad Sci* 1991;626:276–83
23. Di Lieto A, De Rosa G, Albano G, *et al.* Influence of goserelin depot therapy on epidermal growth factor receptor expression in pelvic endometriosis. *Gynecol Endocrinol* 1997;11:17–20
24. Punnonen R, Pettersson K, Vanharanta R, *et al.* Androgen, estrogen and progestin binding in cytosols of benign gynecologic tumors and tumorlike lesions. *Horm Metab Res* 1985;17:607–9
25. Horie K, Takakura K, Imai K, *et al.* Immunohistochemical localization of androgen receptor in the human endometrium, decidua, placenta and pathological conditions of the endometrium. *Hum Reprod* 1992;7:1461–6
26. Casper RF. Regulation of estrogen/progestogen receptors in the endometrium. *Int J Fertil* 1996; 41:16–21

Resident leukocytes in endometriosis

11

C.A. Witz, N.A. Klein, R.R. Tekmal, T.D. Dey and R.S. Schenken

INTRODUCTION

Leukocytes comprise up to 25% of the cell population in proliferative and secretory endometrial stroma[1,2]. Immunocytochemical studies have shown that the majority of these leukocytes are T cells and macrophages[1–5]. Considerable evidence suggests a paracrine role for resident leukocyte-secreted cytokines in regulating cell growth and differentiation in normal eutopic endometrium (UE). Cultures of endometrial stromal cells produce interferon gamma (IFNγ)[6], interleukin-1 (IL-1)[7,8], and interleukin-6 (IL-6)[7,9], and endometrial receptors to IFNγ[10] and IL-1[6,11] have been demonstrated by immunocytochemistry. IFNγ decreases BrdU incorporation into cultured endometrial epithelial cells[12] and it has been suggested that this antiproliferative effect may be related to the decreased proliferative activity found in the basalis layer of eutopic endometrium (UE)[5].

To assess whether resident T cells and macrophage products may play a role in regulating cell proliferation of endometriosis, we employed a dual-staining immunohistochemical technique with monoclonal antibodies to Ki67 (proliferation marker) and leukocyte markers. To assess whether the IFNγ may affect proliferative activity immunocytochemistry and *in situ* hybridization studies were performed. These studies suggest a possible paracrine role for resident leukocytes and IFNγ in regulating cell proliferation in endometriosis.

MATERIALS AND METHODS

Tissue collection

Endometriotic tissue was obtained from women (aged 22–43) undergoing surgery for pelvic pain or infertility, in the proliferative phase of the menstrual cycle. None of the patients had received recent hormonal therapy. Specimens included biopsies of superficial peritoneal implants, appearing as raised reddish nodules (n=14); ovarian endometriomas (n=14); and superficial ovarian endometriosis (n=3). Control tissue consisted of proliferative (n=9) or secretory (n=8) UE obtained from 17 cycling women (aged 28–45) undergoing diagnostic endometrial aspiration biopsy or hysterectomy for non-endometrial pathology. Tissue was immediately snap-frozen in liquid nitrogen and stored at −70°C until sectioning.

Histology

Serial 4 μm frozen sections were placed on baked glycine-coated slides, air-dried, and fixed for five minutes in acetone at 4°C. Sections were transferred to Tris-buffered saline (TBS; 0.1 M Tris-C1, 0.15 M NaCl, pH 7.4) prior to routine staining with hematoxylin and eosin or immunocytochemistry. Eutopic endometrias were dated histologically according to the criteria of Noyes *et al*[13].

Immunocytochemistry

Sections were first stained for the nuclear proliferation marker Ki67 or IFNγ (DAKO Corporation, Carpinteria, CA), and then for the surface antigen CD45 (leukocyte common antigen; AMAC, Inc., Westbrook, ME), CD3 (T-cell marker; DAKO), or CD11c (tissue macrophage marker; DAKO). Briefly, slides were incubated at 37°C with normal horse serum followed by mouse monoclonal antibody to Ki67 (DAKO) or IFNγ biotinylated anti-mouse secondary antibody, and, finally, avidin-biotin peroxidase complex (Vectastain®, catalogue #PK6102; Vector Laboratories, Inc., Burlingame, CA). Slides were then reacted in a mixture of diaminobenzidine (DAB) and hydrogen peroxide, which yielded a brown nuclear reaction product. After washing, the procedure was repeated with the substitution of one of the leukocyte marker antibodies as the primary antibody, and 4-choloro-1-napthol-H_2O_2 as the chromagen, to produce a blue reaction product. Slides were washed in TBS following each step of the sequence. Sections were lightly counterstained with hematoxylin, coverslipped, and examined by light microscopy. Primary antibodies were used at a dilution of 1:50, and secondary antibody at 1:200. For endometriosis specimens, sections were pre-incubated for 20 minutes with 0.3% hydrogen peroxide in methanol for quenching of endogenous peroxidase activity. Similar quenching of UE specimens did not affect nuclear or membrane staining. Negative controls consisted of substituting TBS or non-immune mouse serum at equivalent protein concentrations for the primary antibody.

Sections were examined under oil immersion. The proportion of cells staining for each of the antigens was obtained by counting a minimum of 500 cells in the stroma or epithelium or a minimum of 100 cells contained in lymphoid aggregates.

Proportions were compared using an unpaired *t*-test and results expressed as mean percentages with standard errors of the mean. Prior to data analysis, a non-linear transformation (arcsine transformation) was performed, which resulted in equal detectability of differences between proportions[14].

IFNγ riboprobes and *in situ* hybridization

Immunocytochemistry was performed with monoclonal antibodies to CD45, CD3 or CD11c as described above. Sections were then fixed with 4% paraformaldehyde for five minutes and processed in *in situ* hybridization. ^{32}P-labeled riboprobes were prepared from plasmid containing the Aval-Hinc II 900 bp fragment of the human IFNγ complementary deoxyribonucleic acid (cDNA) inserted into the pGEM3Z multiple cloning site. Plasmid was linearized with Hind III restriction enzyme and transcribed with T7 RNA polymerase to obtain mRNA-complementary riboprobe (antisense) or plasmid was linearized with EcoR1 and transcribed with SP6 RNA polymerase to obtain mRNA-like (sense) riboprobe using ^{32}P-CTP (New England Nuclear, Wilmington, DE) and a riboprobe kit (Promega Biotec, Madison, WI) according to the manufacturers' suggestions. Prehybridization and hybridization were carried out as described by Singer *et al.*[15], Harper *et al.*[16] and Chan *et al.*[17]. Briefly, sections were washed with RNAase-free TBS for one hour and with PBS for five minutes. Sections were then treated with acetic anhydride followed by Tris-glycine solution and incubated with prehybridization buffer (50% formamide, 0.3 M NaC1, 20 mM Tris-C1 [pH 8.0], 10% dextran sulfate, 10% mM Na pyrophosphate, 1X Denhardt's solution, 100 μg/ml yeast tRNA and 100 μg/ml salmon sperm DNA) for one to two hours at 45°C in a humidified chamber. Hybridization was carried out with the same buffer as above containing $2–3 \times 10^5$ cpm/section of IFNγ riboprobe, sense or antisense, for four to six hours. Slides were washed twice for 10 minutes each with 2 × SSC (1 × SSC = 0.15 M NaC1, 0.015 M Na citrate, pH 7.0). Nonhybridized probe was digested with 50 μg/ml RNAase A in 10 mM Tris-C1, pH 8.0, 0.3 M NaC1, for 30 minutes at 37°C. The slides were then washed twice for 30 minutes each at 45°C with 50% formamide containing 2 × SSC and rinsed with 2 × SSC. After dehydration in graded ethanol solutions, slides were dipped in NTB-2 emulsion (1:1 dilution; Eastman Kodak Co., Rochester, NY). After exposure for 10–15 days at 4°C, slides were developed with Kodak D-19 developer, fixed with Kodak Rapidfix, and counterstained with hematoxylin.

Sections were examined under oil immersion. The proportions of CD45-, CD3-, and CD11c-positive cells expressing mRNA for IFNγ were obtained by counting a minimum of 500 cells in the stroma or epithelium and expressed as a percent of the total. Sections processed for the combination of immunocytochemistry and *in situ* hybridization were compared to sections processed for immunocytochemistry or *in situ* hybridization alone. No significant differences were noted in the proportions and distributions of cells expressing CD antigens and IFNγ mRNA. Means were compared using the non-parametric Mann–Whitney *U* test performed using the computer package, Minitab (Minitab, Inc., State College, PA) on a personal computer. Results are expressed as mean ± standard error of the mean.

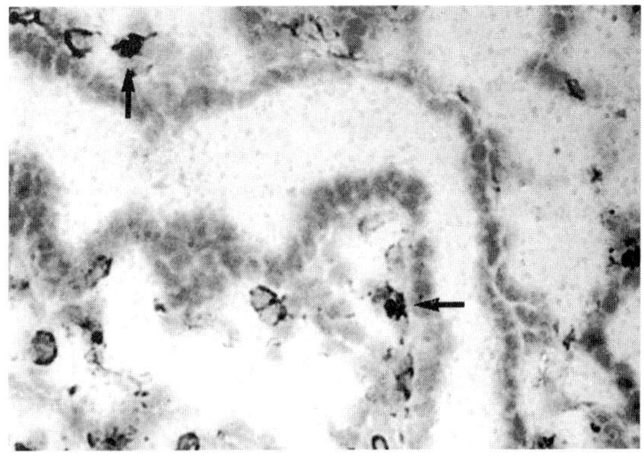

Figure 1 Late secretory endometrium processed for immunocytochemistry and *in situ* hybridization. IFNγ antisense riboprobe (40×); CD45-positive cells also expressing IFNγ mRNA are noted by the arrows

RESULTS

Histologic characteristics

Routine histologic staining of UE tissue revealed normal proliferative and secretory endometria with no evidence of endometriotis or other endometrial pathology. Examination of EE revealed weekly proliferative glands and stroma with surrounding fibrosis and frequent deposits of hemosiderin.

Cell populations and proliferative activity

Cells labeled with CD45, CD3, or CD11c were identified by their plasma membrane reactivity, and proliferating cells were distinguished by nuclear staining (Figure 1). Eutopic endometrium contained CD45+ cells scattered throughout the stroma as well as aggregates of these cells found primarily in the basalis adjacent to glands. Staining with CD3 and CD11c revealed that the majority of the CD45+ cells represented T-cells and macrophages.

Endometriotic tissue contained significantly higher proportions of scattered stromal CD45+, CD3+ and CD11c cells as compared with UE in either the proliferative or secretory phase ($p \leq 0.02$, Table 1). There were no significant differences between peritoneal implants and endometriomas in the proportions of scattered cells expressing each CD marker.

Sections of normal UE demonstrated variable degrees of proliferative activity in both CD-positive and CD-negative cells, as

Table 1 Proportion of scattered stromal cells staining for lymphoid cell antigens. Data are expressed as mean ± SE

Tissue	*% CD45+*	*% CD3+*	*% CD11c+*
Proliferative endometrium ($n = 8$)	7.5 ± 0.8	6.4 ± 0.7	3.8 ± 0.3
Secretory endometrium ($n = 13$)	11.1 ± 1.2	5.0 ± 0.6	4.5 ± 0.3
Endometriosis ($n = 17$)	19.0 ± 1.4†	9.9 ± 0.8†	9.3 ± 1.0†

†Different from proliferative and secretory endometrium, $p \leq 0.02$

evidenced by nuclear staining for Ki67. Dual-staining revealed a low level of proliferative activity in leukocytes scattered throughout the stroma as well as in those found in aggregates located near glands. In UE, the proliferative activity of the scattered leukocytes was greatest in the late secretory phase. In EE, proliferative activity was also noted in the scattered leukocyte population. The percentage of the total stromal cell population composed of proliferating CD45+ cells was similar in UE and EE (0.7% ±0.2 vs. 0.6% ±0.1) although a significantly greater proportion of the CD45-positive cells were proliferating in UE as compared to EE (9.0% ± 2.1 vs. 3.1% ± 1.0; $p = 0.005$).

The percentage of Ki67+ glandular epithelial cells in normal endometrium was significantly greater in the proliferative phase than in the secretory phase (5.7% vs. 3.3%, respectively; $p = 0.03$). Endometriotic tissue contained glands with only occasional cells staining for Ki67 in proportions consistently less than 1%. In endometrium, proliferative activity of CD-negative stromal cells was greater in the proliferative phase than in the secretory phase (8.3% vs. 5.1%, respectively; $p = 0.03$). Minimal CD-negative stromal cell/fibroblast proliferative activity was detected in all endometriosis specimens examined (1.4% vs. 8.3% for proliferative endometriosis, and 5.1% for secretory endometrium; $p < 0.0001$). The percentage of CD45-positive cells staining for IFNγ was significantly greater in EE compared to UE ($p < 0.05$).

All sections stained with TBS or non-immune mouse serum in place of the primary antibody were negative for nuclear or plasma membrane staining. Non-specific staining of hemosiderin deposits in endometriotic tissue was considerably reduced by quenching with 0.03% hydrogen peroxide in methanol prior to immunostaining.

IFNγ *in situ* hybridization

Some cells staining positive for the leukocyte cell markers also expressed IFNγ mRNA, demonstrated by a concentration of black

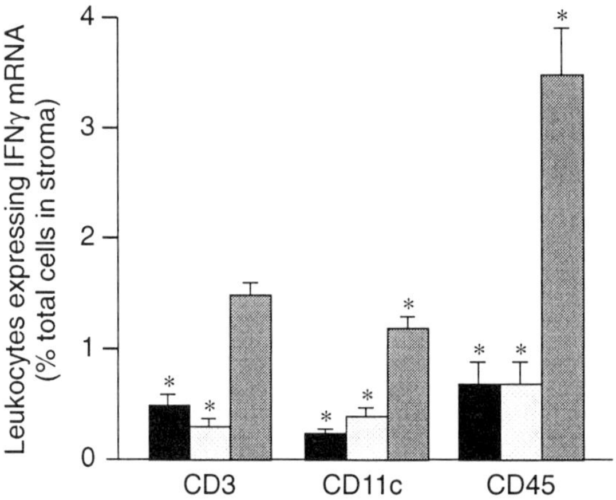

Figure 2 Percentage of CD45-, CD3-, and CD11c-positive cells expressing IFNγ mRNA in UE and EE, expressed as percent of the total cells in the stroma (*$p < 0.01$). ■ proliferative UE; □ secretory UE; □ endometriosis

silver grains overlying the nucleus and cytoplasm in addition to membrane immunostaining (Figure 1). Control sections incubated with the IFNγ sense riboprobe did not show concentrations of black silver grains over cells. This lack of hybridization with IFNγ mRNA indicates the specificity of the riboprobe used. Concentrations of cells in the stroma staining for leukocyte markers and also expressing IFNγ mRNA are shown in Figure 2. The proportion of these dually positive cells was significantly greater in EE than in either proliferative or secretory UE ($p < 0.05$). In addition, we compared the proportion of each leukocyte type expressing IFNγ mRNA (Figure 3). IFNγ mRNA was demonstrated in both CD45-positive cells and T cells and in a smaller proportion of macrophages. Expression of IFNγ mRNA by each of these cell types was greater in EE than in either secretory or proliferative UE ($p < 0.05$).

DISCUSSION

This study establishes the presence of resident leukocytes in endometriotic tissue. As in UE, the majority of these cells are T-cells and

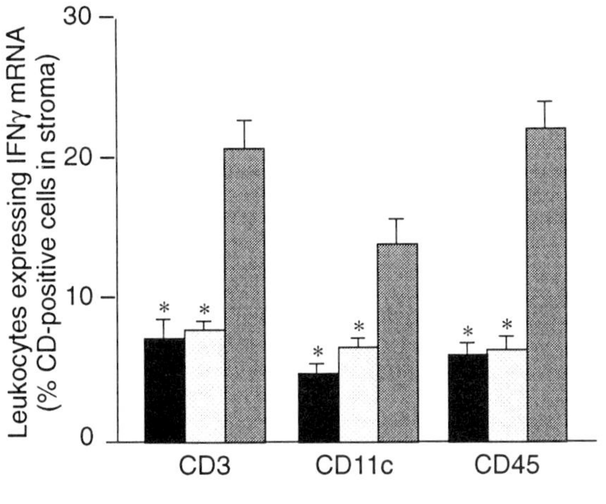

Figure 3 Percentage of leukocytes expressing IFNγ mRNA in UE and EE expressed as the percent of each leukocyte type (*$p < 0.01$). ■ proliferative UE; □ secretory UE; □ endometriosis

macrophages. The presence of leukocytes, both scattered and in aggregates, in normal UE has been well-documented[1–5]. The present study demonstrates that scattered T-cells (CD3+) and macrophages (CD11c+) in EE are present in higher concentrations than in UE.

The observed proliferative activity of both glandular and stromal components is significantly lower in EE than in UE. There is evidence suggesting that inhibitory cytokines decrease proliferative activity of endometrial cellular components. IFNγ decreases Brd-U (a thymidine analog) incorporation into cultured endometrial epithelial cells[12]. IL-1β inhibits ^{3}H-thymidine incorporation into cultured endometrial stromal cells[18]. The possibility that resident leukocytes may provide a source of IFNγ activity is supported by the *in vitro* observation that anti-serum to IFNγ[19] inhibits endometrial T-cell-induced HLA-DR expression in endometrial epithelial cells.

Our findings of IFNγ protein and mRNA in both UE and EE further support a paracrine role for IFNγ in these tissues. We observed that leukocyte IFNγ expression is enhanced in EE as compared to UE. A local antiproliferative effect of IFNγ might contribute to the lower proliferative activity in EE as previously observed by decreased c-myc[20] expression in EE as compared to UE.

Our findings of endometrial macrophage expression of IFNγ mRNA have not been described previously. Although T cell production of IFNγ has been extensively studied, IFNγ production has also been demonstrated in macrophages and natural killer (NK) cells. Macrophages isolated from mouse spleen, bone marrow and peritoneum[21,22], and purified alveolar macrophages from patients with sarcoidosis[23] and normal subjects[24] produce IFNγ in culture. The monoclonal antibody to CD11c may have some cross-reactivity with granulocytes, including NK cells[25]. Indeed, a recent study using several CD antibodies suggests that IFNγ is produced by polymorphonuclear neutrophils in UE[26].

In conclusion, we observed that (1) the concentration of scattered LCs is significantly greater in EE versus UE; (2) the proliferative activity of endometrial stromal and epithelial cells is significantly lower in EE vs. UE; (3) the proportion of proliferating CD45+ stromal cells is similar in UE vs. EE; (4) the overall concentration of CD45+ expression IFNγ protein and mRNA is greater in EE vs. UE; and (5) the percentage of each leukocyte type expressing IFNγ mRNA is also greater in EE. We conclude that these findings support a possible paracrine role for resident leukocytes and IFNγ in regulating cell proliferation in endometriosis.

ACKNOWLEDGEMENTS

The authors would like to thank Dr Jeff Hasdey for providing the plasmid construct containing the IFNγ cDNA. We also wish to thank Ms Irma Garcia for her valuable assistance in the preparation of this manuscript.

References

1. Kamat BR, Isaacson PG. The immunocytochemical distribution of leukocytic subpopulations in human endometrium. *Am J Pathol* 1987;127:66–73
2. Marshall RJ, Jones DB. An immunohistochemical study of lymphoid tissue in human endometrium. *Int J Gynecol Pathol* 1988;7:225–35
3. Bulmer JN, Lunny DP, Hagin SV. Immunohistochemical characterization of stromal leukocytes in nonpregnant human endometrium. *Am J Reprod Immunol Microbiol* 1988;17: 83–90
4. Morris H, Edwards J, Tiltman A, *et al.* Endometrial lymphoid tissue: an immunohistologic study. *J Clin Pathol* 1985;38:644–52
5. Tabibzadeh S. Proliferative activity of lymphoid cells in human endometrium throughout the menstrual cycle. *J Clin Endocrinol Metab* 1990; 70:437–43
6. Tabibzadeh S. Cytokine regulation of human endometrial function. *Ann NY Acad Sci* 1991; 622:89–98
7. Semer D, Reisler K, MacDonald PC, *et al.* Responsiveness of human endometrial stromal cells to cytokines. *Ann NY Acad Sci* 1991;622: 99–110
8. Romero R, Wu YK, Brody DT, *et al.* Human decidua: a source of interleukin-1. *Obstet Gynecol* 1989;73:31–4
9. Tabibzadeh SS, Santhanam U, Sehgal PB, *et al.* Cytokine-induced production of IFN-β_2/IL-6 by freshly explanted human endometrial stromal cells: modulation by estradiol-17β. *J Immunol* 1989;142:3134–9
10. Tabibzadeh S. Evidence of T-cell activation and potential cytokine action in human endometrium. *J Clin Endocrinol Metab* 1990;71:645–9
11. Tabibzadeh S, Kaffka KL, Satyaswaroop PG, *et al.* Interleukin-1 (IL-1) regulation of human endometrial function: presence of IL-1 receptor correlates with IL-1 stimulated prostaglandin E_2 production. *J Clin Endocrinol Metab* 1990;70: 1000–6
12. Tabibzadeh SS, Satyaswaroop PG, Rao PN. Antiproliferative effect of interferon-γ in human endometrial epithelial cells *in vitro*: potential local growth modulatory role in endometrium. *J Clin Endocrinol Metab* 1988;67:131–8
13. Noyes RW, Hertig AT. Dating the endometrial biopsy. *Fertil Steril* 1955;1:3–25
14. Cohen J. *Statistical Power Analysis for the Behavioral Sciences.* 2nd edn. Hillsdale, New Jersey: Lawrence Erlbaum Associates, 1988
15. Singer RH, Lawrence JB, Villnave C. Optimization of *in situ* hybridization using isotopic and non-isotopic detection methods. *Bio Techniques* 1986;4:230–50
16. Harper ME, Maselle LM, Gallo RC, *et al.* Detection of lymphocytes expressing human T-lymphotrophic virus type III in lymph nodes and peripheral blood from infected individuals by *in situ* hybridization. *Proc Natl Acad Sci USA* 1986;83: 772–6
17. Chan SH, Perussia B, Gupta JW, *et al.* Induction of interferon-γ production by natural killer stimulatory factor: characterization of the responder cells and synergy with other inducers. *J Exp Med* 1991;173:869–79
18. Van Le L, Oh ST, Anners JA, *et al.* Interleukin-1 inhibits growth of normal human endometrial stromal cells. *Obstet Gynecol* 1992;80:405–9
19. Tabibzadeh SS, Gerber MA, Satyaswaroop PG. Induction of LHA-DR antigen expression in endometrial epithelial cells *in vitro* by recombinant γ-interferon. *Am J Pathol* 1986;125: 90–6
20. Schenken RS, Johnson JV, Riehl RM. C-myc proto-oncogene polypeptide expression in endometriosis. *Am J Obstet Gynecol* 1991;164: 1031–6
21. Neumann C, Sorg C. Immune interferon. I. Production by lymphokine-activated murine macrophages. *Eur J Immunol* 1977;7:719–25
22. Olstad R, Degre M, Seljelid R. Production of immune interferon (type II) in cocultures of mouse peritoneal macrophages and syngeneic tumor cells. *Scand J Immunol* 1981;13:605–8
23. Robinson BWS, McLemore TL, Crystal RG. Gamma interferon is spontaneously released by alveolar macrophages and lung T lymphocytes in patients with pulmonary sarcoidosis. *J Clin Invest* 1985;75:1488–95
24. Nugent KM, Glazier J, Monick MM, *et al.* Stimulated human alveolar macrophages secrete interferon. *Am Rev Respir Dis* 1985;131:714–18
25. Lanier U, Arnaout MA, Schwarting R, *et al.* p150/95, third member of the LFA-1/CR_3 polypeptide family identified by anti-leu M5 monoclonal antibody. *Eur J Immunol* 1985;15:713–18
26. Yeaman GR, Collins JE, Currie JK, *et al.* IFN-γ is produced by polymorphonuclear neutrophils in human uterine endometrium and by cultured peripheral blood polymorphonuclear neutrophils. *J Immunol* 1998;160:5145–53

Immune reaction

12

H. Ota, S. Igarashi, J. Hatazawa and T. Tanaka

INTRODUCTION

Endometriosis is an enigmatic disease. It is well known that endometriosis is often associated with infertility and miscarriage. Yet, the precise mechanism leading to infertility is still obscure. Until recently, a majority of people have focused on the immunological factors of peritoneal fluid in reproductive failure, while few people have paid attention to the role of endometrium in endometriosis.

It is generally believed that endometriosis is provoked by the presence of ectopic endometrium. It is also known that endometriosis is associated with various autoimmune phenomena. These abnormal immune phenomena appear to play a pivotal role in infertility in endometriosis. Thus, the question arises whether the immune system in endometrium is also activated in endometriosis. Secondly, is the immune system in endometrium involved in infertility in endometriosis? The purpose of this article is to review the available information regarding the involving factors in immune reactions in endometriosis and discuss the critical role of the immune system in endometrial function (Figure 1).

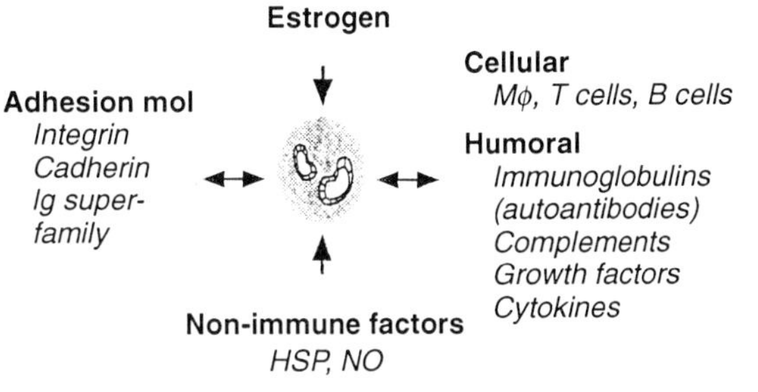

Figure 1 Involving factors in immune reactions in the endometrium in endometriosis. Mϕ, macrophage; HSP, heat shock protein; NO, nitric oxide

CELL SURFACE ANTIGENS

HLA antigens

Several studies indicate that most autoimmune diseases are associated with organ-specific autoantibodies in peripheral blood[1]. It is believed that the expression of class II antigen is a key process for the production of autoantibodies. Several reports indicate the increased expression of the HLA-DR antigen in target organs in Graves' disease and diabetes mellitus[2,3]. Exaggerated expression of the complex molecules of antigen peptides and HLA molecules in target cells are first recognized by macrophages, which activate T cells thereafter.

In the human endometrium, HLA antigens are expressed throughout the menstrual cycle[4]. We have reported the increased expression of HLA antigens in eutopic and ectopic endometria, particularly in glandular epithelial cells, in endometriosis (Figure 2)[5]. These facts suggest that the endometrium, especially the ectopic endometrium and liberated substances from the tissues, are recognized by macrophages, which would in turn activate helper T cells and stimulate B cells to produce antibodies. Thus, the expression of class II antigen in endometrial cells appears to play a critical role in immune reactions in endometriosis.

Integrins

It is known that several adhesion molecules are expressed in the human endometrium: integrins[6], cadherins and immunoglobulin superfamilies. Several reports indicate the abnormal expression of β1 or β3 integrins in

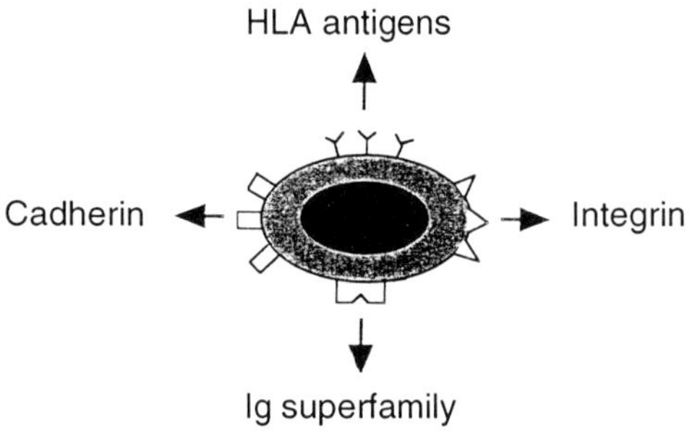

Figure 2 Expression of cell surface antigens in the endometrium

the endometrium in endometriosis[7]. Of the integrins, β1-integrins are typified by very late activation (VLA) antigen molecules. Both integrins are present in the endometrium and the expression is different in each phase of the menstrual cycle. Lessey and his colleagues[8] reported that the expression of VLA-4 was significantly reduced in endometriosis compared with fertile controls. Ligands for VLA-4 are fibronectin, which is produced in endometrial stromal cells and works as a 'molecular glue' during embryo implantation. Furthermore, another report indicates an aberrant expression of integrins in the endometrium in endometriosis, in which a lack of αvβ3-integrin expression (vitronectin receptor) is found during the implantation window in patients with endometriosis[9]. These facts suggest that the integrin–fibronectin/vitronectin system plays a central role in embryo implantation.

Cadherin

E-cadherin mediates cell–cell interaction, and cells adhere preferentially to cells that express the same cadherin. Cadherins are distributed widely among animals and play a significant role in morphogenetic events during embryogenesis[10]. Cadherin is also expressed in the cell-to-cell boundaries of the endometrium[11]. We have reported that the expression of E-cadherin in the endometrium was higher in the secretory phase than in the proliferative phase[12], although there is another report that the expression was unchanged during the cycle[13]. Furthermore, the expression of E-cadherin in the endometrium in endometriosis was significantly higher throughout the menstrual cycle compared to those in the controls. It still remains unclear why expression in some of the adhesion molecules is suppressed and that in other molecules is exaggerated in the endometrium in endometriosis. Further studies are needed to elucidate the exact role of these adhesion molecules in the endometrium in endometriosis.

Immunoglobulin superfamilies

The initiation of a specific immune response is believed to require not only activation through antigen-specific receptors on T cells and B cells but also antigen-independent interactions between accessory molecules. Such molecules belonging to immunoglobulin (Ig) superfamilies are lymphocyte-function-associated antigen-2 (LFA-2; CD2), LFA-3, and intercellular adhesion molecule-1 (ICAM-1), which enhance the avidity of interactions between T cells and antigen-presenting cells, and are potentially involved in signal transduction across the T cell membrane.

LFA-1, a member of the integrin family, is expressed in the majority of leukocytes. ICAM-1, a ligand of LFA-1, is expressed in stromal cells and endovascular cells in the human endometrium[14]. Tabibzadeh and Poubouridis[15] reported positive staining of ICAM-1 in glandular and luminal epithelial cells in the endometrium. It is also clear that LFA-2 binds to LFA-3 with high affinity, and can mediate the adhesion of lymphocytes via interaction with LFA-3. We have shown that the adhesion molecules, LFA-1 and LFA-2 on T cells, and ICAM-1 on the glandular cells, in the endometria in endometriosis were strongly stained[16]. Taken together, these findings indicate that two accessory pathways, LFA-1/ICAM-1 and LFA-2/LFA-3, are probably stimulated in endometriosis. Thus, three distinct pathways of cell–cell interactions, TCR/HLA,

LFA-1/ICAM-1 and LFA-2/LFA-3, would strongly enhance the effect of antigen presentation, leading to abnormal immune phenomena in endometriosis.

CELLULAR FACTORS

Macrophages

As already mentioned, class II antigens are strongly expressed in glandular cells and endometriotic cells in endometriosis. This fact suggests that endometriotic tissues activate the autoimmune system in the disease. Nonetheless, how macrophages are activated and autoantibodies are produced are still not clearly understood. Macrophages are widely distributed throughout the human body. They have various functions: phagocytosis, presenting antigens to lymphocytes, and initiating antigen-specific immune responses. The antigen-presenting cell function of macrophages is mediated by class II MHC, such as HLA-DR.

In endometriosis, macrophages in peritoneal fluid are greater in number and are activated[17]. Macrophages secrete various cytokines such as interleukin-1 and tumor necrosis factor. In endometriosis, these cytokines impede conception via several mechanisms, e.g., sperm phagocytosis and sperm motility, which interfere with fertilization and implantation[18]. We have reported an increased number of macrophages in eutopic and ectopic endometria in endometriosis[19]. Thus, it is possible that macrophages cause reduced fertility in patients with endometriosis.

T cells

A number of leukocytes have been found scattered in the stroma of eutopic endometria. There are several studies on T cell subpopulations in endometriosis. We reported that the number of cells in T cell subsets and macrophages in endometrial tissue from fertile patients showed no cycle-dependent differences[20]. Witz *et al.*[21] found that CD4, CD8, and VLA-1 positive T cells, a marker of activated T cells, were increased in endometrial tissues in patients with endometriosis. These findings support the hypothesis that immune cells are activated in the endometrium of patients with endometriosis.

Human T cell receptors are subdivided into two subtypes, αβT cells and γδT cells. γδT cells have no known ligand and have been found to express neither CD4 nor CD8 molecules, and they recognize antigens without MHC restriction. γδT cells are located in the skin, small intestine, lung, uterus and ovary and function primarily in epithelial immunity. We have found that γδT cells are increased in eutopic and ectopic endometria in endometriosis[16]. Furthermore, it is also known that γδT cells are increased in several autoimmune diseases. Why is the number of γδT cells higher in the endometrium in endometriosis? It has been confirmed that γδT cells are increased at the site of tissue damage in some types of inflammation of the bowel. Similarly, bleeding and/or necrosis occur in endometriotic tissues in endometriosis, which lead to inflammatory reactions and consequently stimulate macrophages and γδT cells.

B cells

There are several reports that B cells in peritoneal fluid are significantly elevated in women with endometriosis. Only a few studies have been conducted on the distribution of B cells in the endometrial stroma[21,22]. Witz *et al.*[21] stained the CD22-positive cells in the endometrium and found no cyclical changes during the menstrual cycle, but noted that the number of B cells tended to increase in the endometriosis group compared with that of the control.

HUMORAL FACTORS

Autoantibodies or immunoglobulins

It is well known that various autoantibodies, particularly those for phospholipids, are highly positive in peripheral blood in endometriosis or adenomyosis[23–25]. El-Roeiy *et al.*[26] reported a reduction of autoantibodies during danazol treatment in endometriosis patients with positive autoantibodies. We also found in adenomyosis that the number of cases with positive autoantibodies is drastically reduced in a time-dependent fashion after hysterectomy or during danazol treatment[25]. Thus, it is plausible that the production of these autoantibodies is induced by the presence of endometriotic tissues.

The autoantibodies belong to either the IgG, IgM or IgA group. There is a report that in endometriosis levels of IgG and IgM are high in autoantibody-positive patients compared with those in autoantibody-negative patients[27].

Several immunohistochemical studies also showed increased positive staining for IgG in the glandular epithelium in endometriosis[28,29].

Complements

A complement is a complex arrangement of interacting proteins that react with immunoglobulins to complete an antigen-antibody response. Assuming the immune system is activated in endometriosis, it appears possible that the complement components are involved in the system, adhering to the endometrial cells. We have found that in normal fertile women the deposition of complement components is rare, while the deposition of complement components C3 or C4 in endometriosis is high, 42 and 58%, respectively[29]. Deposition of the complements is also found in the endometrium in endometriosis. These facts further suggest that the complement system is involved in the abnormal immune response, inducing deposition of the complements in the endometrium in endometriosis.

INTRACELLULAR RESPONSES

Heat shock proteins

Heat shock proteins (HSPs) are constitutively expressed in human organs. They play an essential role as molecular chaperones in the folding of newly synthesized proteins in cells.

We have reported the strong expression of HSPs, particularly HSP27, in endometriosis[30]. There is a study showing that HSP70 is strongly expressed in infertile women, including those with endometriosis, compared with controls[31]. Substantial evidence of the participation of HSPs in various autoimmune diseases has been reported in the literature. How HSPs are involved in abnormal autoimmune phenomena thus becomes a question. It is possible that HSPs act as a molecular chaperone in cells. An increase in intracellular HSPs might be implicated in the immune response mediated by macrophages and/or T cells in endometriosis.

GASEOUS FACTORS

Nitric oxide

It has already been reported that miscarriage rates in patients with endometriosis are high, ranging from 11 to 63% and averaging 37%[32]. Treatment with danazol in endometriosis patients reduces the abortion rate to an average of 11%. Thus, the question becomes: What are the mechanisms that cause infertility or induce early miscarriage in endometriosis? One possibility is that nitric oxide, a potential vasodilator, might be involved in the mechanisms. Recent reports indicate that endothelial nitric oxide synthase, originally identified in vascular endothelial cells, is present in glandular epithelial cells in the endometrium[33,34]. It is of interest that the expression of endothelial nitric oxide synthase in the endometrium varies with the menstrual cycle, and was most marked in the mid-secretory phase in fertile women[35]. In contrast, the expression of the enzyme in endometriosis is persistently marked over the control levels throughout the menstrual cycle. Several studies *in vitro* indicate that nitric oxide affects human spermatozoa[36] or rat embryo[37]. In our preliminary study, we found that the treatment with nitric oxide donor, molsidomine, during the mouse preimplantation phase, markedly reduced the pregnancy rate in a dose-dependent manner. These facts suggest that optimal levels of nitric oxide are critical for sperm function and normal embryonic development. Examining the endometrial environment in endometriosis shows that various immune parameters differ widely from those in normal fertile women, as mentioned in this article. These abnormal immune responses might eventually stimulate macrophages and/or endometrial cells to produce persistently a large amount of nitric oxide and impede fertilization and/or implantation (Figure 3).

CONCLUSION

In endometriosis, a series of immune responses are activated, i.e. a strong expression of cell surface antigens, an increase in immune cells, and deposition of immunoglobulins and complement components. Endometrial cells are under immunological stress, protecting themselves by exposing heat-shock proteins. Furthermore, activated immune cells secrete various cytokines or growth factors, which stimulate the expression of cell surface antigens, forming an immunological 'vicious cycle' (Figure 4). Nitric oxide also seems to be involved in the cycle. Further studies are needed to provide the information that will enable us to restore the normal endometrial function and to improve fecundity in patients with endometriosis.

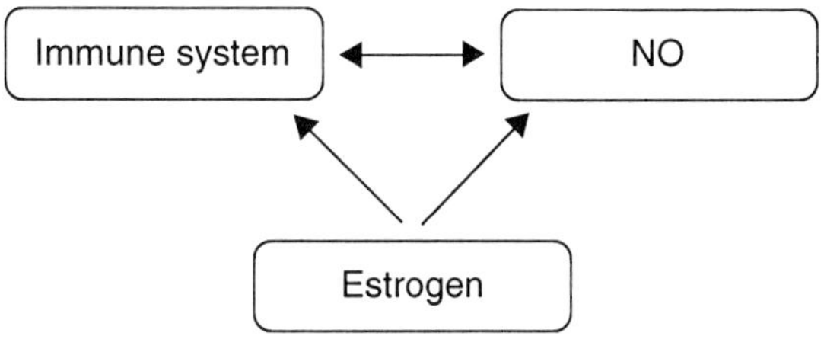

Figure 3 Involvement of nitric oxide in endometrial dysfunction

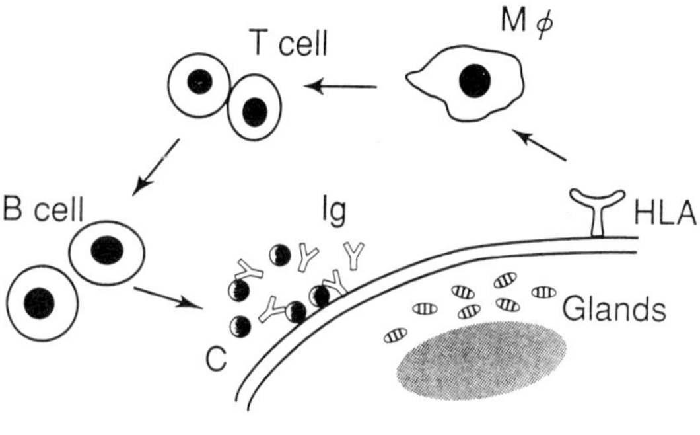

Figure 4 Immunological 'vicious cycle' in the endometrium in endometriosis. C, complement; Ig, immunoglobulin; Mϕ, macrophage

References

1. Shoenfeld Y, Isenberg D. Autoimmune diseases – clinical features and animal models. In Turk JL, ed. *The Mosaic of Autoimmunity*. New York: Elsevier Science, 1989;13–51
2. Hanafusa T, Pujol-Borrell R, Chiovato R, *et al.* Aberrant expression of HLA-DR antigen on thyrocytes in Graves' disease: relevance for autoimmunity. *Lancet* 1983;2:1111–15
3. Bottazzo GF, Dean BM, McNally JM, *et al. In situ* characterization of autoimmune phenomena and expression of HLA molecules in the pancreas in diabetic insulitis. *N Engl J Med* 1985;313:353–60
4. Tabibzadeh SS, Bettica A, Gerber MA. Variable expression of Ia antigens in human endometrium and in chronic endometritis. *Am J Clin Pathol* 1986;86:153–60
5. Ota H, Igarashi S. HLA-DR expression in endometriotic tissue in patients with endometriosis and adenomyosis. *Fertil Steril* 1993;60:834–8
6. Lessey BA, Damjanovich L, Coutifaris C. *et al.* Integrin adhesion molecules in the human endometrium. *J Clin Invest* 1992;90:188–95
7. Tabibzadeh S. Pattern of expression of integrin molecules in human endometrium throughout the menstrual cycle. *Hum Reprod* 1992;7:876–82
8. Lessey A, Castelbaum AJ, Sawin SW, *et al.* Aberrant integrin expression in the endometrium of women with endometriosis. *J Clin Endocrinol Metab* 1994;79:643–9

9. Lessey BA, Castelbaum AJ, Buck CA, *et al.* Further characterization of endometrial integrins during the menstrual cycle and in pregnancy. *Fertil Steril* 1994;62:497–506
10. Shirayoshi Y, Okada TS, Takeichi M. The calcium-dependent cell-cell adhesion system regulated inner cell mass formation and cell surface polarization in early mouse development. *Cell* 1983;35:631–8
11. Inoue M, Ogawa H, Miyata M, *et al.* Expression of E-cadherin in normal, benign, and malignant tissues of female genital organs. *Am J Clin Pathol* 1992;98:76–80
12. Ota H, Tanaka T. Integrin adhesion molecules in the endometrial glandular epithelium in patients with endometriosis or adenomyosis. *J Obstet Gynecol Res* 1997;23:485–91
13. Van der Linden PJQ, De Goeij AFPM, Dunselman GAJ, *et al.* Expression of cadherins and integrins in human endometrium throughout the menstrual cycle. *Fertil Steril* 1995;63:1210–16
14. Tawia SA, Beaton LA, Rogers PAW. Immunolocalization of the cellular adhesion molecules, intercellular adhesion molecule-1 (ICAM-1) and platelet endothelial cell adhesion molecule (PECAM), in human endometrium throughout the menstrual cycle. *Hum Reprod* 1993;8:175–81
15. Tabibzadeh S, Poubouridis D. Expression of leukocyte adhesion molecules in human endometrium. *Am J Clin Pathol* 1990;93:183–9
16. Ota H, Igarashi S, Tanaka T. Expression of γδT cells and adhesion molecules in endometriotic tissue in patients with endometriosis and adenomyosis. *Am J Reprod Immunol* 1996;35:477–82
17. Haney AF, Muscato JJ, Weinberg JB. Peritoneal fluid cell populations in infertility patients. *Fertil Steril* 1981;35:696–8
18. Hahn DW, Carraher RP, Foldesy RG, *et al.* Experimental evidence for failure to implant as a mechanism of infertility associated with endometriosis. *Am J Obstet Gynecol* 1986;155:1109–13
19. Ota H, Igarashi S, Maki M. Distribution of tissue macrophages in uterine muscle layers in patients with adenomyosis. *Med Sci Res* 1991;19:473–4
20. Ota H, Igarashi S, Hayakawa M, *et al.* Effect of danazol on the immunocompetent cells in the eutopic endometrium in patients with endometriosis: a multicenter cooperative study. *Fertil Steril* 1996;65:545–51
21. Witz CA, Montoya IA, Dey TD, *et al.* Characterization of lymphocyte subpopulations and T cell activation in endometriosis. *Am J Reprod Immunol* 1994;32:173–9
22. Klentzeris LD, Bulmer JN, Warren MA, *et al.* Lymphoid tissue in the endometrium of women with unexplained infertility: morphometric and immunohistochemical aspects. *Hum Reprod* 1994; 9:646–52
23. Gleicher N, El-Roeiy A, Confino E, *et al.* Is endometriosis an autoimmune disease? *Obstet Gynecol* 1987;70:115–22
24. Ota H. Autoantibody sensitivity in the diagnosis of endometriosis and adenomyosis. *Jpn J Fertil Steril* 1991;36:799–804
25. Ota H, Maki M, Shidara Y, *et al.* Effects of danazol at the immunological level in patients with adenomyosis, with special reference to autoantibodies: a multi-center cooperative study. *Am J Obstet Gynecol* 1992;167:481–6
26. El-Roeiy A, Dmowski WP, Gleicher N, *et al.* Danazol but not gonadotropin-releasing hormone agonists suppresses autoantibodies in endometriosis. *Fertil Steril* 1988;50:864–71
27. El-Roeiy, A, Gleicher N, Friberg J, *et al.* Correlation between peripheral blood and follicular fluid autoantibodies and impact on *in vitro* fertilization. *Obstet Gynecol* 1987;70:163–70
28. Weed JC, Arquembourg PC. Endometriosis: can it produce an autoimmune response resulting in infertility? *Clin Obstet Gynecol* 1980;23:885–93
29. Ota H, Maki M. Content of immunoglobulin G and complement components C3 and C4 in endometriotic tissue or endometrium in women with adenomyosis or endometriosis. *Med Sci Res* 1990;18:727–8
30. Ota H, Igarashi S, Hatazawa J, *et al.* Distribution of heat shock proteins in eutopic and ectopic endometrium in endometriosis and adenomyosis. *Fertil Steril* 1997;68:23–8
31. Nip MMC, Miller D, Taylor PV, *et al.* Expression of heat shock protein 70 kDa in human endometrium of normal and infertile women. *Hum Reprod* 1994;9:1253–6
32. Daya S. Endometriosis and spontaneous abortion. In Coutinho EM, Spínola P, de Moura LH, eds. *Progress in the Management of Endometriosis.* Carnforth, UK: The Parthenon Publishing Group, 1995:61–8
33. Tseng L, Zhang J, Peresleni T, *et al.* Cyclic expression of endothelial nitric oxide synthase mRNA in the epithelial glands of human endometrium. *J Soc Gynecol Invest* 1996;3:33–8
34. Telfer JF, Irvine GA, Kohnen G, *et al.* Expression of endothelial and inducible nitric oxide synthase in non-pregnant and decidualised human endometrium. *Mol Hum Reprod* 1997;3:69–75
35. Ota H, Igarashi S, Hatazawa J, *et al.* Endothelial nitric oxide synthase in the endometrium during the menstrual cycle in patients with endometriosis and adenomyosis. *Fertil Steril* 1988;69: 303–8
36. Rosselli M, Dubey RK, Imthurn B, *et al.* Effects of nitric oxide on human spermatozoa: evidence that nitric oxide decreases sperm motility and induces sperm toxicity. *Hum Reprod* 1995;10: 1786–90
37. Lee QP, Juchau MR. Dysmorphogenic effects of nitric oxide (NO) and NO-synthase inhibition: studies with intra-amniotic injections of sodium nitroprusside and NG-monomethyl-L-arginine. *Teratology* 1994;49:452–64

Role of monocyte chemotactic protein-1 in the pathophysiology of endometriosis

13

A. Akoum, A. Boucher, C. Jolicoeur, R. Drouin, A. Lemay, R. Maheux, M. Villeneuve and J. Mailloux

INTRODUCTION

Endometriosis is a common gynecologic disease affecting women in their reproductive age. It is generally associated with pelvic pain and infertility, but can also be asymptomatic and found in women undergoing laparoscopy for tubal ligation. Its actual prevalence among the general population is difficult to ascertain, but estimates suggest that the reproductive health of as many as 1% to 10% of women is affected by this disorder[1].

Endometriosis implants are commonly found on the organs of the pelvis and the diagnosis is made by laparoscopy. One of the most predominant hypotheses to explain endometriosis is that put forward by Sampson in 1927, who defined the disease as an ectopic growth of endometrial tissue that can reach the peritoneal cavity by tubal reflux (retrograde menstruation)[2]. This phenomenon is, however, common to all menstruating women and we have as yet no plausible explanation on how these cells could implant and proliferate ectopically only in certain women. Women may have a genetic predisposition to develop the disease[3,4]. Hormonal factors might also be involved in the maintenance and development of endometriotic lesions. Both eutopic and ectopic endometrial tissue depend on ovarian steroids[5] and the medical treatment of endometriosis is based on the suppression of ovarian function[6]. In recent years host immunological dysfunction has been invoked as a causal factor in the development of this disorder, and it may be a cause of pain and reduced fecundity in these patients.

Numerous studies have also focused on the role of monocytes/macrophages in the pathogenesis of endometriosis. Available data indicate that patients with endometriosis have an increased number of activated peritoneal macrophages[7,8]. Peripheral blood monocytes also seem to be more activated in women with endometriosis and secrete elevated levels of interleukin-1 (IL-1)[9,10]. They also show an altered expression of integrin molecules that play an active role in monocyte trafficking, adhesion, signal transduction and activation[11]. Furthermore, monocytes from patients with endometriosis have been shown to stimulate endometrial cell proliferation *in vitro*, while those of normal fertile women suppress the proliferation of endometrial cells[12]. Monocytes/macrophages play a central role in the maintenance of humoral and cell-mediated immunity, and through a panoply of secretory products they can play a significant role in the pathogenesis of endometriosis. These cells secrete growth factors that can stimulate endometrial cell proliferation[13,14] and numerous embryotoxic cytokines[15,16] and lymphokines that can activate B cells and autoantibodies production[17]. In this regard, it is worthy of note here that, according to numerous data, the levels of many cytokines such as IL-1[15,18], tumor necrosis factor α (TNFα)[16,18], IL-6[19], the protein regulated on activation normal T expressed and secreted (RANTES)[20], IL-8[21], transforming growth factor beta (TGFβ)[22] have been found to be elevated in the peritoneal fluid (PF) of patients suffering from endometriosis, which strongly supports the presence of an intra-peritoneal inflammation associated with endometriosis.

MONOCYTE CHEMOTACTIC PROTEIN-1 (MCP-1) AND ENDOMETRIOSIS

Concentration and biological activity in the peritoneal fluid and the peripheral blood

Monocyte chemotactic protein-1, a potent mediator of monocyte recruitment and activation[23,24], belongs to a newly characterized superfamily of small molecular weight cytokines whose major properties are to induce leukocyte chemotaxis with various degrees of cellular specificity[23]. We and others have found that patients with endometriosis have an increased level of MCP-1 in the PF as compared to normal women having no laparoscopical evidence of endometriosis[25,26]. We have also shown that patients with endometriosis had increased monocyte chemotactic activity in their PF in the early stages of the disease (stages I and II), and that MCP-1 may contribute significantly to the monocyte chemotactic activity observed[25]. We then evaluated MCP-1 in the peripheral blood (PB) of patients and found elevated levels in the early and most active stages of the disease[27]. Such a result is in keeping with new findings indicating that endometriosis would not only be a local condition restricted to the peritoneal environment but could also be associated with systemic abnormalities in immune functions.

Secretion by ectopic and eutopic endometrial cells

Other data from our laboratory showed that endometriotic cells are capable of producing MCP-1 in response to pro-inflammatory cytokines (IL-1 and TNFα)[28], which are present in elevated levels in the PF of patients. More interestingly, we subsequently found that cytokine-stimulated eutopic endometrial cells also produce MCP-1, and such a secretion was greater in cells from women with endometriosis than in cells from women having a normal gynecological status at laparoscopy[29].

These results make plausible MCP-1 as an important cell mediator involved in the activation of peripheral blood monocytes and peritoneal macrophages observed in endometriosis patients. They also give rise to the key question of whether, in the presence of disease, such an upregulation of MCP-1 expression may occur *in vivo* and could be encountered *in situ* in the intrauterine endometrium.

In situ expression in the endometrium

This was investigated in endometrial biopsies from women with and without endometriosis by immunohistochemistry and *in situ* hybridization[30].

Our results showed that women with endometriosis have a higher level of MCP-1 expression in the endometrium as compared to normal women, both at the level of the protein (Table 1) and the mRNA (Table 2). The highest level of MCP-1 expression was observed in endometrial glands, although a low level of expression could also be observed in the stroma.

At the protein level, MCP-1 expression was elevated in the initial stages of the disease, particularly in stage II, and decreased in more advanced stages (III–IV). The expres-sion of MCP-1 mRNA was also significantly elevated in the initial stages (I and II), but remained high in more severe disease compared to control. Such a discrepancy in MCP-1 protein and mRNA expression is difficult to explain with certainty, but it might be due to a reduced translation of MCP-1 and/or to a probable degradation of the protein in the endometrium in the more advanced stages of the disease. On the other hand, our results would suggest that endometriosis is more active in the early stages. Some studies have documented that PF inflammation is inversely related to the extent of visible endometriosis[31], and that less extensive disease may be more biochemically active than older implants[32].

Table 1 Number of normal and endometriosis subjects according to the intensity of MCP–1 protein staining in the endometrium

	Stroma					*Glands*				
	Intensity of staining					*Intensity of staining*				
	0	*1*	*2*	*3*	*p value*	*0*	*1*	*2*	*3*	*p value*
Controls	14	8	–	–		7	14	1	–	
Endometriosis (total)	18	29	–	–	0.0518*	2	23	16	6	0.0001*
Stage I	8	10	–	–	0.7107*	1	9	7	1	0.0048*
Stage II	3	14	–	–	0.0144*	–	8	4	5	0.0006*
Stage III– IV	7	5	–	–	0.7809*	1	6	5	–	0.0321*
Controls										
Proliferative phase	5	4	–	–		3	6	–	–	
Secretory phase	9	4	–	–	0.5482§	4	8	1	–	0.7515§
Endometriosis										
Proliferative phase	7	10	–	–		1	11	4	1	
Secretory phase	11	19	–	–	0.7724§	1	12	12	5	0.0760§

* Comparison with controls, *p* values corrected by the Bonferroni procedure; § comparison of the proliferative phase with the secretory phase

Table 2 Number of normal and endometriosis subjects according to the intensity of MCP–1 mRNA staining in the endometrium

	Stroma					*Glands*				
	Intensity of staining					*Intensity of staining*				
	0	*1*	*2*	*3*	*p value*	*0*	*1*	*2*	*3*	*p value*
Controls	11	11	–	–		–	18	4	–	
Endometriosis (total)	20	19	8	–	0.2453*	1	11	27	8	0.0001*
Stage I	6	11	1	–	0.7056*	1	4	11	2	0.0054*
Stage II	13	2	2	1	0.6327*	–	7	9	1	0.0261*
Stage III–IV	1	6	5	–	0.0036*	–	–	7	5	0.0001*
Controls										
Proliferative phase	4	5	–	–		–	7	2	–	
Secretory phase	7	6	–	–	0.7001§	–	11	2	–	0.7267§
Endometriosis										
Proliferative phase	5	7	5	–		–	4	10	3	
Secretory phase	15	12	3	–	0.0864 §	1	7	17	5	0.0804§

* Comparison with controls, *p* values corrected by the Bonferroni procedure; § Comparison of the proliferative phase with the secretory phase

However, it has also been reported that the concentrations of chemokines, such as interleukin-8 and RANTES (regulated on activation normal T expressed and secreted), correlate with the severity of the disease[20,21].

MCP-1 expression was higher in endometriosis patients than in control subjects both in the proliferative and the secretory phases of the menstrual cycle. Within the endometriosis group, however, there was a marked trend for an increased expression in the secretory phase, either at the level of the

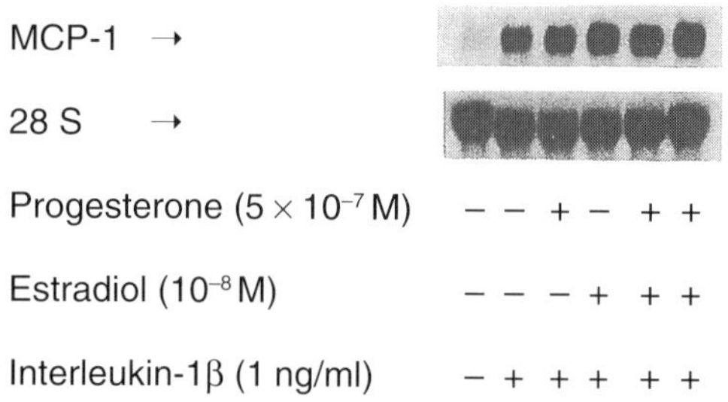

Figure 1 Effect of ovarian hormones estradiol (10^{-8} M) and progesterone (5×10^{-7} M) on MCP-1 mRNA synthesis by endometrial epithelial cells. Cells were treated with hormones until confluence then with 1 ng/ml IL-1β for an additional 6 hours before being harvested for RNA extraction and Northern blot analysis. Hybridization was performed with a ^{32}P-labeled MCP-1 cDNA probe, and also with a ^{32}P-labeled 28S cDNA probe to ensure equal RNA loading

protein or the mRNA. These results reveal a process of cell activation which occurs throughout the menstrual cycle in the endometrium of patients, but is amplified in the secretory phase. Moreover, an intense MCP-1 immunostaining was frequently located in the lumen of endometrial glands in the secretory phase, indicating an increased release of MCP-1 at this period of the cycle, and suggesting a hormonal influence.

Regulation of MCP-1 expression by ovarian hormones

Cultures of endometrial epithelial cells from women with endometriosis were treated until confluence with estradiol, progesterone, or with estradiol followed by progesterone before being exposed or not to IL-1β for a predetermined dose and time. As shown in Figure 1, treatment of cells with estradiol (10^{-8} M) increased MCP-1 mRNA synthesis induced by IL-1 β (1 ng/ml). In addition, treatment with both estradiol (10^{-8} M) and progesterone (5×10^{-7} M) amplified even more this expression. This seemed not to be due to an increased mRNA stability, but rather to a higher level of transcription as observed by run-off analysis (data not shown).

In summary, we found elevated concentration and biological activity of MCP-1 in the peritoneal fluid and the peripheral blood of patients with endometriosis. This potent monocyte chemotactic and activating factor is secreted by ectopic endometrial cells and shows an upregulated expression in the eutopic endometrium of endometriosis patients. In addition, according to our most recent data, estradiol upregulates MCP-1 mRNA synthesis by endometrial epithelial cells of women with endometriosis and exerts a synergistic stimulatory action with progesterone. Taken together, these findings make plausible MCP-1 as a key effector cell mediator involved in the pathogenesis of the disease and strongly argue in favor of the presence of pathophysiological changes in the eutopic endometrium of patients with endometriosis. They also reveal for the first time a hormonal control of MCP-1 expression in eutopic endometrial cells of women with endometriosis.

References

1. Barbieri RL. Etiology and epidemiology of endometriosis. *Am J Obstet Gynecol* 1990;162:565
2. Sampson JA. Peritoneal endometriosis due to the menstrual dissemination of endometrial tissue into the peritoneal cavity. *Am J Obstet Gynecol* 1927;14:422–69
3. Frey CH. The familial occurence of endometriosis. *Am J Obstet Gynecol* 1957;73:418
4. Malinak LR, Buttram VC Jr, Elias S. Heritable aspects of endometriosis II. Clinical characteristics of familial endometriosis. *Am J Obstet Gynecol* 1980;137:332
5. Dizerega GS, Barger DL, Hodgen GD. Endometriosis: role of ovarian steroids in initiation, maintenance and suppression. *Fertil Steril* 1980; 33:649–53
6. Rock JA, Markham SM. Pathogenesis of endometriosis. *The Lancet* 1992;340:1264–71

7. Haney AF, Muscato JJ, Weinberg JB. Peritoneal fluid cell populations in infertility patients. *Fertil Steril* 1981;35:696–8
8. Halme J, Becker S, Hammond MG, *et al.* Increased activation of pelvic macrophages in infertile women with mild endometriosis. *Am J Obstet Gynecol* 1983;145:333–7
9. Dmowski WP, Gebel HM, Braun DP. The role of cell-mediated immunity in pathogenesis of endometriosis. *Acta Obstet Gynecol Scand* 1994; (Suppl) 159:7–14
10. Zeller JM, Hening I, Radwanska E, *et al.* Enhancement of human monocyte and peritoneal macrophage chemiluminescence activities in women with endometriosis. *Am J Reprod Immunol* 1987;13:78
11. Gebel HM, Rana N, Braun PB, *et al.* Differential expression of VLAb1 (CD29) on monocytes from patients with endometriosis. *Am J Reprod Immunol* 1995;34:317–22
12. Braun DP, Muriana A, Gebel HM, *et al.* Monocyte-mediated enhancement of endometrial cell proliferation in women with endometriosis. *Fertil Steril* 1994;61:78–82
13. Halme J, White C, Kauma S, *et al.* Peritoneal macrophages from patients with endometriosis release growth factor activity *in vitro*. *J Clin Endocrinol Metab* 1988;66:1044–9
14. Olive DL, Montoya I, Riehl RM, *et al.* Macrophage-conditioned media enhance endometrial stromal cell proliferation *in vitro*. *Am J Obstet Gynecol* 1991;164:953–8
15. Fakih H, Baggett B, Holtz G, *et al.* Interleukin-1: a possible role in the infertility associated with endometriosis. *Fertil Steril* 1987;47:213–17
16. Eisermann J, Gast MJ, Pineda J, *et al.* Tumor necrosis factor in peritoneal fluid of women undergoing laparoscopic surgery. *Fertil Steril* 1988;50;573–9
17. Badawy SZ, Cuenca V, Freliech H, *et al.* Endometrial antibodies in serum and peritoneal fluid of infertile patients with and without endometriosis. *Fertil Steril* 1990;53:930–2
18. Taketani Y, Kuo TM, Mizuno M. Comparison of cytokine levels and embryo toxicity in peritoneal fluid in infertile women with untreated and treated endometriosis. *Am J Obstet Gynecol* 1992; 167:765–70
19. Rier SE, Parsons AK, Becker JL. Altered interleukin-6 production by peritoneal leukocytes from patients with endometriosis. *Fertil Steril* 1994;61:294–9
20. Khorram O, Taylor RN, Ryan IP, *et al.* Peritoneal fluid concentrations of the cytokine RANTES correlate with the severity of endometriosis. *Am J Obstet Gynecol* 1993;169:1545–9
21. Ryan IP, Tseng JF, Schriock ED, *et al.* Interleukin-8 concentrations are elevated in peritoneal fluid of women with endometriosis. *Fertil Steril* 1995; 63:929–32
22. Oosterlynck DJ, Meuleman C, Waer M, *et al.* Transforming growth factor-β activity is increased in peritoneal fluid from women with endometriosis. *Obstet Gynecol* 1994;83:287–92
23. Schall TJ. Biology of the RANTES/SIS cytokine family. *Cytokine* 1991;3:165–83
24. Leonard EJ, Yoshimura T. Human monocyte chemoattractant protein-1 (MCP-1). *Immunol Today* 1990;11:97–101
25. Akoum A, Lemay A, McColl S, *et al.* Elevated concentration and biological activity of monocyte chemotactic protein-1 in the peritoneal fluid of patients with endometriosis. *Fertil Steril* 1996; 66:17–23
26. Arici A, Oral E, Attar E, *et al.* Monocyte chemotactic protein-1 concentration in peritoneal fluid of women with endometriosis and its modulation of expression in mesothelial cells. *Fertil Steril* 1997;67:1065–72
27. Akoum A, Lemay A, McColl S, *et al.* Increased monocyte chemotactic protein-1 level and activity in the peripheral blood of women with endometriosis. *Am J Obstet Gynecol* 1996;175: 1620–5
28. Akoum A, Lemay A, Brunet C, *et al.* Cytokine-induced secretion of monocyte chemotactic protein-1 by human endometriotic cells in culture. *Am J Obstet Gynecol* 1995;172:594–600
29. Akoum A, Lemay A, Brunet C,*et al.* Secretion of monocyte chemotactic protein-1 by cytokine-stimulated endometrial cells of women with endometriosis. *Fertil Steril* 1995;63:322–8
30. Jolicoeur C, Boutouil M, Drouin R, *et al.* Increased expression of monocyte chemotactic protein-1 in the endometrium of women with endometriosis. *Am J Pathol* 1998;152:125–33
31. Haney AF, Jenkins S, Weinberg JB. The stimulus responsible for the peritoneal fluid inflammation observed in infertile women with endometriosis. *Fertil Steril* 1991;56:408–13
32. Vernon MW, Beard JS, Graves K, *et al.* Classification of endometriotic implants by morphologic appearance and capacity to synthesize prostaglandins. *Fertil Steril* 1986; 46:801–6

Cell adhesion molecules

14

P. Viganò, B. Gaffuri, R. Santorsola, E. Somigliana, M. Busacca, A.M. Di Blasio and M. Vignali

ADHESION MOLECULES: GENERAL VIEW

Cell communication is essential to development, tissue organization and function of all multicellular organisms. Cells communicate with each other and with their environment via soluble mediators and through direct contact. Discovery of cell surface receptors involved in cell–cell, cell–substrate or cell–soluble ligand binding has been a key factor in understanding the mechanisms underlying developmental and immune phenomena. Cell adhesion molecules are cell surface glycoproteins that either extend through the cell membrane or are attached to the membrane by a lipid anchor[1]. Engagement of these surface receptors can transduce a signal leading to cellular events that change the phenotype, movement, gene expression or activation state of the cell. On the other hand, cytoplasmic signals regulate the functional activity and surface expression of these receptors. These molecules thus mediate a dialogue, transferring information in both directions across the membrane. Contrary to earlier notions, there appear to be relatively few kinds of adhesion molecules which mediate developmental and binding events. Over the past few years, four families of adhesion molecules have been described as extensively implicated in a network of cell–cell and cell–matrix interactions (Table 1).

Immunoglobulin superfamily

The immunoglobulin superfamily includes both antigen-specific receptors, such as the T-cell receptor, as well as antigen-independent receptors and their counter-receptors, such as CD2 and lymphocyte function associated molecule-3 (LFA-3). Members of the family share the immunoglobulin domain, composed of 90–100 amino acids arranged in a sandwich of two sheets of anti-parallel β-strands, which is usually stabilized by a disulphide bond at its center. They bind soluble and cell surface ligands and function in cell activation, differentiation and cell–cell interaction. Neural cell adhesion molecule (NCAM) was the first cell adhesion molecule to be isolated and characterized and it was demonstrated in neural tissues, muscle, glia and other specialized locations. The resemblance of NCAM to immunoglobulins, the transplantation antigens and other members of the immunoglobulin superfamily prompted the suggestion that the evolutionary precursor of NCAM gave rise to the immune system. Convincing support for this hypothesis has come from the identification of NCAM-like molecules in the nervous systems of insects which have no adaptive immune system[2].

Integrin family

This consists of at least 14 α/β heterodimers divided into subfamilies according to distinct β subunits. Each subfamily has distinct structural and functional characteristics. The β1 or very late activation antigens (VLA) subfamily contains at least six distinct members and is found on a variety of cell types. The β2 subfamily, or leukocyte integrins, contains three members (LFA-1,

Table 1 Families of adhesion molecules and their counter-receptors

Adhesion molecule	*Synonyms*	*Counter-receptor*
Ig superfamily		
ICAM-1	CD54	LFA-1, Mac-1
PECAM-1	CD31	homotypic
VCAM-1	CD106	VLA-4, α4β7
NCAM	CD56	homotypic, heparan sulfate
HLA-DR		TCR/CD4
LFA-3	CD58	CD2
Integrin family		
LFA-1	αLβ2	ICAM-1, ICAM-2
Mac-1	αMβ2	C3bi, ICAM-1, factor X
P150,90	αXβ2	C3bi
VLA-1	α1β1	Laminin, collagen
VLA-2	α2β1	Laminin, collagen
VLA-3	α3β1	Laminin, collagen, fibronectin
VLA-4	α4β1	Fibronectin, VCAM-1
VLA-5	α5β1	Fibronectin
VLA-6	α6β1	Laminin
	α6β4	Laminin
	αvβ3	Vitronectin, fibronectin, fibrinogen
	αvβ5	Vitronectin
GpIIb/IIIa	αIIbβ3	Fibrinogen, factor VIII
Selectin family		
E-selectin	ELAM-1	SialyLewis^X antigen
L-selectin	LAM-1, Mel-14	HEV
P-selectin	CD62, PADGEM	SialyLewis^X antigen
Cadherin family		
E-cadherin		homotypic
N-cadherin		homotypic
P-cadherin		homotypic
uvomorulin		homotypic
LCAM		homotypic

Mac-1 and p150,75) exclusively expressed on leukocytes and the β3 subfamily or cytoadhesin family has two members (Vitronectin receptor and platelet glycoprotein IIb/IIIa) expressed primarily on endothelial cells and platelets. Recently, four additional β subunits have been defined. Integrin family members engage in heterophilic interactions with cell surface ligands and extracellular matrix components including fibronectin, collagen, laminin and vitronectin. Thus, they are of great significance in embryogenesis, growth and repair and homeostasis. The leukocyte integrins have been shown to have a critical role in inflammatory and immune responses. An important characteristic of integrins is that they exist in active and inactive states. An activated cell can transmit a signal from its cytoplasm that modifies the conformation of the extracellular domains of integrins on the cell membrane, increasing the affinity of integrins for their ligands. This family is phylogenetically ancient; α/β heterodimers have been defined in Drosophila, Xenopus and chicken[2–4].

Selectin family

Three selectin family molecules, endothelial cell adhesion molecule-1 (ELAM-1, E-selectin), leukocyte adhesion molecule (LAM-1, Mel-14, L-selectin) and CD62, also known as platelet activation-dependent granule-external membrane protein (PADG-EM, P-selectin), have been implicated in a number of leukocyte adhesion phenomena including leukocyte homing to lymphoid tissue. All these molecules have an NH_2-terminal domain of 117–120 amino acids, which is homologous to C-type lectins, followed by a single epidermal growth factor precursor motif of 34–40 amino acids and two to nine short consensus repeats of 62 amino acids. Cell surface expression of these molecules is inducible with cytokines or procoagulant factors, suggesting a role in inflammatory processes and coagulation[2]. Importantly, selectins are involved in the 'rolling' of leukocytes against the vascular endothelium prior to integrin binding and activation of the migratory activity, so that the leukocyte can migrate into the extracellular space at the site of inflammation.

Cadherin family

The cadherin family mediate cell–cell interactions and require calcium for their homophilic binding activity and biochemical integrity. Each cadherin type has a unique but wide tissue distribution that may vary during different stages of development. Cadherins are important constituents of adherens junctions where they are responsible for cytoskeletal organization. Furthermore, they seem to play an important role in invasive processes and metastasis of tumor cells. They are each made as a larger precursor with a signal sequence and about 100 amino acids that are cleaved off before expression on the cell surface. E-cadherin is expressed in all proliferating epithelial cells derived from ectoderm and endoderm; N-cadherin is found in the nervous system, heart and lens; P-cadherin is found in placenta and V-cadherin in endothelial cells[5–7].

INTEGRINS AND CADHERINS IN ENDOMETRIUM AND ENDOMETRIOSIS: CYCLIC CHANGES AND SYNCHRONIZED EXPRESSION

Integrins

According to Lessey *et al.*, integrins may participate in the establishment of an endometrial period of receptivity, the so called 'implantation window', during which embryonic development and uterine receptivity become carefully synchronized to allow a successful implantation[8,9]. Indeed, epithelial distribution of $\alpha 1\beta 1$, $\alpha V\beta 3$ and $\alpha 4\beta 1$, was found to change with the advancement of the menstrual cycle, and their coexpression occurs only during a 4-day midluteal period[9]. The 4-day interval (days 20 to 24) of the coexpression of these three molecules is thought to correspond precisely to the putative window of implantation in the human[9]. Thus, these data suggest that integrins may play a crucial role in nidiation and maintenance of early pregnancy. Clinical observations of a marked loss of glandular $\beta 3$ integrin during the putative window of implantation in patients with 'out of phase' biopsies[10], in certain patients with minimal or mild endometriosis[11] and in some women with unexplained infertility[10] are consistent with this hypothesis. In particular, in endometriosis, loss of timely $\beta 3$ expression may identify a subgroup of patients affected by the disease whose infertility relates to abnormal endometrial function[11]. It is noteworthy that, probably owing to the different degree of sensitivity that has characterized studies performed by immunohistochemistry, not all the authors agree with the results obtained by Lessey *et al.*[9]; according to the study of van der Linden *et al.*[12], except for integrin $\alpha 2\beta 1$, the expres-sion of other $\beta 1$ molecules was not dependent upon the phase of the cycle. Moreover, Klentzeris *et al.* reported that most $\beta 1$ integrins could be identified in endometrium from fertile women throughout the luteal phase but failed to detect $\alpha5\beta1$ in any endometrial specimens[13]. Finally, both Sillem *et al.*[14] in an *in vitro* system and Hii and Rogers[15] did not observe any difference in glandular $\alpha V\beta3$ expression between women with and without endometriosis. In contrast, Hii and Rogers[15] showed a significant increase in the percentage of vessels expressing $\alpha V\beta3$ in the endometrium of women with endometriosis, which is consistent with an increased endometrial angiogenesis. Thus, although some findings need to be further clarified through more extensive clinical observations, a greater understanding of the role of integrins in uterine receptivity and implantation will probably provide new insights into cellular and biological mechanisms related to endometriosis establishment.

Immunohistochemical analysis showed that all the integrins detected on endometrium can be detected on endometriotic lesions thus enforcing the hypothesis that the endometrium is the progenitor of endometriosis and suggesting that these molecules could also be involved in the attachment of endometrial tissue fragments to the peritoneum[16]. No difference in integrin expression between eutopic and ectopic endometrium biopsied synchronously from patients with endometriosis was seen in a comparative study by Bridges *et al.*[17], while Beliard *et al.* reported that expression of fibronectin receptors was lower in eutopic than in ectopic glands[18].

Cadherins

E- and P-cadherin expression was found on endometrial samples[12,16] while cells from menstrual effluent and retrogradely shed endometrium revealed E-cadherins to a lesser extent[16]. It has been proposed that a reduced pattern of this adhesion molecule could be the result of the proteolytic activity accompanying menstrual shedding of endometrium[16]. No major differences in cadherin expression were found between patients with and without endometriosis, suggesting that this molecule does not play a prominent role in the development of the disease[16].

ADHESION MOLECULES OF THE IMMUNOGLOBULIN SUPERFAMILY IN ENDOMETRIUM: IMPLICATIONS FOR INTERACTION WITH CELLS OF THE IMMUNE SYSTEM

The presence and distribution of many molecules of the immunoglobulin superfamily on human endometrium throughout the menstrual cycle have been extensively documented. In particular, expression of intercellular adhesion molecule (ICAM)-1[19–21], platelet endothelial cell adhesion molecule (PECAM)[20], HLA-DR[19] and LFA-3[22] has been associated with the presence, aggregation and preferential distribution of lymphoid cells in endometrium. Variations in the distribution of expression of these antigens have been suggested as important mechanisms by which the migration of leukocytes from the circulation across the endothelial cell barrier is regulated in human endometrium[19,20]. Focal enhancement of expression of these molecules adjacent to lymphoid aggregates[19] and the ability of cytokines to induce them[21,23] enforce this view.

Moreover, these endometrial immunoglobulin-like molecules have also been implicated in the interaction between endometrial cells and the peritoneal immune system[21]. Indeed, several authors have been arguing about the importance of an immunological peritoneal clearance system in the etiopathogenesis of endometriosis[24]. This physiological clearance may be one of the situations in which the immune system can recognize and eliminate misplaced autologous cells and prevent uncontrolled growth of self aberrant tissue in ectopic locations. As a result, endometrial cells which reach the peritoneal cavity by retrograde menses could be eliminated by immune cells. Macrophages and immune cells which exert a non-MHC restricted cytotoxicity such as natural killer

(NK) cells and NK-like T cells have been suggested to be involved in the effective elimination of ectopic endometrial cells thus impairing their ectopic implantation and growth. Moreover, a defect in this immune recognition has been claimed as a key mechanism in the initiation and progression of endometriosis[24–26].

The β2 integrin/intercellular adhesion molecule (ICAM)-1 pathway

Endometrial cells which reach the peritoneal cavity by retrograde menses may interact with local immunologically active cells through specific receptor-ligand interactions which are also subjected to cytokine modulation.

We have previously demonstrated that lymphocyte adhesion to endometrial cells is β2 integrin-1/ICAM-1 pathway-dependent as an anti ICAM 1 antibody is able to inhibit the interaction between NK cells and endometrial targets[21]. ICAM-1, which is expressed at high density on endometrium[21], is a 90-kDa glycoprotein which is a member of the immunoglobulin superfamily of adhesion molecules. In general, ICAM-1 is expressed on hemopoietic and non-hemopoietic cells including leukocytes, fibroblasts, endothelial and epithelial cells. Its induction is an important means of regulating inflammatory responses. In the absence of an inflammatory response, ICAM-1 is expressed on only a few cell types.

Therefore, since ICAM-1-mediated interaction seems to be critical to immune recognition of endometrial cells, our efforts have been directed toward the analysis of the mechanisms and cytokines that might regulate this interaction.

Regulatory effect of the soluble form of ICAM-1

Interestingly, a shedding form of ICAM-1 has recently been identified and characterized in at least three molecular forms with molecular masses of about 240, 430 and more than 500 kDa. Endometrial cells are also constitutively able to release the soluble form of ICAM-1 (sICAM-1)[27]. The circulating ICAM-1 retained the ability to bind to the β2 integrin and thus competes with the cell-bound molecule for binding to the same receptor on immune cells. As a consequence, sICAM-1 disturbs the efficient attack of CD8-lymphocytes and NK cells against their targets and effective immunological reaction is prevented. Consistent with this observation, a direct correlation was found between levels of sICAM-1 released by endometrial cells and the inhibition of NK cell-mediated lysis[27]. Interestingly, higher concentrations of this soluble protein have been detected in medium conditioned by endometrial cells obtained from patients with advanced stages of endometriosis when compared to women without the disease[27]. Finally, we set up experiments to examine whether differences in sICAM-1 release might exist between 24 paired samples of eutopic and ectopic endometrium biopsied synchronously in the same patients. Both eutopic and ectopic endometrial stromal cells were cultured for 48 hours at a density of 3×10^5/ml. As shown in Figure 1, ectopic cells in culture released significantly higher levels of sICAM-1 when compared to eutopic samples. Therefore, in disease-affected women, ectopic cells are a source of sICAM-1 even more potent than eutopic endometrium. As sICAM-1 is able to interfere with ICAM-1-mediated immune functions, it is tempting to speculate that shedding of sICAM-1 from cells derived from endometriosis implants might be one of the determinants for spreading potential.

Regulatory effect of interleukin (IL)-1β

IL-1β is one of the inflammatory cytokines of macrophage origin which has been demonstrated to be increased in peritoneal fluid of women with endometriosis[24]. Therefore, it is of utmost interest to evaluate whether this cytokine might modulate the ICAM-1 system in endometrium. In a previous study, we demonstrated that exposure of endometrial stromal cells to recombinant IL-1β resulted

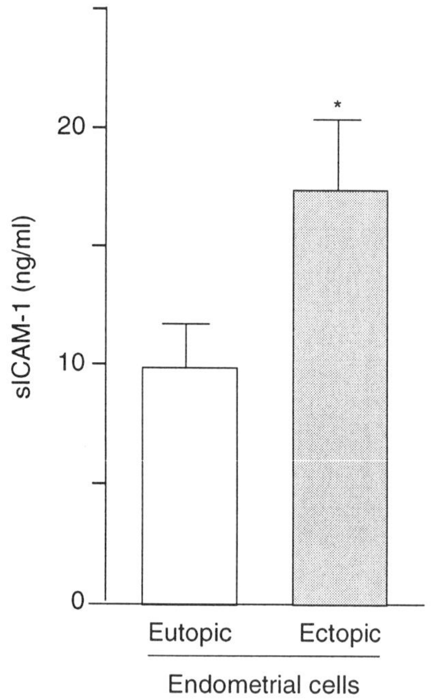

Figure 1 Eutopic and ectopic cell release of sICAM-1. Forty-eight-h conditioned media were harvested from cultures containing 3×10^5 cells/ml derived from 24 samples of eutopic endometrial cells and 24 samples of ectopic cells and tested for their content of sICAM-1 by a specific ELISA. Data are expressed as mean ± SEM. *p<0.05 vs eutopic samples

in a 5–10-fold increase in ICAM-1 expression[21]. To evaluate whether sICAM-1 shedding could also be modulated by the cytokine, endometrial stromal cells were treated for 48 hours with and without different concen-trations of IL-1β. As shown in Figure 2, IL-1β (0.5 ng/ml) led to a 2 to 3-fold increase in levels of sICAM-1. Given the ability of IL-1β to modulate endometrial surface and soluble forms of ICAM-1, we cannot exclude that this specific cytokine may be involved in the regulation of ICAM-1-mediated functions in peritoneal cavity.

Regulatory effect of interleukin (IL)-12

IL-12, formerly termed natural killer cell stimulatory factor, is a major factor in the regulation of NK cell cytotoxic activity. IL-12 is a heterodimeric molecule produced by monocyte-macrophages and dendritic cells. It exerts pleiotropic effects particularly on NK but also on T and B cells including induction of transcription and secretion of cytokines, enhancement of cytotoxicity and induction of proliferation. The IL-12 heterodimer is composed of two disulphide-linked chains, p35 and p40, encoded by separate genes. Simultaneous expression of the two genes is required for production of the biologically active IL-12 heterodimer. All the cell types producing the biologically active p75 heterodimer also produce a large excess of the free p40 chain. The physiological significance of the overproduction of the free p40 chain still needs to be elucidated although some evidence indicates that natural p40 acts as a physiological antagonist of IL-12. We have previously measured concentrations of IL-12 and its free p40 subunit in peritoneal fluid of 33 patients with endometriosis and 40 women without laparoscopic evidence of the disease[28]. Similar concentrations of IL-12, but significantly higher levels of the antagonist free p40 are present in peritoneal fluid of patients with endometriosis as compared to women without the disease. Given the variety of effects exerted on NK cells by IL-12, we reasoned that IL-12 may be a specific factor able to correct the NK cell defect in

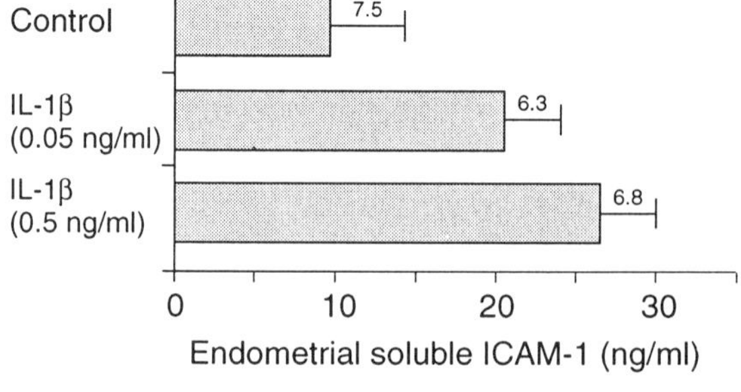

Figure 2 Effect of IL-1β on sICAM-1 release by endometrial cells in culture. Subconfluent endometrial cells were treated with or without IL-1β for 48 h. The culture media were collected and sICAM-1 was quantified by ELISA. Data are expressed as mean ± SEM of five separate experiments

endometriosis. Therefore we pretreated NK cells with different concentrations of heterodimeric IL-12 for 24 hours (Figure 3).

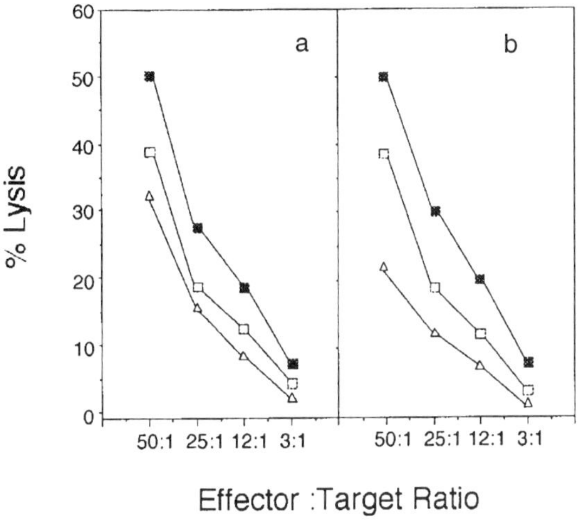

Figure 3 Effect of IL-12 on NK cell-mediated lysis of autologous endometrial stromal cells. Two representative experiments are shown. NK cells and autologous endometrial samples were obtained from a woman with stage III endometriosis (b) and from a woman without evidence of the disease (a). NK cells were incubated with medium alone (△), IL-12 (3 ng/ml; □) or IL-12 (10 ng/ml; ■) for 24 h. Cytotoxicity at various E/T ratios was then tested in a standard 4 h-^{51}Cr-release assay using autologous endometrial stromal cells as targets.

In women with and without endometriosis, addition of IL-12 to NK cells caused an enhancement of cytotoxicity but it should be noted that, in endometriosis patients, in which the unstimulated NK cell activity is lower, IL-12 is able to restore normal levels of cytotoxicity. Therefore, IL-12 may be considered a good candidate for controlling the cytolytic arm of the initial immunosurveillance toward endometrial antigens.

SUMMARY

Cell adhesion molecules are expressed in all tissues and cells potentially involved in the pathogenesis of endometriosis. Specifically, alterations in the expression of these molecules have been suggested to be involved in defective ability of the immune system to eliminate regurgitated endometrial cells, persistence of endometriotic lesions and decreased uterine receptivity in patients with endometriosis. Studies are in progress to evaluate the regulatory action of cytokines and factors commonly present in uterine and peritoneal environments on adhesion molecule expression. A better understanding of these regulatory mechanisms may lead to novel strategies for the treatment of patients with endometriosis.

References

1. Cunningham BA. Cell adhesion molecules and the regulation of development. *Am J Obstet Gynecol* 1991;164:939–48
2. Springer TA. Adhesion receptors of the immune system. *Nature* 1990;346:425–34
3. Larson RS, Springer TA. Structure and function of leukocyte integrins. *Immunol Rev* 1990;114: 181–206
4. Hemler ME. VLA proteins in the integrin family: structure, functions and their role on leukocytes. *Ann Rev Immunol* 1990;8:365–81
5. Takeichi M. Cadherins: a molecular family important in selective cell-cell adhesion. *Ann Rev Biochem* 1990;59:237–52
6. Takeichi M. The cadherins: cell-cell adhesion molecules controlling animal morphogenesis. *Development* 1988;102:639–55
7. Frixen UH, Behrens J, Sachs M, *et al.* E-cadherin mediated cell-cell adhesion prevents invasiveness of human carcinoma cells. *J Cell Biol* 1991; 113:173–85
8. Lessey BA, Damjanovich L, Coutifaris C, *et al.* Integrin adhesion molecules in the human endometrium. Correlation with the normal and abnormal menstrual cycle. *J Clin Invest* 1992; 90:188–95
9. Lessey BA, Castelbaum AJ, Buck CA, *et al.* Further characterization of endometrial integrins during the menstrual cycle and in pregnancy. *Fertil Steril* 1994;62:497–506
10. Lessey BA, Castelbaum AJ, Sawin SW, *et al.* Integrins as a marker of uterine receptivity in women with primary and unexplained infertility. *Fertil Steril* 1995;63:535–42

11. Lessey BA, Castelbaum AJ, Sawin SW, *et al.* Aberrant integrin expression in the endometrium of women with endometriosis. *J Clin Endocrinol Metab* 1994;79:643–9
12. van der Linden PJQ, de Goeij AFPM, Dunselman GAJ, *et al.* Expression of cadherins and integrins in human endometrium throughout the menstrual cycle. *Fertil Steril* 1995;63:1210–16
13. Klentzeris LD, Bulmer JN, Trejdosiewicz LK, *et al.* Beta-1 integrin cell adhesion molecules in the endometrium of fertile and infertile women. *Hum Reprod* 1993;8:1223–30
14. Sillem M, Prifti S, Rabe T, *et al.* Endometrial integrin expression is independent of estrogen or progestin treatment *in vitro. Fertil Steril* 1997;67:877–82
15. Hii LLP, Rogers PAW. Endometrial vascular and glandular expression of integrin $\alpha V\beta 3$ in women with and without endometriosis. *Hum Reprod* 1998;13:1030–5
16. van der Linden PJQ, de Goeij AFPM, Dunselman GAJ, *et al.* Expression of integrins and E-cadherin in cells from menstrual effluent, endometrium, peritoneal fluid, peritoneum and endometriosis. *Fertil Steril* 1994;61:85–90
17. Bridges JE, Prentice A, Roche W, *et al.* Expression of integrin adhesion molecules in endometrium and endometriosis. *Br J Obstet Gynaecol* 1994;101: 696–700
18. Beliard A, Donnez J, Nisolle M, *et al.* Localization of laminin, fibronectin, E-cadherin, and integrins in endometrium and endometriosis. *Fertil Steril* 1997;67:266–72
19. Tabibzadeh SS, Poubouridis D. Expression of leukocyte adhesion molecules in human endometrium. *Am J Clin Pathol* 1990;93:183–9
20. Tawia SA, Beaton LA, Rogers PAW. Immunolocalization of the cellular adhesion molecules Intercellular Adhesion Molecule-1 (ICAM-1) and Platelet Endothelial Cell Adhesion Molecule (PECAM) in human endometrium throughout the menstrual cycle. *Hum Reprod* 1993;8:175–81
21. Viganò P, Pardi R, Magri B, *et al.* Expression of Intercellular Adhesion Molecule-1 (ICAM-1) on cultured human endometrial stromal cells and its role in the interaction with natural killers. *Am J Reprod Immunol* 1994;32:139–45
22. Busacca M, Viganò P, Magri B, *et al.* The adhesion molecules on human endometrial stromal cells. Immunological implications. *Ann NY Acad Sci* 1994;734:43–6
23. Tabibzadeh SS, Gerber MA. Induction of HLA-DR antigen expression in human endometrial epithelial cells *in vitro* by recombinant γ-interferon. *Am J Pathol* 1986;125:90–6
24. Ho H-N, Wu M-Y, Yang Y-S. Peritoneal cell immunity and endometriosis. *Am J Reprod Immunol* 1997;38:400–12
25. Oosterlynck DJ, Cornillie FJ, Waer M, *et al.* Women with endometriosis show a defect in natural killer activity resulting in a decreased cytotoxicity to autologous endometrium. *Fertil Steril* 1991;56:45–51
26. Viganò P, Vercellini P, Di Blasio AM, *et al.* Deficient anti-endometrium lymphocyte-mediated cytotoxicity in patients with endometriosis. *Fertil Steril* 1991;56:894–9
27. Somigliana E, Viganò P, Gaffuri B, *et al.* Endometrial stromal cells as a source of intercellular adhesion molecule (ICAM)-1 molecules. *Hum Reprod* 1996;11:1190–4
28. Mazzeo D, Viganò P, Di Blasio AM, *et al.* Interleukin-12 and its free p40 subunit regulate immune recognition of endometrial cells: potential role in endometriosis. *J Clin Endocrinol Met* 1998;83:911–16

Synthesis and secretion of a haptoglobin-like protein by peritoneal endometriotic lesions

15

K.L. Sharpe-Timms, M. Piva, E.A. Ricke, K.E. Cox and R.L. Zimmer

INTRODUCTION

Endometriotic lesions are comprised of endometrial epithelial glands and stroma which are histologically similar yet biochemically different from their uterine counterparts[1]. Unique biochemical characteristics of ectopic endometriotic tissues may be involved in the pathogenesis, growth and remodeling, and pathophysiologies of endometriosis. These atypical characteristics may also facilitate development of novel diagnostic and therapeutic methods for endometriosis, which currently requires costly and invasive surgical procedures often leading to a counterproductive period of infertility[2,3]. Of particular interest is the complex, endometriosis-associated secretory glycoprotein discovered by our laboratory which we called endometriosis protein-I (ENDO-I)[4,5]. ENDO-I is differentially expressed by endometriosis, and limited NH_2-terminal amino acid sequence analysis and cDNA analysis demonstrate ENDO-I is a haptoglobin-like protein. Identification of localized production of haptoglobin-like ENDO-I by endometriotic lesions in the peritoneal cavity is intriguing, particularly in view of the recent identification of angiogenic and highly immunosuppressive qualities of haptoglobin (Hp).

MATERIALS AND METHODS

Endometriosis was surgically induced in mature female Sprague-Dawley rats (250 g) as previously described[7], used routinely by our laboratory[4,6,8–15] and approved by our institutional animal care and use committee. For most experiments, rats were euthanized at 4 weeks post surgical induction of endometriosis. In some experiments, rats were killed at 36 hours, 2 weeks and 4 weeks after the surgical induction of endometriosis.

Human tissues and fluids were obtained from randomly selected, informed volunteer patients routinely presenting to the physicians in the department of obstetrics and gynecology at the University of Missouri School of Medicine as approved by the institutional review board–health sciences section as previously described[5]. Peritoneal endometriotic implants, including red petechia, reddish-brown lesions and black-blue lesions were elevated with biopsy forceps and the area circumscribed by either laser or sharp dissection. The date of the patient's last menstrual period and use of any medication were recorded. Endometrial dating and the presence of endometriosis were histologically confirmed by the pathology department at the University of Missouri School of Medicine.

Endometriotic tissue explant cultures were performed as previously described[4,5]. *De novo* synthesized and secreted radiolabeled endometriotic lesion glycoproteins were purified from endometriotic tissue explant culture media using lectin Sepharose chromatography and further resolved by two-dimensional sodium dodecyl sulfate polyacrylamide gel electrophoresis (two-dimensional SDS–PAGE)[6]. Presence of ENDO-I was documented by fluorography and quantified by computer assisted image analysis[4,5]. Endometriosis secretory glycoproteins isolated in this fashion were then transferred to PVDF membranes and used to obtain limited NH_2-terminal ENDO-I protein sequence data by automated Edman degradation, and to study immunoreactivity using Western blot analysis[6].

Rat and human ENDO-I partial cDNAs were obtained using 3' RACE procedure (Gibco BRL; Gaithersburg, MD)[6,15,16]. Poly A enriched mRNA was isolated from tissues using the Invitrogen Micro-FastTrack kit (San Diego, CA) according to manufacturer's instructions. The mRNAs were reversed-transcribed into the corresponding cDNAs using an adapter primer and Super Script II Reverse Transcriptase from the 3' RACE kit. ENDO-I cDNA was specifically amplified using a gene specific primer as forward primer and the universal amplification primer (supplied with the 3' RACE kit) as the reverse primer. Rat and human gene specific primers were designed by back translation of specific amino acids of the Hp β-chain.

3' RACE products were examined on agarose/ethidium bromide gels[17] and the specificity of ENDO-I amplification was tested by Southern blot analysis. Rat ENDO-I gene expression was evaluated in rat endometriotic lesions, uterus and liver. Human ENDO-I gene expression was evaluated in several different tissues from several different patients including peritoneal endometriotic lesions ($n = 8$), eutopic endometrium ($n = 17$: $n = 5$ from women without endometriosis, $n = 8$ with endometriosis, $n = 4$ with adenomyosis), peritoneum from women without visual endometriosis ($n = 4$) and endometrioma ($n = 4$). Semi-quantitative RT–PCR was performed using glyceraldehyde-3-phosphate dehydrogenase (GAPDH) as internal standard. Relative expression was calculated by dividing the density of each ENDO-I band by the density of its corresponding GAPDH band. A logarithmic transformation of the ratio was performed to homogenize variances and normalize the distribution. One way analysis of variance was performed followed by Tukey's *post hoc* test.

Preliminary studies have been undertaken to explore cytokine regulation of ENDO-I mRNA expression using *in vitro* explant culture. ENDO-I mRNA levels in uterine endometrium and ectopic endometriotic tissues from two women were determined by semiquantitative RT–PCR and Southern blot analysis following incubation in the presence or absence of interleukin-6 (IL-6; 100 ng/ml)[16]. Differences between the ENDO-I/GAPDH ratio between samples treated with or without IL-6 were determined using Student's *t* test.

The effects of endometrial and peritoneal cell co-culture on ENDO-I production were also evaluated. Rat cells were obtained following enzymatic digestion of various tissues as previously described[11,18,19]. Isolated cell cultures and co-cultures of uterine, peritoneal, heart and liver cells were constructed. *De novo* synthesized and secreted radiolabeled proteins in the culture media were separated by two-dimensional SDS–PAGE, visualized by fluorography and analyzed by computer assisted image analysis. The cells were harvested and routinely prepared for evaluation by light and transmission electron microscopy.

RESULTS

ENDO-I is a complex, acidic, secretory glycoprotein which appears as two rows of 10–12 isoforms as visualized by two-dimensional SDS–PAGE and fluorography (Mr 40–55 kD, pI 4.0–5.2; Figure 1). We have demonstrated that ENDO-I is a glycoprotein by virtue of its multiple isoform appearance, its ability to incorporate [^{3}H]-glucosamine and its ability to bind to wheat germ lectin, which recognizes N-acetylglucosamine and terminal sialic acid residues[4–6].

We have reported that rat endometriotic lesions collected four weeks after surgical induction of endometriosis and human endometriotic lesions collected during all stages of the reproductive cycle, but not uterine endometrial tissues, synthesize and secrete ENDO-I *in vitro*[4,5]. As determined by

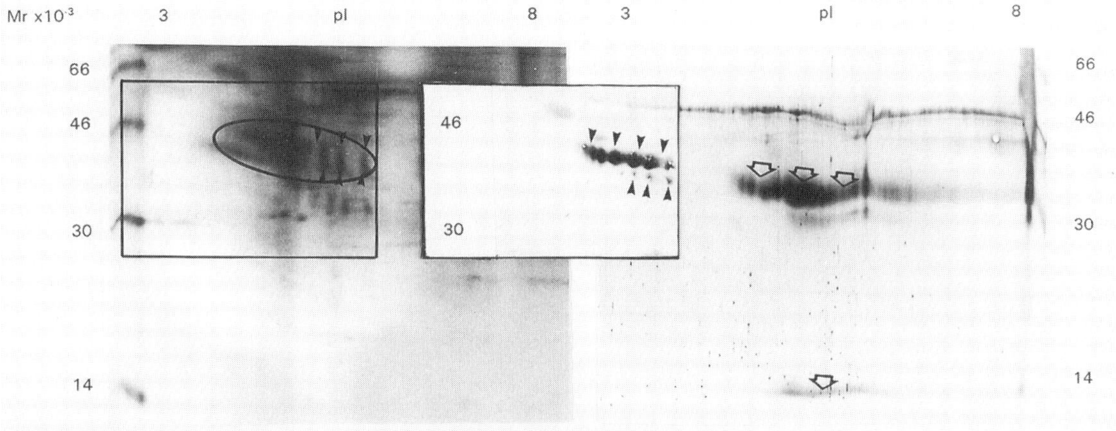

Figure 1 Human endometriotic lesion secretory glycoproteins compared to haptoglobin (Hp). (**a**) *De novo* synthesized and secreted human endometriotic lesion secretory glycoproteins were partially purified, isolated by two-dimensional SDS–PAGE and transferred to PVDF membranes. Visualization of radiolabeled ENDO-I (Mr > 40 kDa; oval) in a fluorograph of the membrane confirmed the presence of *de novo* synthesized ENDO-I in the culture medium. The box area was cut from the membrane and immunostained using the polyclonal anti-Hp antibody. (**b**) Insert shows that the polyclonal anti-Hp antibody recognized six of the multiple isoforms of the top row (arrowheads) and three to four of the isoforms of the bottom row (arrowheads) of *de novo* synthesized ENDO-I observed in the fluorographs. (**c**) Two-dimensional SDS–PAGE separation and Western blot analysis (using the polyclonal anti-Hp antibody) of human hepatic Hp showing the β-chain of human Hp migrated to 35 kDa (three open arrows) and the α-chain migrated to approximately 18 kDa (one open arrow). Note that the β-chain of human Hp (c) migrates to a lower position than ENDO-I (b). No protein was visualized corresponding to the Hp α-chain in the separation of the ENDO-I glycoproteins (a)

computer assisted image analysis of two-dimensional SDS–PAGE autoradiograph images of endometriosis secretory proteins, we have recently observed that rat endometriotic lesions collected 36 hours post-surgical induction failed to produce ENDO-I *in vitro* (mean ± SEM optical density [OD] from four different autoradiographs from four different rats = 7.8 ± 3.3 = background) as compared to rat endometriotic lesions collected 2 weeks (OD = 5324.0 ± 347.7) or 4 weeks (OD = 6381.0 ± 187.9) post-surgical induction, which produced significant amounts of ENDO-I *in vitro* (Cox and Sharpe-Timms, unpublished observations).

Analysis of three of the multiple rat ENDO-I isoforms yielded 16 amino acids, 15 of which were identified: IIGGSMDAKGSFPXQA (X=residue not called)[6]. Comparing this deduced amino acid sequence with amino acid sequences in data banks, we found that the 15 called ENDO-I amino acid residues share 100% sequence homology with the NH_2-terminal of the β-chain of hepatic Hp.

Using two-dimensional SDS–PAGE Western blot analysis we found that specific subsets of the *de novo* synthesized and secreted rat and human ENDO-I isoforms share antigenicity with a polyclonal Hp antibody (Dako, Carpinteria, CA; Figure 1) whereas a monoclonal Hp antibody (Sigma Chemical Co., St. Louis, MO) did not recognize any ENDO-I isoforms[6]. Neither the polyclonal Hp antibody nor the monoclonal Hp antibody detected any protein in the two-dimensional SDS–PAGE separations of *de novo* synthesized endometriotic lesion proteins, which matched the molecular size and isoelectric point coordinates of the Hp α-chains (Figure 1). Both the polyclonal Hp antibody and the monoclonal Hp antibody in question recognize both the α-chains and the β-chains of rat serum Hp and human serum Hp at concentrations similar to those of ENDO-I present in two-

Table 1 Relative ENDO-I transcript expression level (ENDO-I:GAPDH ratio) in pelvic endometriosis, eutopic endometrium, peritoneum and endometrioma. ENDO-I gene expression was studied by semi-quantitative RT–PCR. Relative expression was calculated by dividing the density of each ENDO-I band by the density of its corresponding GAPDH band. Ratios are shown as raw data. Statistical analysis was performed following logarithmic transformation of the ratios to homogenize variances and normalize the distribution. One way analysis of variance was performed followed by Tukey's *post hoc* test

	Number	*Median ENDO-I/GAPDH*	*25%*	*75%*	*p value**
Pelvic endometriosis	8	1.33	0.84	3.49	< 0.001
Eutopic endometrium	17	0.05	0.03	0.08	NS
Peritoneum	4	0.10	0.05	0.15	NS
Endometrioma	4	0.06	0.04	0.10	NS

*ENDO-I expression was significantly greater in pelvic endometriosis than in other tissues tested. No difference was observed between eutopic endometrium, peritoneum nor endometrioma

dimensional SDS–PAGE electrophoretic separations of partially purified ENDO-I. Collectively, the fact that ENDO-I (Mr 40–55 kD) is between 5–20 kD larger than the β-chain of hepatic Hp β-chain (M = 35)[20], and the differences in immuno-reactivity noted between Hp and ENDO-I provide strong evidence that ENDO-I is structurally similar but not identical to hepatic Hp.

A 950 bp transcript was amplified from rat endometriotic tissue and from liver but not from uterus[6]. Rat ENDO-I cDNA was almost identical (99.8%) to the rat hepatic Hp β-chain over an 859 bp overlap (nucleotides 102–958) that corresponds to the coding sequence and the 3' untranslated region of the message. Only one nucleotide was different between rat ENDO-I and Hp cDNAs, nucleotide 476 of the ENDO-I PCR fragment was a G residue whereas the corresponding nucleotide in rat Hp was a C.

A 950 bp transcript was also amplified from human endometriotic tissues[15]. As with the rat, human ENDO-I cDNA was almost identical (99.4%) to the human hepatic Hp β-chain over a 873 bp overlap (nucleotides 368–1222) which corresponds to the coding sequence and 3' untranslated region[15]. Downstream of the last nucleotide of the 3' untranslated region, several adrenylate residues corresponding to the poly A tail of the mRNA were detected. This finding ruled out genomic contamination. The four ASN N-glycosylation sites of the β-chain of hepatic Hp are also present in ENDO-I.

The highest ENDO-I relative transcript level was present in pelvic ectopic endometrium and was significantly higher than the average level of ENDO-I transcript in all eutopic endometrial samples combined, peritoneum and endometrioma ($p < 0.01$; Table 1)[15]. No statistical difference was detected between eutopic endometrium, peritoneum and endometrioma. While red petechial peritoneal endometriotic lesions expressed sufficient ENDO-I transcript for detection and quantification by this methodology, ENDO-I transcript was barely detectable in ovarian endometrioma and not detectable in black lesions.

Our preliminary studies of the effects of IL-6 on ENDO-I expression demonstrated that IL-6 increased the relative amount of ENDO-I transcript 29-fold in uterine endometrium from women with endometriosis ($p < 0.001$) and twofold in peritoneal endometriosis as compared to the same samples cultured without IL-6 (Figure 2). Further studies with additional samples are being performed to confirm these observations.

Cell morphology, proliferation and *de novo* synthesis and secretion of ENDO-I were affected by the type of cells co-cultured. Peritoneal mesothelial cells augmented

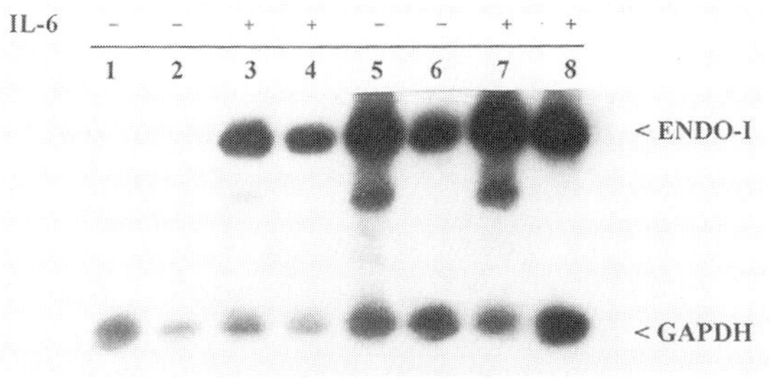

Figure 2 RT–PCR analysis of ENDO-I expression by eutopic endometrium from women with endometriosis (UE-E) and pelvic endometriotic lesions (PE). Two UE-E samples were incubated without (–; lanes 1 and 2) and with 100 ng/ml of human recombinant interleukin-6 (IL-6) (+; lanes 3 and 4). Two PE samples were incubated without (–; lanes 5 and 6) and with 100ng/ml of IL-6 (+; lanes 7 and 8). Total RNA was isolated and mRNAs were reverse transcribed. ENDO-I cDNA was amplified using a gene specific primer. The amplified bands were resolved by agarose electrophoresis, transferred to membranes and analyzed by Southern blot analysis. A 250 bp DNA fragment spanning from nucleotide 39 to nucleotide 288 of human ENDO-I cDNA sequence was labeled by PCR and used as a hybridization probe. Lanes 1, 3 and 5, 7, and lanes 2, 4 and 6, 8 are matching samples from two different patients

proliferation and induced cellular aggregation of uterine stromal cell monolayers, and peritoneal subserosal cells amplified proliferation and induced an irregular, compacted morphology in uterine epithelial cells[11]. Ultrastructurally, peritoneal cells co-cultured with uterine cells developed numerous secretory vesicles which contained electron dense material (Figure 3)[18]. ENDO-I was found in the culture media of isolated peritoneal cells but not isolated uterine cells. A dramatic upregulation of ENDO-I production was found when uterine cells were co-cultured on basal layers of peritoneal cells. No ENDO-I was found in culture media from liver or heart cells cultured either on plastic or on basal layers of peritoneal cells.

DISCUSSION

Interestingly, we have shown endometriosis synthesizes and secretes a protein which is structurally similar to hepatic Hp. Hepatic Hp is an acute phase protein composed of two α- and two β-polypeptide chains which exhibit considerable polymorphism[21]. Haptoglobin α-subtypes vary genetically, immunologically and functionally in a variety of physiological and pathological conditions[22–25]. In certain disease states, alterations in Hp glycosylation occur on the Hp β-chain at four distinct asparagine residues (ASN 23, 46, 50, 80)[22, 26]. Total serum concentrations of Hp may also change in association with inflammation, infection, trauma and disease[25, 27].

To date, limited information about glycosylation of Hp-like ENDO-I is available, although it is known that the four ASN-sites of the Hp β-chain have been conserved. Studies are ongoing to define unique ENDO-I glycosylation patterns. This information will help determine the unique nature of ENDO-I and establish its potential for a minimally-invasive serum marker for the disorder. We are also studying the possibility that women with endometriosis may express a unique hepatic Hp phenotype which imparts a genetic predisposition to develop endometriosis.

Although the most recognized site of Hp synthesis and secretion is the liver, extrahepatic sites of Hp production have been reported. Significant amounts of Hp mRNA have been detected in adipose and lung tissues in mice and baboons which are dramatically upregulated upon induction of inflammation[28–30]. A 42 kD rabbit endometrial epithelial cell glycoprotein produced during the receptive phase to embryo implantation[31] and a bovine oviductal fluid glycoprotein[32] also share limited NH_2-terminal amino acid sequence homology with the β-chain of Hp. O'Bryan and colleagues[33] purified a 67 kD protein from Sertoli cell-enriched culture media that consisted of two dissimilar subunits of 9 kD (α-chain) and 24 kD (β-chain) on SDS–PAGE under reducing conditions. Sequence analysis of the 9 kD subunit revealed NH_2-terminal sequence identity with the Hp α-chain. Our work demonstrates that endometriosis also synthesizes and secretes a Hp-like protein, yet further studies will have to

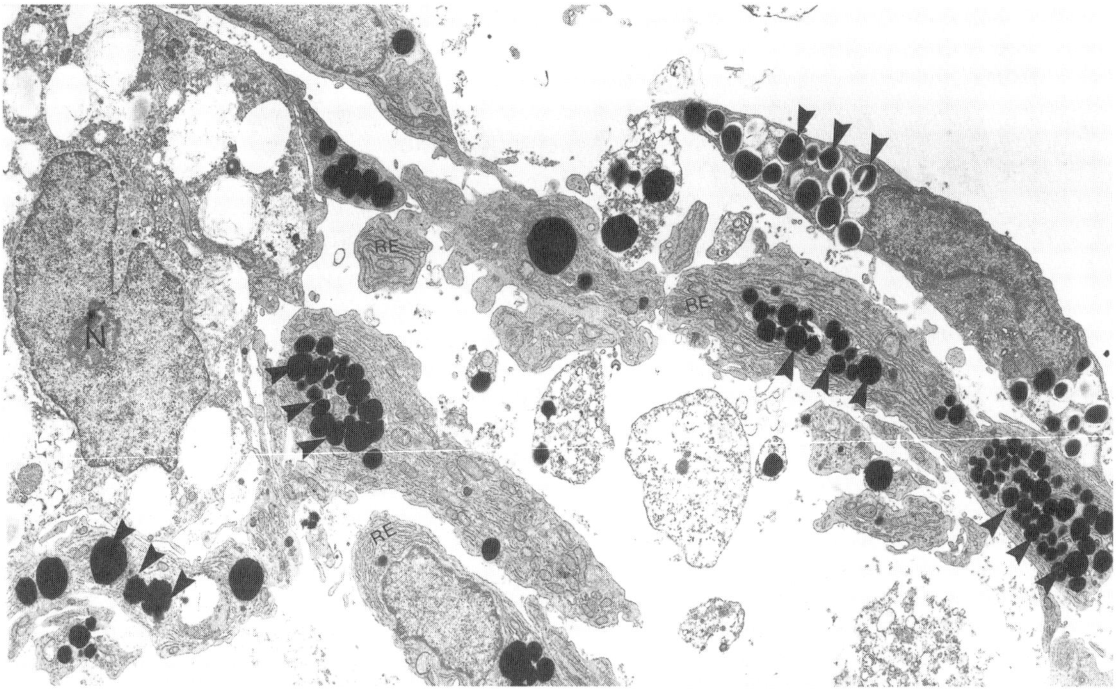

Figure 3 Representative transmission electron micrograph of uterine cell/peritoneal cell co-cultures. The scant cytoplasm of the peritoneal cells contained numerous ribosomes and rough endoplasmic reticulum (RE) with dilated cisternae. The nuclei were large, occupying most of the cytoplasm, and had an even distribution of chromatin except at their periphery where chromatin formed a narrow, dense band on the inner aspect of the nuclear membrane. Prominent nucleoli (N), a distinguishing feature of the peritoneal cells, were observed. Strikingly, peritoneal cells co-cultured with endometrial cells developed numerous secretory vesicles (triple arrow heads) containing electron-dense material in the cytoplasm

be performed to confirm any similarities or differences between ENDO-I and these Hp-like proteins.

The fact that ENDO-I is not found in explant culture media from endometriotic lesions collected 36 hours after surgical-induction of endometriosis but subsequently appears in explant culture of lesions collected at two and four weeks post-induction suggest that regulatory mechanisms of ENDO-I expression differ from mechanisms regulating hepatic Hp or other extra-hepatic Hp production. In the liver, Hp steady state mRNA levels rise sharply in response to induced inflammation within 24 hours and decrease to basal levels by 48 hours after induced inflammation (inflammation induced by laparotomy)[33, 34]. By contrast, Hp mRNA levels in the testis decrease by more than two-fold and Hp expression by the lung remains unchanged in response to induced inflammation[33, 35]. Although the mechanisms regulating ENDO-I expression remain to be determined, the fact that ENDO-I is not produced in response to laparotomy-induced inflammation, as is hepatic Hp, demonstrates that production of ENDO-I does not occur as an acute phase response to inflammation.

In addition to its well-known function as a carrier of hemoglobin, potential roles for Hp in local defense mechanisms and angiogenic stimulation of endothelial cell differentiation and vascularization have been described[25, 27]. For example, using an established *in vitro* model of angiogenesis and an *in vivo* angiogenesis model, Hp was identified as an angiogenic factor in sera from patients with systemic vasculitis[36]. Thus, it is possible that Hp-like ENDO-I could be responsible for vascularization of endometriotic lesions.

In association with certain inflammatory states and with certain cancers, hepatic Hp has also been found to exhibit immunomodulatory activity[22,23,37–40]. While the mechanism of Hp immunomodulation is unknown, Hp has been shown to bind to immune cells including monocytes, granulocytes, $CD8^+$ T cells, natural killer cells and macrophages via the αMβ2 integrin receptor (also called CD11b/CD18 or MAC-1)[39,40] and may thereby regulate immune function by acting as a natural antagonist for receptor-ligand activation of the immune system[41]. Haptoglobin has been shown to inhibit macrophage phagocytic function[42] and stimulate macrophage production of prostaglandins, which in turn suppresses lymphocyte function[38]. Several types of malignant cells produce increased levels of a differentially glycosylated form of Hp that renders it 100- to 1000-fold more immunosuppressive than normal liver-derived Hp in the systemic circulation[22,23,43,44]. Thus, Hp-like ENDO-I could bind to immune cells in the lesion or in the peritoneal cavity and evoke local immunosuppression thereby allowing development of ectopic endometriotic lesions or eliciting some of the aberrant immune phenomena noted in women with this disorder.

In summary, we propose that serum concentrations and/or glycosylation patterns of ENDO-I may ultimately be valuable for nonsurgical diagnosis of endometriosis. In addition, if ENDO-I is structurally unique and specific to endometriotic lesions, an autologous antigen mediated immunotherapy which produces humoral or cellular responses against ENDO-I, and the tissue expressing it, may be developed. Development of novel, less invasive methodologies for diagnosis and treatment of endometriosis could reduce or eliminate the need for invasive surgical procedures and thereby reduce expenditure of health care budgets. Further, it is possible that unique patterns of ENDO-I glycosylation could impart unique functions or increase functions (angiogenic, immunomodulatory or unknown) several-fold as compared to hepatic Hp. We, therefore, hypothesize that Hp-like ENDO-I modulates the pathogenesis of endometriosis by enhancing angiogenesis and by suppressing activity of peritoneal immune cells to prevent cell mediated cytotoxicity of ectopic endometrial tissue. Ongoing studies in our laboratory propose to analyze ENDO-I's angiogenic and immunomodulatory properties, which may for the first time offer an explanation for anomalies of the immune system and neovascularization associated with endometriosis.

ACKNOWLEDGEMENT

This research has been supported by the National Institutes of Health Institute of Child Health and Human Development grant number 29026.

References

1. Sharpe-Timms KL. Basic Research in Endometriosis. *Obstet Gynecol Clin N Am* 1997;24:269–90
2. Meldrum DR. Clinical management of endometriosis with luteinizing hormone-releasing hormone analogues. *Semin Reprod Endocrinol* 1985;3:371–5
3. Barbieri RL. Gonadotropin-releasing hormone agonists and estrogen-progestogen replacement therapy. *Am J Obstet Gynecol* 1990;162:593–5
4. Sharpe KL, Vernon MW. Polypeptides synthesized and released by rat endometriotic tissue differ from those of the uterine endometrium in culture. *Biol Reprod* 1993;48:1334–40

5. Sharpe KL, Zimmer RL, Griffin WT, *et al.* Polypeptides synthesized and released by human endometriosis tissue differ from those of the uterine endometrium in culture. *Fertil Steril* 1993;60:839–51
6. Sharpe-Timms KL, Piva M, Ricke EA, *et al.* Endometriosis synthesizes and secretes a haptoglobin-like protein. *Biol Reprod* 1998;58: 988–94
7. Vernon MW, Wilson EA. Studies on the surgical induction of endometriosis in the rat. *Fertil Steril* 1985;44:684–94
8. Sharpe KL, Bertero MC, Lyon BP, *et al.* Follicular atresia and infertility in rats treated with a gonadotropin-releasing hormone (GnRH) antagonist. *Endocrinology* 1990;127:25–31
9. Sharpe KL, Bertero MC, Vernon MW. Rapid regression of endometriosis by a new gonadotropin-releasing hormone antagonist in rats with surgically induced disease. In Chada DP, Buttram VC, eds. *Current Concepts in Endometriosis.* New York: Alan R. Liss, Inc., 1990;444–58
10. Sharpe KL, Bertero MC, Vernon MW. Detection of a progesterone-induced, secretory protein synthesized by the uteri but not the endometriotic implants of rats with induced endometriosis. *Fertil Steril* 1991;55:403–10
11. Sharpe KL, Zimmer RL, Khan RS, *et al.* Proliferative and morphogenic changes induced by the co-culture of rat uterine and peritoneal cells: a cell culture model for endometriosis. *Fertil Steril* 1992;58:1220–9
12. Wright JA, Sharpe-Timms KL. Gonadotropin-releasing hormone agonist (GnRHa) therapy reduces postoperative adhesion formation and reformation following adhesiolysis in rat models for adhesion formation and endometriosis. *Fertil Steril* 1995;63:1094–100
13. Sharpe-Timms KL, Penney LL, Zimmer RL, *et al.* Partial purification and amino acid sequence analysis of endometriosis protein-II (ENDO-II) reveals homology with tissue inhibitor of metalloproteinase-1 (TIMP-1). *J Clin Endocrin Metab* 1995;80:3784–7
14. Sharpe-Timms KL, Zimmer RL, Jolliff WJ, *et al.* Gonadotropin-releasing hormone agonist (GnRHa) therapy alters activity of plasminogen activators (PA), matrix metalloproteinase (MMP) and of their inhibitors (PAI and MMPI) in rat models for adhesion formation and endometriosis: potential GnRHa-regulated mechanisms reducing adhesion formation. *Fertil Steril* 1998;69:916–23
15. Piva M, Sharpe-Timms KL. Peritoneal endometriotic lesions differentially express a haptoglobin-like gene. *Mol Hum Reprod* 1999;5: 71–8
16. Piva M, Knittig RA, Griffin WT, Sharpe-Timms KL. Interleukin-6 (IL-6) up regulates expression of endometriosis Protein-I (ENDO-I) mRNA, a haptoglobin-like gene that is differentially expressed by pelvic endometriosis. 54th Annual Meeting of the American Society of Reproductive Medicine 1998b; 0-171
17. Sambrook J, Fritsch EF, Maniatis T. *Molecular Cloning. A Laboratory Manual,* 2nd edn. Cold Spring Harbor Laboratory Press, 1989
18. Zhang YL, Zimmer RL, Sharpe-Timms KL. Synthesis and secretion of endometriosis protein-I (ENDO-I) by peritoneal cells is augmented by coculture with endometrial cells. *Soc Study Reprod* 1996; P-90
19. Zhang YL, Sharpe-Timms KL. Co-culture of endometrial with peritoneal cells alters secretory activity: an electron microscopy study. *Am Soc Reprod Med* 1996; P-107
20. Goldstein LA, Heath EC. Nucleotide sequence of rat haptoglobin cDNA. Characterization of the αβ-subunit junction region of prohaptoglobin. *J Biol Chem* 1984;259:9212–17
21. Turner GA. Haptoglobin. A potential reporter molecule for glycosylation changes in disease. *Adv Exp Med Biol* 1995;376:231–8
22. Oh SK, Very DL, Walker J, *et al.* An analogy between fetal haptoglobin and a potent immunosuppressant in cancer. *Cancer Res* 1987;47:5120–6
23. Oh SK, Kim SH, Walker JE. Interference with immune response at the level of generating effector cells by tumor-associated haptoglobin. *J Nat Canc Inst* 1990;82:934–40
24. Myrick JE, Caudill SP, Hubert IL, *et al.* Identification of haptoglobin alpha-2FF variants in mid-trimester maternal serum as potential markers for Down syndrome. *Appl Theor Electrophoresis* 1990;1:233–41
25. Langlois MR, Delanghe JR. Biological and clinical significance of haptoglobin polymorphism in humans. *Clin Chem* 1996;42:1589–1600
26. van Dijk W, Turner GA, Mackiewicz A. Changes in glycosylation of acute-phase proteins in health and disease: occurrence, regulation and function. *Glycosylation Dis* 1994;1:5–14
27. Dobryszycka W. Biological functions of haptoglobin – new pieces to an old puzzle. *Euro J Clin Chem Clin Biochem* 1997;35:647–54
28. Friedrichs WE, Navarijo-Ashbaugh AL, Bowman BH, *et al.* Expression and inflammatory regulation of haptoglobin gene in adipocytes. *Biochem Biophys Res Comm* 1995;209:250–6
29. Martinez A, Jansen L, Buchanan JM, *et al.* A human (3.3 kb) haptoglobin-CAT transgene is modulated in lungs of transgenic mice by inflammation. *Biochem Biophys Res Comm* 1995; 208:309–15
30. Yang FM, Friedrichs WE, Navarijo-Ashbaugh AL, *et al.* Cell type-specific and inflammatory-induced expression of haptoglobin gene in lung. *Lab Invest* 1995;73:433–40
31. Hoffman LH, Winfrey VP, Blaeuer GL, *et al.* A

haptoglobin-like glycoprotein is produced by implantation-stage rabbit endometrium. *Biol Reprod* 1996;55:176–84

32. Way AL, Zaczek DJ, Killian GJ. Presence of a haptoglobin-like protein in bovine oviductal fluid (ODF). *Biol Reprod* 1997;56:134 (Abstract 207)
33. O'Bryan MK, Grima J, Mruk D, *et al.* Haptoglobin is a Sertoli cell product in the rat seminiferous epithelium: its purification and regulation. *J Androl* 1997;18:637–45
34. Baumann H, Prowse KR, Marinkovic S, *et al.* Stimulation of hepatic acute phase response by cytokines and glucocorticoids. *Ann NY Acad Sci* 1989;577:280–95
35. Pajovic S, Jones VE, Prowse KR, *et al.* Species-specific changes in regulatory elements of mouse haptoglobin genes. *J Biol Chem* 1994;269;2215–24
36. Cid MC, Grant DS, Hoffman GS, *et al.* Identification of haptoglobin as an angiogenic factor in sera from patients with systemic vasculitis. *J Clin Invest* 1993; 91:977–83
37. Baseler MW, Burrell R. Acute phase reactants in experimental inhalation lung disease. *Proc Soc Exp Biol* 1981;111:49–55
38. Baseler MW, Burrell R. Purification of haptoglobin and its effects on lymphocyte and alveolar macrophage responses. *Inflammation* 1983;7:387–400
39. El Ghmati SM, Van Hoeyveld EM, Van Strijp AG, *et al.* Identification of haptoglobin as an alternative ligand for CD11b/CD18. *J Immunol* 1996;156:2542–52
40. Relman D, Tuomanen E, Falkow S, *et al.* Recognition of a bacterial adhesion by an integrin: macrophage CR3 (alpha M beta 2, CD11b/CD18) binds filamentous hemagglutinin of *Bordetella pertussis. Cell* 1990;61:1375–82
41. Kohler W, Prokop O. Relationship between haptoglobin and Streptococcus pyrogenes T4 antigens. *Nature* 1978;271:373
42. Oh SK, Ross S, Walker JM, *et al.* Role of a SER immune suppressor in immune surveillance. *Immunology* 1988;64:73–9
43. Thompson S, Turner GA. A new method for the analysis of blood serum glycoproteins using Sepharose-coupled lectins and its application in human disease. In Bog-Hansen TC, Freed DLJ, eds. *Lectins – Biology, Biochemistry, Clinical Biochemistry.* Vol 6. St. Louis: Sigma Chemical Co., 1988:453–7
44. Elg SA, Carson LE, Fowler JM, *et al.* Ascites levels of haptoglobin in patients with ovarian cancer. *Cancer* 1993;71:3938–41

Paracrine growth factors in endometriosis: evidence for a role of the IGF/IFGPB-3/ protease system of the peritoneal fluid in tissue remodeling

16

A. Lemay, A. Akoum and M. Koutsilieris

The appearance and development of endometriosis have been related to the secretion of female sex hormones, mainly estradiol. Since endometriosis is clinically absent before menarche and when present is no more manifest after menopause, a crucial role was assigned to the sex steroid hormones. The suppression of ovarian steroids production by GnRH agonist downregulation of the gonatrophs is actually effective not only in relieving pain but in causing regression of active lesions[1]. However, there is a wide heterogeneity in the macroscopic and microscopic development of lesions[2]. The endometriotic cells frequently do not differentiate in synchrony with the endometrium. The number of estrogen and progesterone receptors is often low in endometriosis lesions and there is a lack of cyclic variation in their concentrations as compared to that in the corresponding endometrium[3]. Moreover, it has been elegantly documented that endometrial fragments can be transplanted on the peritoneum of castrated monkeys although sex steroid hormone replacement has facilitated the development of endometriotic implants[4].

It is now well appreciated that growth substances acting in an autocrine and/or paracrine regulatory fashion can mediate the effects of steroid hormones on target tissues[5,6]. According to the retrograde menstruation theory, regurgitated endometrial cells or tissue debris could implant and grow on the various surfaces of the pelvic cavity (Figure 1). Recent studies have indicated that the peritoneal fluid contains several mitogens and proteases which could reflect immuno-inflammatory changes and tissue remodeling taking place in the pelvic cavity.

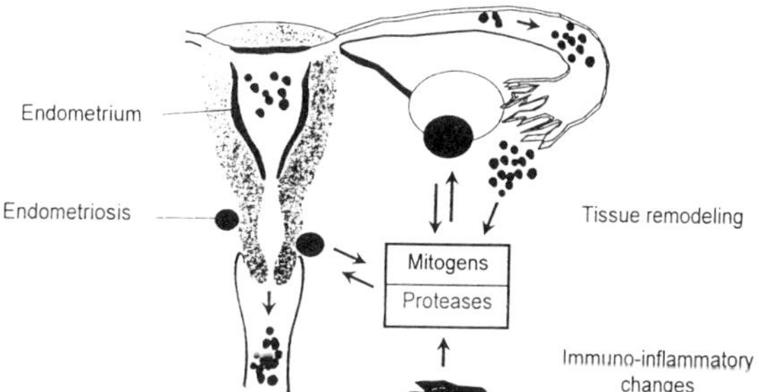

Figure 1 Peritoneal fluid paracrine factors in endometriosis. The mitogenic activity of the peritoneal fluid is related to proteases originating from macrophages but also from endometrial derived cells or other cells present in the peritoneal cavity. These mitogenic and proteolytic activities would reflect tissue remodeling and immuno-inflammatory changes taking place in the peritoneal cavity

This paper briefly outlines the recent observations regarding tissue and peritoneal growth factors as they could relate to tissue remodeling in the pathophysiology of endometriosis; it also summarizes our previous and recent data implicating the IGF/IGFBP-3/protease of the peritoneal fluid as a paracrine system that could play a strategic role in the development of this condition.

EXPRESSION AND SECRETION OF GROWTH FACTORS BY ENDOMETRIAL AND ENDOMETRIAL-DERIVED CELLS

In the last few years, several growth factors including IGFs have been assessed in the endometrium[7, 8]. The receptors, regulatory proteins, cellular localization and steroid dependence of several of these proteins have also been studied. More recent data also report the tissue distribution of epidermal growth factor (EGF), transforming growth factors α (TGF-α) and TGF-β, acidic and basic fibroblast growth factors (FGFa, FGFb) and vascular endothelial growth factor (VEGF) in endometriotic tissues[9–12]. These growth factors can stimulate the proliferation of stromal cells in culture prepared from eutopic endometrial tissue. Moreover, stromal and/or epithelial cells can secrete TGF-β, VEGF and platelet derived growth factor (PDGF) and the release of these mitogens can be modified by estrogens and progesterone[12–14]. Recent studies in fact report that the peritoneal fluid contain IGFs, EGF, FGF, TGF-β and VEGF[15,16]. Endometriosis patients have higher levels of TGF-β, VEGF and macrophage colony stimulating factor (M-CSF) in their peritoneal fluid as compared to that of control women requesting tubal ligation and having a normal pelvis[12,16,17]. Although growth factors detected in the peritoneal fluid could originate from macrophages[17–21] or from other cells in the pelvic cavity, they may well come from endometriotic cells and/or endometrial cells regurgitated through the Fallopian tubes.

EXPRESSION AND SECRETION OF PROTEASES BY ENDOMETRIAL AND ENDOMETRIAL-DERIVED CELLS

Using techniques of immunohistochemistry, *in situ* hybridization and Northern blot analysis, Southern blot analysis and reverse transcriptase polymerase chain reaction (RT–PCR), several proteases have been documented as being expressed in the eutopic endometrium and ectopic endometriotic implants[22–25]. As measured by an immunoradiometric method cathepsin D level was significantly higher in endometriotic tissue than in the endometrium[26]. Endometrial stromal cells can also release several matrix metalloproteases[27–28]. The secretion of proteases is generally decreased by progesterone and increased by cytokines such as interleukin-1α (IL-1α) and tumor necrosis factor-α (TNF-α)[29–31]. Progesterone also decreases the secretion of plasminogen activator inhibitor (PAI) and tissue inhibitor of metalloprotease-3 (TIMP-3)[32]. Endo-II, a protein released in culture media by rat endometriotic tissue, was partially purified and revealed to have homology with TIMP-1[33]. It is also interesting to consider that plasminogen activators have previously been found to be elevated in the peritoneal fluid of patients with endometriosis[34].

The observations reported above are in line with the concept that proteases are coupled with growth factors in tissue remodeling (Figure 2). It is readily apparent that several growth factors and proteases which are stored or fixed on the extracellular matrix or anchored in precursor form in the cell membrane can take part in the lysis of stroma and proliferation of cells during tissue implantation and proliferation in several physiological and pathological conditions, for example embryonic pattern formation and tumor progression[35,37]. Endometrial matrix metalloproteases have recently been shown to be involved with hormones and growth factors

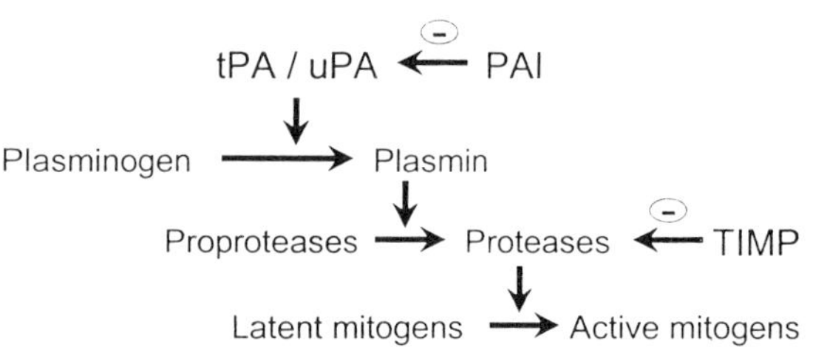

Figure 2 Cascade of proteases and mitogens in tissue remodeling. Several proteases and mitogens present in the peritoneal fluid are fixed on extracellular matrix or anchored in a precursor form in the cell membrane and can take part in the lysis of stroma and proliferation of cells during the process of tissue remodeling in endometriosis

in the process of normal menstruation[38,39]. It is then likely that similar interactions could exist between growth factors and proteases in the process of tissue remodeling in endometriosis.

IDENTIFICATION OF PERITONEAL FLUID MITOGENIC IGFBP-3 FRAGMENTS

One approach to look at the tissue remodeling in endometriosis was to characterize the mitogenic activity of the peritoneal fluid. Early studies indicated that the peritoneal fluid contains macrophage-derived growth factor(s) (MDGF). Addition of conditioned media from cultured macrophages increased [^{3}H]thymidine incorporation in NIH-3T3 mouse embryo fibroblasts[18–20]. A similar observation reported [^{3}H]thymidine incorporation in endometrial stromal cells at a higher rate in endometriosis patients than in controls[19]. A recent study corroborated these observations for the peritoneal fluid from mild endometriosis but rather an inhibitory effect from that of severe endometriosis[20]. Interestingly, this stimulatory effect was partially prevented by preincubating the cells with an anti-IGF receptor type I[40].

These results prompted our studies on the characterization of peritoneal fluid mitogenic activity. In initial experiments, NIH/3T3 mouse embryo fibroblasts, human endometrial adenocarcinoma cells and primary cultures of rabbit epithelial and stromal cells were used to assess the effect of individual peritoneal fluid on [^{3}H]thymidine incorporation into cellular DNA[41]. The rate of [^{3}H]thymidine incorporation into cellular DNA of all cell types was significantly higher compared with that in controls when increasing amounts of proteins from peritoneal fluid were added to culture media.

A purification scheme was elaborated for the characterization of growth factors from endometrial cell types. In an initial study, peritoneal fluid was collected from women with laparoscopic evidence of endometriosis. Peritoneal fluid material was retained on and eluted from carboxymethyl sepharose, heparin/sepharose, cartridges of C18 silica and reverse-phase high performance liquid chromotography (rHPLC) columns in sequence. At the rHPLC stage, discrete protein peaks were found showing mitogenic activity for fibroblasts and rabbit endometrial epithelial cells[42]. Unfortunately, there was not enough material to achieve identification of the rHPLC-recovered material.

The purification scheme described above was applied to a larger amount of peritoneal fluid coming from women without evidence of endometriosis at laparoscopy. Stromal and epithelial cells isolated from human endometrium then available were used to assess the proliferative effects of peritoneal extracts. Analysis of the purified material on sodium dodecyl sulfate polyacrylamide gel electrophoresis (SDS–PAGE) revealed four protein bands with relative molecular weights of 17 000–18 000, 20 000, 25 000 and 30 000. After the first step of purification on rHPLC, we obtained the four ultraviolet peaks detected by SDS–PAGE in the eluates of the Sep-Pak column. All four eluates showed mitogenic activity on human epithelium-derived endometrial cells[43]. The peaks separated by SDS–PAGE were transferred to an Immobilon-p membrane for microsequencing. The N-terminal sequences of these peptides matched the 162–171, 162–180, 162–167 and 162–171 amino acids of IGFBP-3. The common start of these peptides isolated from the peritoneal fluid of healthy women was identical to the N-terminal truncated forms of IGFBP-3 previously detected in rat serum. This part of the IGFBP-3 molecule is highly preserved in the IGFBP-3 of different species and contains N-linked glycosylation sites, suggesting an important role in the structure-function of IGFBP-3. These results indicate that the peritoneal fluid contains N-terminal truncated fragments of the IGFBP-3 which have a mitogenic effect on primary culture of epithelial cells isolated from the human endometrium. Our results are in good agreement with the recent data from Giudice and colleagues[40] showing the presence of IGFBP-3 protease activity in the peritoneal fluid of healthy women as compared to no appreciable amounts of enzyme activity in paired serum samples.

Insulin-like growth factor binding proteins (IGFBPs) are multifunctional proteins that regulate not only the transport of IGFs but also their presentation to the cell surface receptors. At least six IGFBPs have been found and several of these exist in multiple forms owing to glycosylation and/or phosphorylation. IGFBP-3, the major serum carrier of the IGFs, exist in serum primarily as a 150-kDa ternary complex comprised of IGFBP-3, an acid labile subunit and IGF peptide. According to Giudice *et al.*[40], peritoneal fluid concentrations of IGFBP-3, measured by immunoassay, were approximately 60% of paired serum levels. Western immunoblotting of column fractions revealed immunoactive IGFBP-3 forms of 37–43 kDa and 28 kDa in serum and almost exclusively the 28 kDa band in the peritoneal fluid, suggesting that IGFBP-3 in peritoneal fluid was proteolytically processed. Western ligand immunoblots and ligand blots also indicated a significant decrease in a 27 kDa species in endometriosis[44].

In order to evaluate fragments of IGFBP-3, a small peptide (P23) corresponding to the common sequence of the four truncated forms of IGFBP-3 has been synthesized. A polyclonal antibody has also been generated against this peptide in the rabbit and purified by affinity. This antibody has been used to probe IGFBP-3 fragments after separation and enrichment of proteins contained in pooled peritoneal fluid by preparative isoelectric focusing. As indicated in Figure 3, the anti-P23 antibody could reveal fragments between 20 and 25 kDa in pooled fractions C (pH 6.1 to 6.7) only in the peritoneal fluid from patients having endometriosis as compared to the same fractions obtained from control women without the disease. We have not been able to purify these fragments yet in order to probe their action on endometrial-derived cells. However, preliminary information indicates that the P23 peptide shows 30 to 40% of the mitogenic activity obtained with IGF-1 on NIH-3T3 mouse fibroblasts and KLE

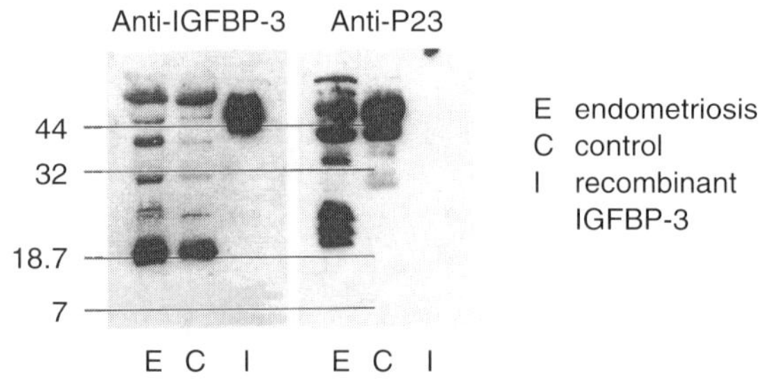

Figure 3 Immunoblot detection of IGFBP-3 and its fragments in enriched fractions prepared by isoelectric focusing. The anti P23 antibody generated against a synthetic peptide reveals fragments between 20 and 25 kDa only in the peritoneal fluid from patients having endometriosis as compared to the same fraction obtained from a group of control women without the disease

endometrial adenocarcinoma cells. Thus, this distinct profile of IGFBP-3 fragments in the peritoneal fluid of patients having endometriosis and the mitogenic activity related to the fragments would indicate a role of an IGF/IGFBP-3/protease system in tissue remodeling in endo-metriosis.

CO-DETECTION OF MITOGENIC UROKINASE AND PROTEOLYTIC ACTIVITIES OF IGFBP-3

Considering the potential role of IGFBP-3 protease and our previous findings of mitogenic activity of N-terminal truncated forms of IGFBP-3 in the peritoneal fluid, it appeared pertinent to provide evidence for a probable link between the mitogenic and proteolytic activities of the peritoneal fluid. In order to rapidly evaluate these two types of activity, we have used the isoelectric focusing procedure[45]. After an initial focusing between pH3 and 10, and a second focusing between pH5 and 8, the mitogenic activity was mainly found to be associated with fractions corresponding to pH7.10 ± 0.02. To evaluate the proteolytic ac-tivity, proteins of each fraction were incubated with [^{125}I]-labeled IGFBP-3 in the presence or absence of diisopropylfluorophosphate (DPF) as a protease inhibitor. Proteins were then separated on

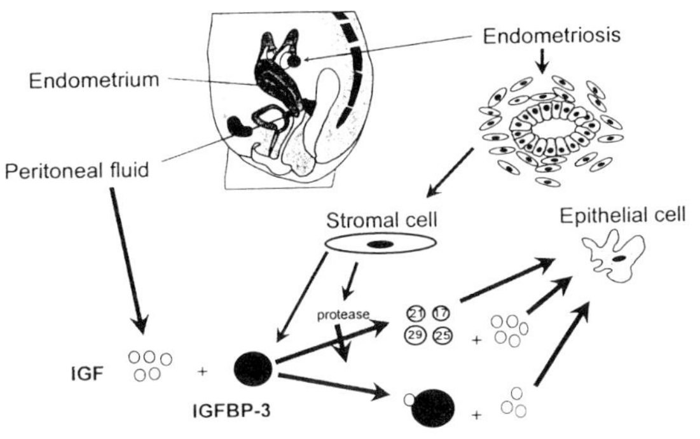

Figure 4 Peritoneal fluid IGF/IGFBP-3/protease system in endometriosis. A significant proteolytic degradation of IGFBP-3 in the peritoneal fluid results in a reduction of its binding affinity for IGFs, with possibly more potent IGF variants and direct mitogenic activity of IGFBP-3 fragments on epithelial cells derived from the endometrium

SDS–PAGE. In fractions 13 and 20, showing elevated mitogenic activity, there was an important decrease of the band having a mass of 29 000 kDa, with the appearance of strong signals mainly for the bands with masses of 14 000 and 18 000. In these two fractions the proteolysis of IGFBP-3 was almost completely prevented by the addition of DFP in the incubation medium. The finding of this experiment, of mitogenic activity associated with proteolysis of IGFBP-3 in common fractions, is further evidence for the hypothesis that the mitogenic activity is related to the fragmentation of IGFBP-3.

Similar pooled fractions prepared by isoelectric focusing were further passed through a Sep-Pak column and proteins electro-phoresed on SDS gel. Immunoblotting was performed using monoclonal anti-IGFBP-3 and anti-urokinase antibodies. The antibody reactions were revealed by a second antibody labeled with peroxidase and enhanced chemoluminescence. Urokinase was detected in the same fractions showing IGFBP-3 fragments, mitogenic and proteolytic activities (data not shown). These observations indicate that the mitogenic activity found in the peritoneal fluid of women having endo-metriosis would be related at least in part to the proteolysis of IGFBP-3, this hydrolysis being probably related to the activation of the plasminogen/plasmin cascade by urokinase.

The IGF/IGFBP-3/protease system shown in Figure 4 was previously demonstrated in the serum of pregnant women. There is a significant proteolytic degradation of IGFBP-3 in the peritoneal fluid, giving differences in measurement of IGFBP-3 by ligand blotting and Western immunoblotting. The physiological implications of IGFBP-3 degradation by protease have been presented by Binoux and associates[46] and Lamson and colleagues[47]. Proteolysis of IGFBP-3 results in a reduction of its binding affinity for IGFs and in an increase in the dissociation rate of bound IGFs, thus increasing the bioavailability of IGFs. One study reported that Des (1-3) IGF-1, a more potent IGF variant and extracted from a variety of tissues including the uterus[42] can also be generated in the serum by an acid protein[48]. We have previously reported that urokinase-type plasminogen activator stimulates osteoblasts in PA-III cell-induced osteoblastic cell metastases via an IGF-1 dependent mechanism[49]. Our finding that N-terminal truncated fragments of IGFBP-3 have apparent direct mitogenic activity on epithelial cells derived from human endometrium suggests other mechanisms of action of the IFG system. Receptors for IGFBP-3 have been found in Hs578T human breast cancer cells[50]. Recent data also indicate that IGFBP-3 can mediate direct stimulatory or inhibitory effects on several cell lines by IGF independent mechanisms and specific binding sites[51]. There could also be changes in receptor response to altered IGFBP-3. The elucidation of these putative mechanisms requires further characterization of IGFBP-3 fragments *in vitro* using cell culture systems.

IMMUNOHISTOCHEMISTRY OF THE IGFBP-3 IN EUTOPIC ENDOMETRIAL AND ECTOPIC ENDOMETRIOTIC TISSUE BIOPSIES

Our data and the literature suggest that IGFBP-3, as part of an IGF/IGFBP-3/protease

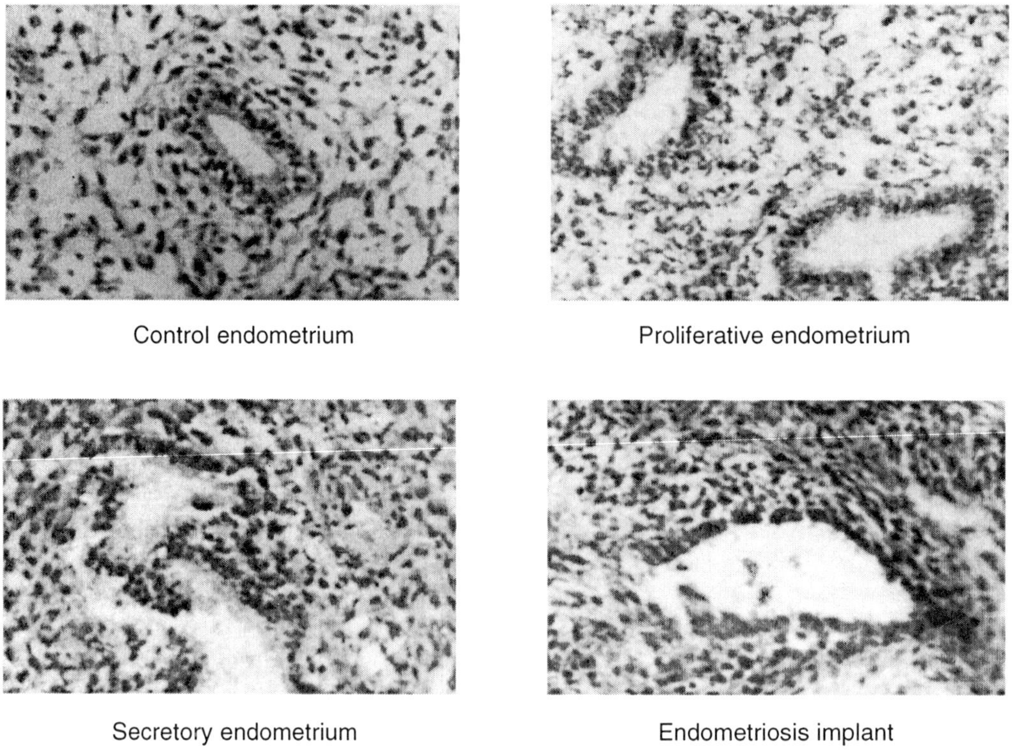

Figure 5 Immunohistochemistry of IGFBP-3 in the endometrium and endometriosis lesion. Positive immunostaining with anti IGFBP-3 was observed both in the stroma and the epithelial glands mostly during the secretory phase. The immunostaining in endometriotic tissue is much more intense, indicating increased expression

system could be involved in the implantation and development of endometriosis. According to the retrograde menstruation theory, IGFBP-3 in the PF could come at least in part from endometrial cells regurgitated through the Fallopian tubes at the time of menses or directly from endometriotic implants. The mRNA expression and protein synthesis of IGFBP-3 have already been reported in the endometrium of normal women[52,53]. However, the presence of IGFBP-3 in endometriosis lesions and in the endometrium of patients with endometriosis has not been documented. It was then of interest to look for the expression of IGFBP-3 in endometrial tissue and endometriotic biopsies obtained at laparoscopy from healthy women and from women with endometriosis. The expression of IGFBP-3 was assessed by immunohistochemistry using a purified polyclonal goat anti-IGFBP-3 antibody, biotin conjugated mouse anti-goat antibody, streptavidin peroxidase and diaminobenzidin as chromogen. In the endometrium, positive immunostaining was observed both in the stroma and the epithelial glands mostly during the secretory phase (Figure 5). An increased expression of IGFBP-3 was noticeable in patients presenting with endometriosis as shown in Figure 6. The IGFBP-3 immunostaining in the endometriotic tissue was marked in 90% of the glands and 70% of the stroma without apparent differences related to the cycle phase. These findings provide additional evidence for the involvement of IGFBP-3 in the pathophysiology of endometriosis. IGFBP-3 found in the peritoneal fluid would arise at least in part from endometrial cells regurgitated through the Fallopian tubes or directly from endometri-

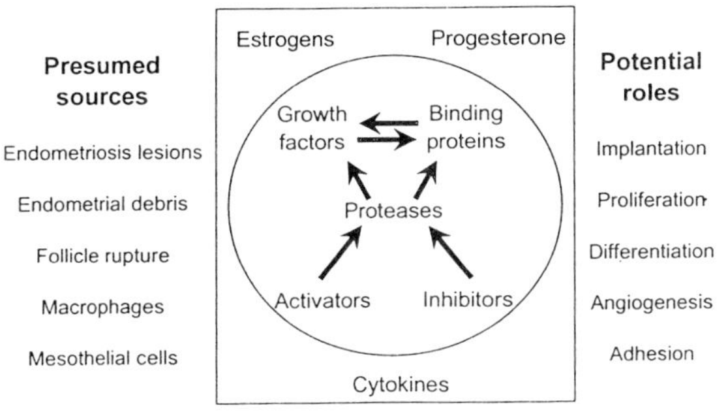

Figure 6 Peritoneal growth factors and tissue remodeling in endometriosis. Interactions between growth factors, binding proteins and proteases are influenced at several levels by sex steroid homones and cytokines. These factors originate from several presumed sources and have potential roles at several steps in the development of the disease

otic implants. As part of an IGF/IGFBP-3/ protease system, the increased expression of IGFBP-3 might be related to more active tissue remodeling in endometriosis, especially in endometriotic lesions.

POTENTIAL ROLES OF IGF/IGFBP-3/ PROTEASE IN TISSUE REMODELING IN ENDOMETRIOSIS

Based on data in the literature and on our recent experimental observations, the mitogenic activity of the peritoneal fluid would be related at least in part to an IGF/ IGFBP-3/protease system. The proteolysis of IGFBP-3 is associated with increased mitogenic activity. This effect could be due to increased bioavailability of insulin-like growth factors but also to intrinsic mitogenic properties of the IGFBP-3 fragments. Further studies are required to better understand the relationship between peritoneal fluid mitogens and proteases. The actual data also indicate that the proteolysis of IGFBP-3 results from urokinase activation of plasmin and matrix metalloproteases. Other growth factors could also be activated by this cascade of proteases[6]. It is readily apparent that these interactions between growth factors, binding proteins and proteases are influenced at several levels not only by estrogens and progesterone but also by numerous cytokines actually found to be associated with the immuno-inflammatory changes taking place in the peritoneal fluid in endometriosis. Mitogens, proteases, sex steroids and cytokines are present in endometrial debris and follicular fluid spilling into the peritoneal cavity in the cycling woman and would contribute to the initiation or the perpetuation of the pathophysiological change. These biomolecular changes in peritoneal fluid would reflect tissue remodeling involved in implantation, proliferation, differentiation, angiogenesis or adhesion formation. IGFBP-3 protease, activity which has been observed initially in the serum of women with normal pregnancy[54], has already been documented in several other physiological situations such as the seminal plasma of normal men[55] and the embryonic cavities in early human pregnancy[56]. Pathological conditions have been associated with an altered IGF/IGFBP-3/protease system in the serum of patients with diabetes[57], breast cancer[58], in the cerebrospinal fluid of subjects with central nervous system tumors or meningitis[59] and in the synovial fluid of cases of arthritis[60]. Very recent data report changes in receptor expression of EGF, in pelvic endometriosis and in peritoneal fluid concentration of TIMP-1 following GnRH agonist suppressive treatment[61,62]. The eventual evaluation of alterations in growth factors and proteases appears promising for a better understanding of the physiopathology of the disease and should be helpful for the development of new strategies for its diagnosis and management.

References

1. Lemay A. La place de la suppression ovarienne dans le traitement de l'endométriose. *Ref Gynecol Obstet* 1993;1:243-25U
2. Schweppe KW. Endometriotic lesions: location, gross histologic and structural aspects. In Chadha DR,Buttram VC Jr, eds. *Current concepts in endometriosis, progress in clininal and biological research.* New York: AR Liss Inc. 1990;323:33–47
3. Spinola PG. Steroid receptors in endometriosis. In Coutinbo EM, ed. *Progress in the management of endometriosis. Part Publish Internat Congr Syny and Services Series* 1995;11:123–27
4. DiZerega GS, Barber DL, Hodgen GD. Endometriosis: role of ovarian steroids in initiation, maintenance and suppression. *Fertil Steril* 1984;33:649–53
5. James R, Bradshaw RA. Polypeptide growth factors. *Ann Rev Biochem* 1984;53:259–68
6. Brigstock DR. Growth factors in the uterus. *Baillièr's Clin Endo Metab* 1991;5:791–808
7. Giudice LC. Growth factors and growth modulators in human uterine endometrium: their potential relevance to reproductive medicine. *Fertil Steril* 1994;61:1–17
8. Smith SK. The endometrium and endometriosis. In Thomas EJ, Rock JA, eds. *Modern Approaches to endometriosis.* Dordrecht: Kluwer Acad Publ 1991:57–77
9. Simms JS, Chigini N, Williams RS, *et al.* Identification of epidermal growth factor, transforming growth factor-alpha, and epidermal growth factor receptor in surgically induced endometriosis in rats. *Obstet Gynecol* 1991;83:455–61
10. Chegini N, Gold IL, Williams RS. Localization of transforming growth factor beta isoform TFG-β1, TGF-β2, and TGF,β3 in surgically induced endometriosis in the rat. *Obstet Gynecol* 1994; 83:455–61
11. Ferriani RA, Charnock-Jones DS, Prentice A, *et al.* Immunohistochemical localization of acidic and basic fibroblast growth factors in normal human endometrium and endometriosis and the detection of their mRNA by polymerase chain reaction. *Hum Reprod* 1993;8:11–16
12. Shifren JL, Tseng JF, Zaloudek CJ, *et al.* Ovarian steroid regulation of vascular endothelial growth factor in the human endometrium: implications for angiogenesis during the menstrual cycle and in the pathogenesis of endometriosis. *J Clin Endocrinol Metab* 1996;81:3112–18
13. Tan XM, Zhao Y, Rossi MJ, *et al.* Expression of transforming growth factor-β (TGFβ)isoforms and TGFβ type II receptor messenger ribonucleic acid and protein, and the effect of TGFβs on the endometrial stromal cell growth and protein degradation *in vitro.Endocrinology* 1994;135:450–9
14. Arici A, MacDonald PC, Casey ML. Modulation of the levels of transforming growth factor β messenger ribonucleic acids in human endometrial stromal cells. *Biol Reprod* 1996;54:463–9
15. Ramey JW, Archer DF.Peritoneal fluid: its relevance to the development of endometriosis. *Fertil Steril* 1993;60:1–14
16. Oosterlynck DJ,MeulemanC,Waer M, *et al.* Transforming growth factor-β activity is increased in peritoneal fluid from women with endometriosis. *Obstet Gynecol* 1994;83:287–92
17. Weinberg JB,Haney AF, Xu FJ, *et al.* Peritoneal fluid and plasma levels of human macrophage colony-stimulating factor in relation to peritoneal fluid macrophage content.*Blood* 1991;78:513–16
18. Halme J, Kauma WS, Estes J, *et al.* Peritoneal macrophages from patients with endometriosis release growth factor activity *in vitro. J Clin Endocrinol Metab* 1988;66:1044–9
19. Surrey ES, Halme J. Effect of peritoneal fluid from endometriosis patients on endometrial stromal cell proliferation *in vitro. Obstet Gynecol* 1990;76:792–7
20. David L, Olive MD, Iris Montoya, *et al.* Macrophage-conditioned media enhance endometrial stromal cell proliferation *in vitro. Am J Obstet Gynecol* 1991;164:953–8
21. Meresman GF, Barnanao RI, Tanenbaum A, *et al.* Effect of peritoneal fluid from patients with mild and severe endometriosis on endometrial stromal cell proliferation. *Arch Gynecol Obstet* 1997;259:109–15
22. Rodgers WH, Osteen KG, Matrisian LM, *et al.* Expression and localization of matrilysin, a matrix metalloproteinase, in human endometrium during the reproductive cycle. *J. Obstet Gynecol* 1993;168:253–60
23. Head JR, MacDonald PC, Casey ML. Cellular localization of membrane metalloendopeptidase (enkephalinase) in human endometrium during the ovarian cycle. *J Clin Endocrinol Metab* 1993; 76:769–76
24. Fernandez-Shaw S, Marshall JM, Hicks B, *et al.* Plasminogen activators in ectopic and uterine endometrium. *Fertil Steril* 1995;63:45–51
25. Osteen KG, Rodgers WH, Gaire M, *et al.* Stromal epithelial interaction mediates steroidal regulation of metalloproteinase expression in human endometrium. *Proc Natl Acad Sci USA* 1994;91: 10129–33

26. Bergqvist A, Ferno M, Mattson S. A comparison of cathepsin D levels in endometriotic tissue and in uterine endometrium. *Fertil Steril* 1996;65: 1130–4
27. Rawdanowicz TJ, Hampton AL, Nagase H, *et al.* Matrix metalloproteinase production by cultured human endometrial stromal cells: identification of interstitial collagenase, gelatinase-A, 1β gelatine-B, and stromelysin-1 and their differential regulation by interleukin-1α and tumor necrosis factor-α. *J Clin Endocriol Metab* 1994;79:530–6
28. Martelli M, Capana A, Bischof P. Sécrétion de matrixines par l'endométre humain. *Gynecol Obstet* 1993;1:200–13
29. Bruner KL, Rodgers WH, Gold LI, *et al.* Transforming growth factor β mediates the progesterone suppression of an epithelial metalloproteinase by adjacent stroma in the human endometrium. *Proc Natl Acad Sci USA* 1995;92:7362–6
30. Casey ML, MacDonald PC. Transforming growth factor-β inhibits protesterone-induced enkephalinase expression in human endometrial stromal cells. *J Clin Endocrinol Metab* 1996;81: 4022 7
31. Casslen B, Nordengren J, Gustavsson B, *et al.* Progesterone stimulates degradation of urokinase plasminogen activator (u-PA) in endometrial stromal cells by increasing its inhibitor and surface expression of the u-PA receptor. *J Clin Endocrinol Metab* 1995;80:2776–84
32. Higuchi T, Kanzaki H, Nakayama H, *et al.* Induction of tissue inhibitor of metalloproteinase 3 gene expression during *in vitro* decidualization of human endometrial stromal cells. *Endocrinology* 1995;136:4973–81
33. Sharpe-Timms KL, Penney LL, Zimmer RL, *et al.* Partial purification and amino acid sequence analysis of endometriosis proteinII (Endo-II) reveales homology with tissue inhibitor of metalloproteinase-I(TIMP-I). *J Clin Endocrinol Metab* 1995;80:3784–7
34. Astedt B, Nordenskjold F. Plasminogen activators in endometriosis. *Acta Obstet Gynecol Scand Suppl* 1984;123:23–4
35. Feige JJ. La crinopexe: un modèle décrivant les mécanismes qui régissent la disponibilité des facteurs de croissance. *Med Sci* 1992;2:805–10
36. Hicht PM, Anderson KV. Extracellular proteases and embryonic pattern formation. *Trends Cell Biol* 1992;2:197–202
37. Blasi F. Urokinase and urokinase receptor: a paracrine/autocrine system regulating cell migration and invasiveness. *Bio Essays* 1993;2: 105–11
38. Solamonsen LA, Woolley DE. Matrix metalloproteinoses in normal menstruation. *Hum Reprod* 1996; (Suppl. 2):124–33
39. Casey L, MacDonald PC. The endothelin-parathyroid hormone-related protein vasoactive peptide system in human endometrium: modulation by transforming growth factor-β. *Hum Reprod* 1996;11(Suppl.2): 62–82
40. Giudice LC, Dsupin BA, Gargosky SE, *et al.* The insulin-like growth factor system in human peritoneal fluid: its effects on endometrial stromal cells and its potential relevance to endometriosis. *J Clin Endocrinol Metab* 1994;79:1284–93
41. Koutsilieris M, Allaire-Michaud L, Fortier M. Mitogens for endometrial-like cells can be detected in human peritoneal fluid. *Fertil Steril* 1991;56:888–93
42. Koutsilieris M, Allaire-Michaud L, Fortier M, Lemay A. Mitogen(s) for endometrial-like cells can be detected in human peritoneal flud. *Fertil Steril* 1991;59:93–7
43. Koutsilieris M, Akoum A, Lazure C, *et al.* N-terminal truncated forms of insulin-like growth factor binding protein-3 in the peritoneal fluid of women without laparoscopic evidence of endometriosis. *Fertil Steril* 1995;63:314–21
44. Taskin O, Giudice L, Mangal R, *et al.* Insulin-like growth factor binding proteins in peritoneal fluid of women with minimal and mild endometriosis. *Hum Reprod* 1996;11:1741–6
45. Koutsilieris M, Lavergne E, Lemay A. Association of protease activity against IGFBP-3 with peritoneal fluid mitogens: possible implications for the ectopic growth of endometrial cells in women with endometriosis. *Anticancer Res* 1997;17:1239–44
46. Binoux M, Hossenlopp P, Lassarre C, *et al.* Degradation of IGF binding protein-3 by proteases: physiological implications. In Spencer BM, ed. *Proceedings of the 2nd International Symposium on Insulin-Like Growth Somatomedins.* New York: Elsevier Science Publishing Co, Inc., 1991;329–36
47. Lamson G, Giudice LC, Cohen P, *et al.* Proteolysis of IGFPB-3 may be a common regulatory mechanism of IGF action *in vivo*. *Growth Regulation* 1993;3:91–5
48. Ogasawara M, Karey KP, Marquardt H. Identification and purification of truncated insulin-like growth factor I from porcine uterus. Evidence for high biological potency. *Biochemistry* 1989;28: 2710–2721
49. Koutsilieris M, Frenette G, Lazure C, *et al.* Urokinase-type plasminogen activator: a paracrine factor regulating the bioavailability of Igs in PA-III cell-induced osteoblastic metastases. *Anticancer Res* 1993;13:481–6
50. Oh Y, Muller HL, Lamson G, Rosenfeld RG. Insulin-like growth factor (IGF)-independent action of IGF-binding protein-3 in Hs578T human breast cancer cells. *J Biol Chem* 1993;268: 14964–71

51. McCusker RH, Busby WH, Dehoff MH, *et al.* Insulin-like growth factor (IGF) binding to cell monolayers is directly modulated by the addition of IGF-binding proteins. *Endocrinology* 1991;129: 939–49
52. Giudice LC, DsupinBA, Jin IH, *et al.* Differential expression of messenger ribonucleic acids encoding insulin-like growth factors and their receptors in human uterine endometrium and decidua. *J Clin Endocrinol Metab* 1993;76:1115–22
53. Zhou A, Dsupin BA, Guidice LC, *et al.* Insulin-like growth factor system gene expression in human endometrium during the menstrual cycle. *J Clin Endocrinol Metab* 1994;79:1723–34
54. Giudice LC, Farrel EM, Pham H, *et al.* Insulin-like growth factor binding proteins in maternal serum throughout gestation and in the puerperium: effects of a pregnancy-associated serum protease activity. *J Clin Endocrinol Metab* 1990;71:806–16
55. Cohen P, Graves HCP, Peehl DM, *et al.* Prostate specific antigen (PSA) is an insulin-like growth factor binding protein-3 in embryonic cavities in early human pregnancy: their potential relevance to maternal-embryonic and fetal interactions. *J Clin Endocrinol Metab* 1992;75:1046–53
56. NoNoshita LD, Wathen NC, Dsupin BA, *et al.* Insulin-like growth factors (Igs), IGF-binding proteins(IGFBPs), and proteolyzed IGFBP-3 in embryonic cavities in early human pregnancy: their potential relevance to maternal-embryonic and fetal interactions. *J Clin Endocrinol Metab* 1994;79:1249–55
57. Bang P, Brismal K, Rosenfeld RG. Increased proteolysis of insulin-like growth factor binding protein-3(IGFBP-3)in non insulin-dependent diabetes mellitus serum, with elevation of a 29 kilodalton (kDa) glycosylated IGFBP-3 fragment contained in the approximately 130-to 150 kDa ternary complex. *J Clin Endocrinol Metab* 1994; 78:1119–27
58. Frost VJ, Helle SI, Lonning PE, *et al.* Effects of treatment with megestrol acetate, aminoglutethimide, or formestane on insulin-like growth factor (IGF) I and II, IGF-binding proteins (IGFBPs), and IGFBP-3; protease status in patients with advanced breast cancer. *J Clin Endocrinol Metab* 1996;81:2216–21
59. Muller HL, Oh Y, Gargosky SE, *et al.* Concentrations of insulin-like growth factor (IGF)-binding protein-3 (IGFBP-3), IGF, and IGFBP-3 protease activity in cerebrospinal fluid of children with leukemia, central nervous system tumour, or meningitis. *J Clin Endocrinol Metab* 1993;77:1113–19
60. Matsumoto T, Gargosky SE, Iwasaki K, *et al.* Identification and characterisation of insulin-like growth factors (IGFs), IGF-binding proteins (IGFBPs), and IGFBP proteases in human synovial fluid. *J Clin Endocrinol Metab* 1996;81:150–5
61. Di Lieto A, De Rosa G, Albano G, *et al.* Influence of goserelin depot therapy on epidermal growth factor receptor expression in pelvic endometriosis. *Gynecol Endocrinol* 1997;11:17–20
62. Kathy L, Sharpe-Timms KL, Keisler Lydia W, *et al.* Tissue inhibitor of metalloproteinase-1 concentrations are attenuated in peritoneal fluid and sera of women with endometriosis and restored in sera by gonatropin-releasing hormone agonist therapy. *Fertil Steril* 1998;69: 1128–34

Matrix metalloproteinases and endometriosis

17

I. Kokorine, M. Nisolle, J. Donnez, C. Singer, C. Galant, Y. Eeckhout, P.J. Courtoy and E. Marbaix

INTRODUCTION

Endometriotic foci are defined histologically by the association of endometrial-like glands and stroma outside the corpus uteri. Some lesions grow, differentiate and bleed like the eutopic endometrium, although not necessarily synchronously, whereas other, deep, endometriotic lesions may invade organs such as the bladder or the colon. During these processes, the extracellular matrix is remodeled, either by mechanisms similar to those involved in the proliferation, angiogenesis and menstrual breakdown of the *functionalis* of the eutopic endometrium, or possibly by processes resembling those responsible for the invasion of cancer cells in the deep lesions. Extracellular matrix remodeling also has to occur at the origin of the endometriotic lesions, be it by implantation of retrograde menstrual fragments[1] or by metaplasia of the mesothelium and its surrounding mesenchyme or of embryonic remnants[2].

The extracellular matrix of peritoneal endometriotic lesions contains types I and III fibrillar collagens, as well as type IV collagen, distributed as in the eutopic endometrium[3]. Enzymes degrading such components of the extracellular matrix of the endometriotic lesions will thus share similarities with those found in the eutopic endometrium, but differences either in the nature or the regulation of these enzymes are also probable because of the variable aspects several lesions may present within the same patient at the same time and because of the invasiveness of some forms of endometriosis. Indeed, endometriotic cells invade collagen gels *in vitro* much better than proliferative eutopic endometrial cells and similarly to a metastatic bladder carcinoma cell line[4].

The enzymes able to degrade the extracellular matrix proteins are classified according to the structure of their catalytic site: the cysteine and the aspartic proteinases are lysosomal enzymes active at acidic pH whereas the serine and the metalloproteinases are active at neutral pH (Table 1). Some enzymes of the latter two groups are stored intracellularly, such as the mast cell tryptase and chymase among serine proteinases and the gelatinase B among metalloproteinases, at least in neutrophils. Others are bound to the cell membrane such as the membrane-type matrix metalloproteinases, but many of them are secreted as zymogens in the extracellular milieu and require activation to be able to degrade their substrate(s). Such is the case for plasmin and plasminogen activators as examples of the serine proteinases, and for most matrix metalloproteinases (MMPs).

MATRIX METALLOPROTEINASES

Among all the enzymes acting on the extracellular matrix, MMPs are likely to be involved in the pathogenesis, the growth and bleeding, and the invasiveness of endometriosis because of their ability to degrade almost all constituents of the extracellular matrix with the notable exception of type VI

Table 1 Classes of proteinases degrading constituents of the extracellular matrix

Classes	*Examples*	*Distribution*	*pH of maximal activity*
Aspartic proteinases	Cathepsin D	Lysosomes	Acidic
Cysteine proteinases	Cathepsins B,L	Lysosomes	Acidic
Metalloproteinases	Interstitial collagenase	Secreted as zymogen	Neutral
	Neutrophil collagenase	Stored in granules	
	Membrane-type MMPs	Exposed on cell surface	
Serine proteinases	Plasmin	Secreted as zymogen	Neutral
	Leucocyte elastase	Stored in granules	
	Plasminogen activators	Bound to cell receptors	

Adapted from Eeckhout[5]

collagen[6,7]. These structurally related proteinases all possess a catalytic domain with a highly conserved zinc-binding site located in a deep cleft within the active domain, as well as an N-terminal prodomain responsible for the latency of the zymogens by blocking the catalytic zinc. All MMPs except matrilysin (MMP-7) further possess a hemopexin-like C-terminal domain thought to participate at the substrate specificities of these enzymes. Various subgroups of MMPs have thus been proposed according to these substrate specificities (Table 2).

Activation of the proMMPs by removal of the prodomain is an important mechanism in the control of the degradation of the extracellular matrix[7]. Physiological activation of proMMPs could result from a tightly controlled proteolytic cascade involving other proteinases such as plasmin, kallikrein and other MMPs which must themselves be activated. Every step within this cascade can be blocked by specific inhibitors such as plasminogen activator inhibitors (PAIs), tissue inhibitors of metalloproteinases (TIMPs) and α2-macroglobulin. Alternatively, free radicals or oxygen species locally produced in inflammatory sites could disrupt the link between the cysteine of a conserved motif within the prodomain and the Zn of the catalytic site, thereby bending away the prodomain and allowing further (auto)catalytic cleavage of the prodomain[8]. Once active, the MMPs can still be completely inhibited by α2-macroglobulin and TIMPs in a stoichiometric manner. Four different TIMPs have been identified, TIMPs-1, -2, -3 and -4, all of which are able to inhibit the activity of any MMP. Whereas TIMPs-1 and -2 diffuse through the extracellular milieu, TIMP-3 appears to stick to the extracellular matrix.

MATRIX METALLOPROTEINASES IN THE EUTOPIC ENDOMETRIUM

Many MMPs as well as TIMPs-1, -2 and α2-macroglobulin are expressed in the human endometrium although with different patterns of expression throughout the menstrual cycle, as shown by Northern blot, *in situ* hybridization and Western blot studies[9–14]. TIMPs-1, -2 and MMP-2 are expressed at all phases of the cycle but show an increased expression around menstruation[9]. In contrast, the expression of MMP-1, MMP-9, MMP-3 and MMP-10 is restricted to the perimenstrual phase whereas MMP-7 and MMP-11, abundantly expressed around menstruation, are also produced, albeit to lower levels, during the proliferative phase of the cycle[9–11]. All MMPs are produced by the stromal cells in the endometrium, except MMP-7 which is expressed by the epithelial cells[10, 12, 15].

The perimenstrual expression and activation of MMPs appear to be related to the fall in plasmatic concentration of progesterone. Indeed, progesterone strongly inhibits the expression and the activation of proMMP-1, proMMP-9, proMMP-3 and

Table 2 Human matrix metalloproteinases

Enzymes	*MMP #*	*Selected substrates and preferences*
Collagenases		
Interstitial collagenase-1	MMP-1	Collagen III>I>II
Neutrophil collagenase-2	MMP-8	Collagen I>III, II
Rodent-type collagenase-3	MMP-13	Collagen II>I=III, proMMP-9
Gelatinases		
Gelatinase A	MMP-2	Gelatins, collagens I, IV, V, VII, X, XI, elastin, fibronectin, laminin, aggrecan
Gelatinase B	MMP-9	Gelatins, collagen IV, V, elastin
Stromelsins		
Stromelysin-1	MMP-3	Aggrecan, fibronectin, laminin, gelatins, collagen IV, proMMP-8, proMMP-9
Stromelysin-2	MMP-10	Aggrecan, fibronectin, collagen IV, proMMP-8
Matrilysin	MMP-7	Aggrecan, fibronectin, laminin, gelatins, collagen IV, elastin, proMMP-9
Membrane-type MMPs		
MT1-MMP	MMP-14	proMMP-2, proMMP-13, collagens I, II, III, fibronectin, laminin
MT2-MMP	MMP-15	proMMP-2
MT3-MMP	MMP-16	proMMP-2
MT4 MMP	MMP-17	Not known
Others		
Stromelysin-3	MMP-11	IGFBP-1
Metalloelastase	MMP-12	Elastin
No name	MMP-19	Not known
Enamelysin	MMP-20	Amelogenin

Adapted from Nagase[7]; IGFBP-1, insulin-like growth factor binding protein-1

proMMP-7 in cultured endometrial explants[16, 17]. In purified stromal cells, progesterone also inhibits the expression of proMMP-1, proMMP-9, proMMP-3 and proMMP-11[17–20]. Conversely, progesterone withdrawal enhances the expression of proMMP-2 in stromal cells previously decidualized[18, 21]. However, progesterone poorly inhibits the expression, but still controls the activation, of proMMP-2 in cultured explants[16].

Endometrial explants cultured without ovarian steroids release high levels of collagenase and gelatinase activities, part of which is spontaneously activated during culture[11, 16, 22]. The release occurs after one-day of tissue culture-lag and can be prevented by addition of physiological concentrations of ovarian steroids, except when the explants are prepared from a menstrual endometrium, in which case the release is high from the first day of culture on. In the latter condition, progesterone cannot inhibit the production of collagenase probably because of the low levels of progesterone receptors in perimenstrual endometria. A similar hormonal regulation was observed in the endometrium of spayed rhesus monkeys treated with estradiol and progesterone implants[23]: removal of the progesterone implant induced the expression of MMP-11 one day later and of MMP-7, MMP-3 and MMP-10 two days after withdrawal. Expression of MMP-3 and MMP-10 largely decreased 2–3 days after their induction whereas expression of MMP-11 and of MMP-7 lasted for up to six days after withdrawal. This pattern of expression reproduces what happens during the human menstrual cycle, i.e. an expression restricted to menstruation for MMP-3 and MMP-10 and extended to the proliferative phase for MMP-7 and MMP-11.

The expression and the activation of endometrial MMPs is thus induced or enhanced upon progesterone withdrawal, as occurs at the end of the menstrual cycle. However, these MMPs are not expressed everywhere in the endometrium. Expression of MMP-1, MMP-9 and MMP-10 remains focal in the perimenstrual endometrium whereas that of MMP-3 is more diffuse[10, 12, 24], thus indicating that additional mechanisms to the progesterone control are involved in the regulation of the expression of these MMPs. In particular, expression of MMP-1 is first restricted to foci of the perimenstrual endometrium preferentially localized in the superficial part of the mucosa, then extends to larger and deeper areas of the tissue as menstruation proceeds[12]. The stromal cells expressing MMP-1 are constantly localized around glands devoid of progesterone receptor immunostaining, suggesting some paracrine interaction between epithelial and stromal cells in the regulation of the expression of MMP-1.

A paracrine regulation was indeed confirmed by culturing isolated purified stromal cells which were unable to produce MMP-1 even in the absence of progesterone, unless cultured with a medium conditioned by purified epithelial cells. Monoclonal antibodies against interleukin-1α could block the induction of MMP-1 expression, whereas antibodies raised against other cytokines were ineffective, indicating that interleukin-1α released by the epithelial cells lacking progesterone receptors can be responsible for the paracrine induction of MMP-1 expression[19]. Similar paracrine mechanisms involving the transforming growth factor-β have been demonstrated in the inhibition of MMP-7 expression by epithelial cells upon progesterone treatment[25].

The prominent perimenstrual production of all MMPs expressed in the human endometrium suggests that these enzymes are involved in the menstrual breakdown of this tissue. Indeed, although the expression of TIMPs-1 and -2 increases at that time of the cycle, uninhibited activity of MMP-1 can be measured in media conditioned by menstrual endometrial explants during the first day of culture and can be extracted from menstrual endometrium[11, 22] (Marbaix *et al.*, unpublished observations), indicating that the expression and the activation of this enzyme override the production of TIMPs at menstruation. Similarly, withdrawal of progesterone from the culture medium of purified stromal cells induces the expression of several MMPs but has no effect on the production of TIMPs[18]. The restricted detection of MMP-1 mRNA and immunolocalization of MMP-1, MMP-9 and MMP-3 to breaking down areas in a menstrual endometrium support their involvement in the degradation of the endometrium[12, 24]. The remarkable distribution of MMP-1 mRNA expressing cells at the edge of menstrual fragments is also suggestive of the digestion of the framework of the extracellular matrix by this proteinase, allowing shedding of tissue pieces[12]. Furthermore, the finding of MMP-1 mRNA and of MMP-1 in the wall of arterioles could be relevant in the origin of menstrual hemorrhages[12, 22]. Finally, the pivotal role of MMPs in the endometrial extracellular matrix breakdown at menstruation was demonstrated *in vitro* by mimicking menstruation in cultured endometrial explants[26]. Complete inhibition of the menstrual matrix breakdown was obtained by culturing explants with specific synthetic inhibitors of metalloproteinases, which abolished the activity of MMPs, or with sex steroids which prevented the expression of MMPs. In contrast, explants cultured without sex steroid and without inhibitor, or with inhibitors of serine, cysteine or aspartic proteinases showed extensive menstrual breakdown.

MATRIX METALLOPROTEINASES IN ENDOMETRIOTIC FOCI

Among MMPs and TIMPs expressed in menstrual endometrium, MMP-1, MMP-3,

Table 3 Relationship between MMP-1 expression, presence of sex steroid receptors and matrix breakdown in endometriotic lesions

Endometriotic lesions		*Ovarian*	*Red peritoneal*	*Black peritoneal*	*Recto-vaginal*
MMP-1 mRNA		4/11	4/13	0/12	0/11
Foci expressing MMP-1 mRNA					
Progesterone receptors	Stromal cells	1/4	1/4		
	Epithelial cells	1†/3*	0/4		
Estrogen receptors	Stromal cells	1/4	2/4		
	Epithelial cells	0/2*	2/4		
Matrix breakdown		3/3*	2/3*		
Tissue without detectable MMP-1 mRNA††					
Progesterone receptors	Stromal cells	8/10	7/10	10/12	10/11
	Epithelial cells	6/7	5/9	8/11	9/11
Estrogen receptors	Stromal cells	9/10	8/10	9/11	11/11
	Epithelial cells	7/7	7/9	8/10	9/11
Matrix breakdown		1/7	2/7	1/10	1/7

Expanded from Kokorine *et al.*[27]. †, Only very few epithelial cells faintly immunostained for progesterone receptor in this area; *, not all 4 cases presenting MMP-1 mRNA could be analysed for this parameter, owing to the small size of the endometriotic focus; ††, analysis includes MMP-1 mRNA negative areas in MMP-l expressing endometriotic lesions; not all parameters could be analysed in each case, because of the small size of some lesions

MMP-7 and TIMP-1 have been disclosed in endometriotic lesions[27–30]. Progesterone seems to be less inhibitory on the expression of MMP-7 in ectopic than in eutopic endometrium, because MMP-7 mRNA was disclosed in epithelial cells of an endometriotic lesion sampled during the secretory phase of the menstrual cycle (at which time it is not detected in the eutopic endometrium)[31]. However, the expression of these MMPs and TIMP is not ubiquitous and remains somehow regulated in endometriosis.

Indeed, MMP-1 mRNA was detected by *in situ* hybridization only in about one third of ovarian and of red peritoneal lesions[27], i.e. endometriotic lesions that are regarded as 'active' because of their proliferative activity and of their more developed vascularization[32]. As in the eutopic endometrium, MMP-1 expression was focal and the detection of stromal cells containing its mRNA increased with the number of hybridized histological sections within a lesion. MMP-1 expression was also related to the breakdown of the extracellular matrix as assessed by silver staining of the collagen-rich 'reticular' fibrils, suggesting a role for MMP-1 in the initiation of bleeding inside the endometriotic foci and/or of tissue shedding and reimplantation of the lesion. Furthermore, MMP-1 expression was also related to the lack of immunostaining for progesterone receptors in the neighbouring epithelial cells (Figures 1–4 and Table 3). However, in contrast with the eutopic endometrium, MMP-1 mRNA was also detected in endometriotic lesions sampled outside menstruation. In black peritoneal or recto-vaginal lesions, so-called 'inactive' lesions, no MMP-1 mRNA could be found even when analysing numerous histological sections by *in situ* hybridization and even when the lesion was sampled around menstruation.

These results indicate that the expression of MMP-1 is not so well regulated in endometriotic lesions as in the eutopic endometrium throughout the menstrual cycle, but that the ovarian steroids, in

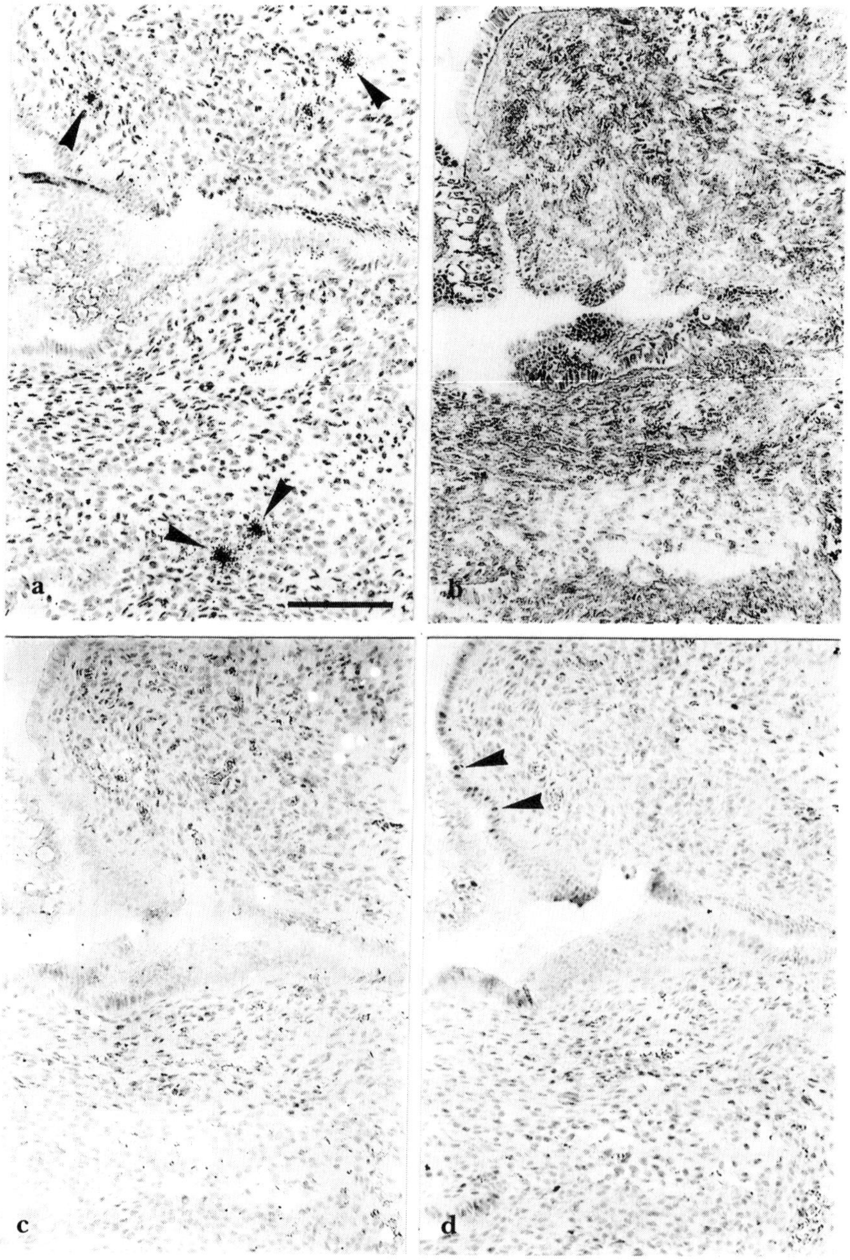

Figure 1 Peritoneal red endometriotic lesion from a 33-year-old woman, sampled during the mid-secretory phase of the menstrual cycle. (a) *In situ* hybridization of MMP-1 mRNA (arrowheads indicate MMP-1 expressing stromal cells); (b) Silver staining of collagen-rich 'reticular' fibers; (c) Immunolabeling of progesterone receptors; (d) Immunolabeling of estradiol receptors (arrowheads indicate some immunostained epithelial cells). Bar: 100 μm

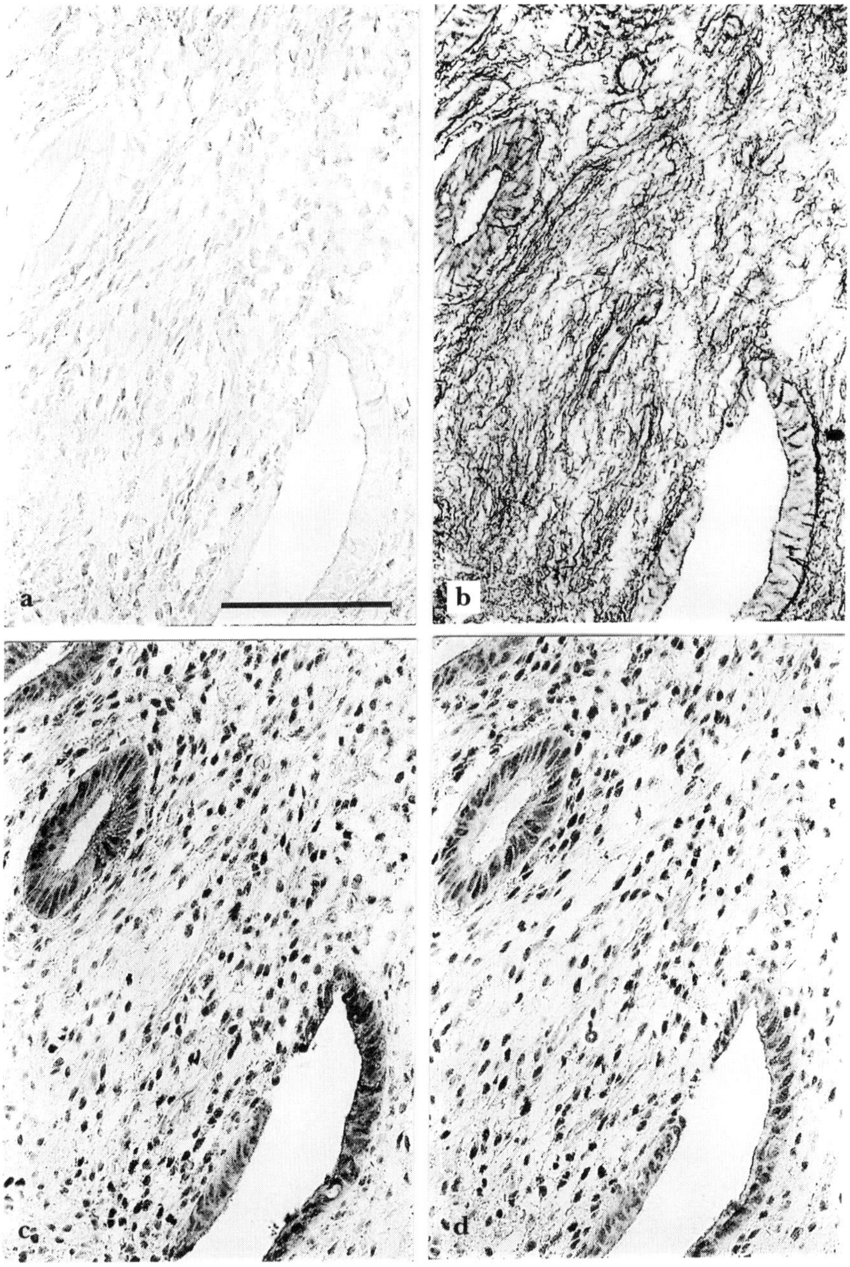

Figure 2 Peritoneal black endometriotic lesion from a 39-year-old woman, sampled at the early proliferative phase of the menstrual cycle. (a) *In situ* hybridization of MMP-1 mRNA; (b) Silver staining of collagen-rich 'reticular' fibers; (c) Immunolabeling of progesterone receptors; (d) Immunolabeling of estradiol receptors. Bar: 100 μm

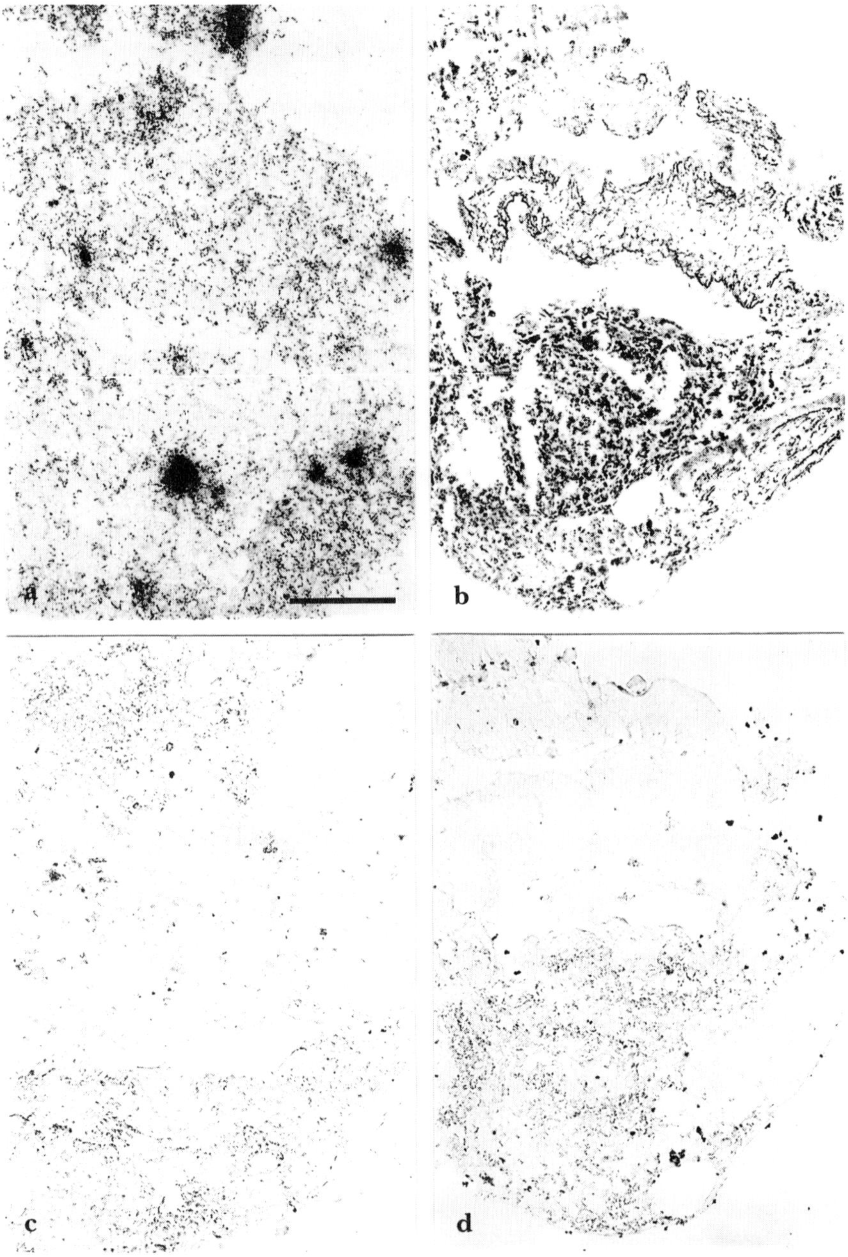

Figure 3 Ovarian endometriotic lesion from a 30 year-old woman, sampled at menstruation. (a) *In situ* hybridization of MMP-1 mRNA; (b) Silver staining of collagen-rich 'reticular' fibers; (c) Immunolabeling of progesterone receptors; (d) Immunolabeling of estradiol receptors. Bar: 100 μm

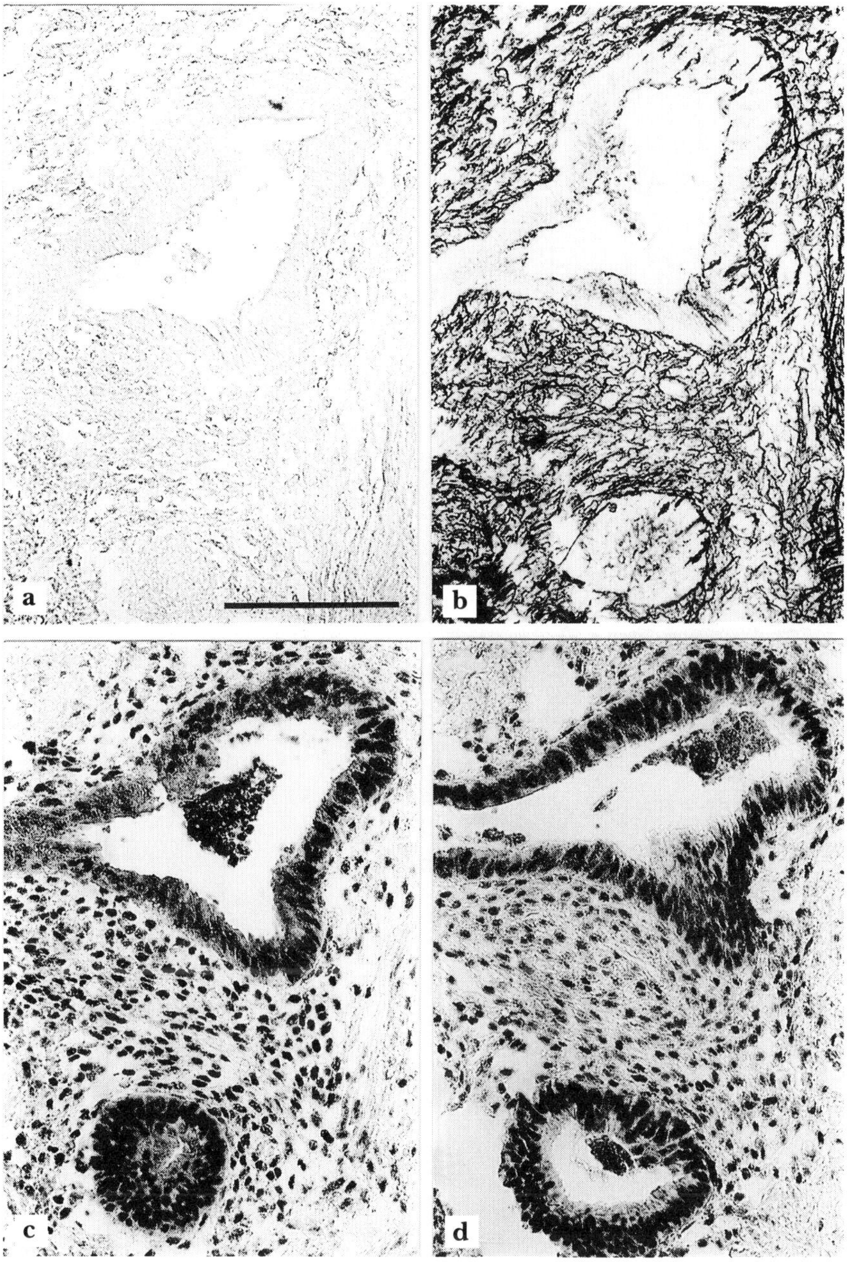

Figure 4 Rectovaginal endometriotic lesion from a 34 year-old woman, sampled at the mid-proliferative phase of the menstrual cycle. (a) *In situ* hybridization of MMP-1 mRNA; (b) Silver staining of collagen-rich 'reticular' fibers; (c) Immunolabeling of progesterone receptors; (d) Immunolabeling of estradiol receptors. Bar: 100 μm

particular progesterone, are still likely to control the expression of MMP-1 at places where the ectopic tissue contains the appropriate receptors. As is the case for the basal layer of the eutopic endometrium, inactive endometriotic lesions possess sex steroid receptors and do not express MMPs, even at menstruation. However, it cannot be excluded that expression of MMP-1 could still occur at sites of matrix breakdown if such lesions were reactivated and started bleeding.

MATRIX METALLOPROTEINASES INVOLVEMENT IN XENOGRAFTS OF ENDOMETRIAL TISSUE

Several studies have been performed to reproduce the implantation of retrograde menstrual fragments generating endometriotic lesions by grafting endometrial tissue into the peritoneal cavity of animals. A role for proteinases in this process was suggested from experiments in which serine proteinase inhibitors lowered the rate of endometriotic-like lesions in monkeys grafted intraperitoneally with fragments from their own endometrium[33].

The involvement of MMPs in the generation of endometriotic lesions upon implantation of menstrual endometrium is strongly supported by experimental grafting of human endometrium into athymic 'nude' mice[34] (Nisolle *et al.*, unpublished observations). Indeed, the establishment of endometriotic-like lesions was suppressed or considerably decreased when the expression of most MMPs in the endometrial fragments was prevented by progesterone, or when the activity of MMPs was specifically inhibited by addition of TIMPs[34]. Similarly, the number of endometriotic-like lesions developing in 'nude' mice was higher when transplanting menstrual endometrial fragments, which abundantly express MMP-1, than when transplanting proliferative endometrial pieces, which express barely detectable MMP-1 mRNA (Nisolle *et al.*, unpublished observations). Interestingly, interleukin-1α (shown to induce the expression of MMP-1 by stromal cells purified from the eutopic endometrium[19]) could override the inhibitory effect of progesterone and promote the implantation of endometrial xenografts[35] whereas transforming growth factor-β could not prevent the implantation of endometrial xenografts into 'nude' mice despite preventing the expression of a MMP (presumably MMP-7)[36].

CONCLUSIONS AND HYPOTHESES

Endometriotic lesions can express at least MMP-1, MMP-3, MMP-7 and TIMP-1 as does the eutopic endometrium at menstruation. The focal expression of MMP-1, restricted to breaking down areas of 'active' lesions, suggests a role for these enzymes in the pathogenesis and the evolution of the disease. The involvement of MMPs in the pathogenesis of endometriosis is further strongly supported by the prevention of endometrial xenografts in 'nude' mice by progesterone, which inhibits the expression of MMPs, or by TIMPs, which inhibit MMPs' activity. However, as retrograde menstruation is physiological[37], it remains to be found why endometriosis develops only in some women whereas they should all have in their peritoneum endometrial debris rich in MMP activity at each menstruation, a problem reminiscent of the 'seed and soil' controversy in cancer metastasis.

As in the eutopic menstrual endometrium, expression (and activation) of MMPs, in particular MMP-1, in endometriotic foci could induce the breakdown of the extracellular matrix and the resulting bleeding, thought to be responsible for the symptomatology of the disease[38]. The focal expression of MMP-1 around glands lacking immunodetectable progesterone receptors is suggestive of a hormonal control of the expression of this MMP and thus of the activity of the endometriotic lesion. However, the reason for the focal absence of progesterone receptors in endometriotic foci is still unknown. We suggest that a better understanding of the regulation of sex steroid receptor expression could help in finding ways to control the expression of MMPs and to prevent bleeding and symptoms from endometriotic lesions.

Bleeding alone cannot explain all the pathology associated with endometriosis. In particular, deep lesions can invade organs such as the recto-vaginal wall, the bladder or the colon (or the uterus itself in adenomyosis) in a manner similar to cancer cells. MMPs have been largely implicated in the invasion process by cancer cells but their role in the invasion by endometriosis remains to be investigated.

ACKNOWLEDGEMENTS

We thank Professor H. Nagase from the Kansas University Medical Center, Kansas City, KS, for the gift of MMP-1 cDNA. We are also grateful to Professor Y. Okada from the Keio University, Tokyo, Japan, and to Dr K. Iwata from Fuji Chemical Industries Ltd., Japan, for the gifts of anti-MMP-1 monoclonal antibodies. Drs E. A. Bone (British Biotech), P. Mitchell (Central Pfizer), C. G. Caillard (Rhone-Poulenc Rorer) and D. Bradshaw (Roche) are thanked for gifts of materials.

M.-Ch. Baelden, Ph. Camby, A. Herssens-Marcelis, S. Lagasse, P. Lefebvre-Lemoine, Y. Marchand, F. N'Kuli, S. Ruttens, P. Vanden Berghe and L. Wenderickx are gratefully acknowledged for technical assistance.

The work was supported by the Belgian Fonds de la Recherche Scientifique Médicale, by the Fonds de Développement Scientifique of the Université Catholique de Louvain, and by Ipsen Biotech, Paris, France. This paper presents research results of the Belgian Programme on Interuniversity Poles of Attraction, Prime Minister's Office, Federal Services of Scientific, Technical and Cultural Affairs, and of Concerted Research Actions of the 'Communauté Française de Belgique'.

References

1. Sampson JA. Peritoneal endometriosis due to menstrual dissemination of endometrial tissue into the pelvic cavity. *Am J Obstet Gynecol* 1927;14:422–67
2. Meyer R. Ueber den Stand der Frage der Adenomyositis und Adenomyome in Allgemeinen und Insbesondere ueber Adenomyositis seroepithelialis und Adenomyometritis sarcomatosa. *Zentralbl Gynakol* 1919;36:743–59
3. Stovall DW, Anners JA, Halme J. Immunohistochemical detection of type I, III, IV collagen in endometriosis implants. *Fertil Steril* 1992;57:984–9
4. Gaetje R, Kotzian S, Herrmann G, *et al.* Invasiveness of endometriotic cells *in vitro*. *Lancet* 1995;346:1463–5
5. Eeckhout Y. Tissue breakdown. In d'Arcangues C, Fraser IS, Newton JR, Odlind V, eds. *Contraception and Mechanisms of Endometrial Bleeding*. Cambridge: Cambridge University Press, 1990:431–9
6. Murphy G. Matrix metalloproteinases and their inhibitors. *Acta Orthop Scand* 1995;66 (Suppl. 266):55–60
7. Nagase H. Activation mechanisms of matrix metalloproteinases. *Biol Chem* 1997;378:151–60
8. Saari H, Suomalainen K, Lindy O, *et al.* Activation of latent human neutrophil collagenase by reactive oxygen species and serine proteases. *Biochem Biophys Res Commun* 1990;171:979–87
9. Hampton AL, Salamonsen LA. Expression of messenger ribonucleic acid encoding matrix metalloproteinases and their tissue inhibitors is related to menstruation. *J Endocr* 1994;141:R1–3
10. Rodgers WH, Matrisian LM, Giudice LC, *et al.* Patterns of matrix metalloproteinase expression in cycling endometrium imply differential functions and regulation by steroid hormones. *J Clin Invest* 1994;94:946–53
11. Marbaix E, Kokorine I, Henriet P, *et al.* The expression of interstitial collagenase in human endometrium is controlled by progesterone and by oestradiol and is related to menstruation. *Biochem J* 1995;305:1027–30
12. Kokorine I, Marbaix E, Henriet P, *et al.* Focal cellular origin and regulation of interstitial collagenase (matrix metalloproteinase-1) are related to menstrual breakdown in the human endometrium. *J Cell Sci* 1996;109:2151–60
13. Hulboy DL, Rudolph LA, Matrisian LM. Matrix metalloproteinases as mediators of reproductive function. *Mol Hum Reprod* 1997;3:27–45
14. Sayegh R, Awwad JT, Maxwell C, *et al.* α2-macroglobulin production by the human

endometrium. *J Clin Endocrinol Metab* 1995;80: 1021–6

15. Rodgers WH, Osteen KG, Matrisian LM, *et al.* Expression and localization of matrilysin, a matrix metalloproteinase, in human endometrium during the reproductive cycle. *Am J Obstet Gynecol* 1993;168:253–60
16. Marbaix E, Donnez J, Courtoy PJ, *et al.* Progesterone regulates the activity of collagenase and related gelatinases A and B in human endometrial explants. *Proc Natl Acad Sci USA* 1992;89:11789–93
17. Osteen KG, Rodgers WH, Gaire M, *et al.* Stromal-epithelial interaction mediates steroidal regulation of metalloproteinase expression in human endometrium. *Proc Natl Acad Sci USA* 1994;91:10129–33
18. Salamonsen LA, Butt AR, Hammond FR, *et al.* Production of endometrial matrix metalloproteinases, but not their tissue inhibitors, is modulated by progesterone withdrawal in an *in vitro* model for menstruation. *J Clin Endocrinol Metab* 1997;82:1409–15
19. Singer CF, Marbaix E, Kokorine I, *et al.* Paracrine stimulation of interstitial collagenase (MMP-1) in the human endometrium by interleukin-1α and its dual block by ovarian steroids. *Proc Natl Acad Sci USA* 1997;94:10341–5
20. Schatz F, Papp C, Toth-Pal E, *et al.* Ovarian steroid-modulated stromelysin-1 expression in human endometrial stromal and decidual cells. *J Clin Endocrinol Metab* 1994;78:1467–72
21. Irwin JC, Kirk D, Gwatkin RBL, *et al.* Human endometrial matrix metalloproteinase-2, a putative menstrual proteinase. Hormonal regulation in cultured stromal cells and messenger RNA expression during the menstrual cycle. *J Clin Invest* 1996;97:438-47
22. Marbaix E, Kokorine I, Donnez J, *et al.* Regulation and restricted expression of interstitial collagenase suggest a pivotal role in the initiation of menstruation. *Hum Reprod* 1996;11(Suppl. 2):134–43
23. Brenner RM, Rudolph L, Matrisian L, *et al.* Non-human primate models: artificial menstrual cycles, endometrial matrix metalloproteinases and s.c. endometrial grafts. *Hum Reprod* 1996;11(Suppl.2):150–64
24. Salamonsen LA, Woolley DE. Matrix metalloproteinases in normal menstruation. *Hum Reprod* 1996;11(Suppl.2):124–33
25. Bruner KL, Rodgers WH, Gold LI, *et al.* Transforming growth factor β mediates the progesterone suppression of an epithelial metalloproteinase by adjacent stroma in the human endometrium. *Proc Natl Acad Sci USA* 1995;92:7362–6
26. Marbaix E, Kokorine I, Moulin P, *et al.* Menstrual breakdown of human endometrium can be mimicked *in vitro* and is selectively and reversibly blocked by inhibitors of matrix metalloproteinases. *Proc Natl Acad Sci USA* 1996;93: 9120–5
27. Kokorine I, Nisolle M, Donnez J, *et al.* Expression of interstitial collagenase (matrix metalloproteinase-1) is related to the activity of human endometriotic lesions. *Fertil Steril* 1997;68: 246–51
28. Osteen KG, Bruner KL, Sharpe-Timms KL. Steroid and growth factor regulation of matrix metalloproteinase expression and endometriosis. *Semin Reprod Endocrinol* 1996;14:247–55
29. Saito T, Mizumoto H, Kuroki K, *et al.* Expression of MMP-3 and TIMP-1 in endometriosis and the influence of Danazol. *Acta Obstet Gynaecol Japonica* 1995;47:495–6
30. Sharpe-Timms KL, Penney LL, Zimmer RL, *et al.* Partial purification and aminoacid sequence analysis of endometriosis protein-II (ENDO-II) reveals homology with tissue inhibitor of metalloproteinase-1 (TIMP-1). *J Clin Endocrinol Metab* 1995;80:3784–7
31. Osteen KG, Bruner KL, Eisenberg E. The disease endometriosis. In Diamond MP, Osteen KG, eds. *Endometrium and Endometriosis*. Malden, MA: Blackwell Science, 1997:20–6
32. Nisolle M, Casanas-Roux F, Anaf V, *et al.* Morphometric study of the stromal vascularization in peritoneal endometriosis. *Fertil Steril* 1993;59:681–4
33. Sillem M, Hahn U, Coddington CC, *et al.* Ectopic growth of endometrium depends on its structural integrity and proteolytic activity in the cynomolgus monkey (*Macaca fascicularis*) model of endometriosis. *Fertil Steril* 1996;66:468–73
34. Bruner KL, Matrisian LM, Rodgers WH, *et al.* Suppression of matrix metalloproteinases inhibits establishment of ectopic lesions by human endometrium in nude mice. *J Clin Invest* 1997;99:2851–7
35. Osteen KG, Bruner KL, Sierra-Rivera E, *et al.* Interleukin-1α opposes progesterone suppression of matrix metalloproteinases in an endometriosis model. *Biol Reprod* 1996;54(Suppl 1):121
36. Osteen KG, Bruner KL, Eisenberg E, *et al.* Progesterone induced transforming growth factor-β (TGF-β) suppresses endometrial metalloproteinases but TGF-β alone cannot block endometriotic-like lesions in nude mice. *Fertil Steril* 1995;64:S35
37. Halme J, Hammond MG, Hulka JF, *et al.* Retrograde menstruation in healthy women and inpatients with endometriosis. *Obstet Gynecol* 1984;64:151–4
38. Brosens I. Endometriosis: a lesion because it is characterized by bleeding. *Am J Obstet Gynecol* 1997;176:263-7

Interleukin-1α opposes suppression of human endometrial matrix metalloproteinases by progesterone in a model of experimental endometriosis

18

K.L. Bruner, N.R. Keller and K.G. Osteen

INTRODUCTION

The human endometrial cycle is dynamic in nature, exhibiting extensive tissue growth, differentiation and breakdown in response to changing levels of ovarian steroids. Estradiol provides the initial stimulus during endometrial growth while rising levels of progesterone promote cellular differentiation in support of pregnancy establishment. Unfortunately, ovarian steroids are also a component of the cellular pathophysiology of endometriosis, a complex disease often resulting from the extra-uterine implantation of endometrial tissue following retrograde menstruation[1,2]. The development of endometriosis appears to be steroid dependent[3] and occurs more frequently in women with increased exposure to estrogens[4]. In contrast to the effects of estrogen, progesterone may act to suppress or inhibit development and progression of endometriosis[5,6]. Additionally, a broad array of locally produced growth factors and immune cytokines acts in concert with steroids to regulate endometrial function[7,8]. As is true for steroids, these locally produced factors can significantly affect the development and progression of endometriosis[9]. However, the precise cellular mechanisms which link either steroid exposure or specific growth factor and cytokine action to the disease processes of endometriosis are not yet established.

Although considered a benign disease, establishment of endometriosis requires the successful ectopic implantation of refluxed menstrual tissue, an invasive event involving active degradation of the extracellular matrix within the peritoneum[10]. The matrix metalloproteinases (MMPs) are recognized to perform matrix degradation and remodeling during many reproductive processes which require the physical breakdown or restructuring of tissue[11]. Among many MMPs found within the reproductive tract, MMPs of the stromelysin family are highly expressed in the endometrium during menstruation and continue to exhibit a more focal pattern of expression during subsequent repair and growth[12, 13]. Although the specific mRNAs of MMP-3, MMP-11 and MMP-7 are detected during the estrogen-dominated proliferative phase, these enzymes cannot be detected when the endometrium is under the influence of progesterone. Both *in vivo* and *in vitro* findings confirm that progesterone suppresses MMP expression either through direct or indirect mechanisms[12–16].

The role that MMP regulation plays in endometriosis is not yet established, but evidence has begun to accumulate from several laboratories which implicates these enzymes in this disease[9,17,18]. Our laboratory has recently provided perhaps the most direct evidence linking progesterone inhibition of MMPs to the prevention of ectopic implantation of human endometrial tissue. Using a nude mouse model of endometriosis[19], either progesterone treatments of human endometrial tissue or treatments with TIMP-1, a natural metalloproteinase inhibitor, can prevent the establishment of ectopic lesions in the peritoneum of recipient mice. Given the collective findings of the above studies, it is tempting to speculate that suppression of MMPs may directly link progesterone action to the observed therapeutic benefits of this steroid in the clinical treatment of endometriosis. However, many women with endometriosis fail to respond significantly to progesterone therapy, perhaps as a consequence of other signal transduction mechanisms which can regulate endometrial MMPs in opposition to the prevailing steroid environment. For example, following tissue injury, locally produced cytokines such as interleukin-1 (IL-1) may transiently up-regulate MMPs in support of normal repair processes[20]. Additionally, IL-1 appears to be critical for normal implantation[21], a process which requires local MMP expression during the progesterone-dominated environment of pregnancy establishment. Outside the uterine corpus, we have reported that IL-1α can stimulate a high level of MMP-7 expression at sites of ectopic pregnancy[22]. The ability of IL-1 to stimulate MMPs in opposition to progesterone may complicate the regulation of MMPs during ectopic implantation of endometrial tissue since this cytokine may be elevated in the peritoneal fluid of women with endometriosis[23].

Clearly, the etiology of endometriosis is multi-faceted and no single regulatory mechanism or single family of molecules can account for the diverse presentation of this complex disease. However, developing a better understanding of the role that MMP regulation plays in endometriosis may provide new insights into the disease process as well as contribute to the development of new therapeutic strategies. In the current study, we present evidence which indicates that normal epithelial cells secrete IL-1α in response to injury and that this cytokine can override progesterone- mediated suppression of MMP-3 and MMP-7. Additionally, we demonstrate that the ability of IL-1α to induce expression of these enzymes in opposition to progesterone action can contribute to the development of experimental endometriosis.

MATERIALS AND METHODS

Acquisition of human tissue

Endometrial tissues were obtained during the proliferative phase (days 9–12) of the menstrual cycle from a donor population (ages 21–45) exhibiting regular menstrual cycles. An endometrial thickness of greater than 9 mm was confirmed by vaginal ultrasound prior to each biopsy, and a serum progesterone level of less than 1.0 ng/ml was necessary for inclusion in this study. Biopsies were obtained from the fundus region of the endometrial cavity with a Pipelle® endometrial suction curette (Unimar, Inc.; Wilton, CT) and immediately washed in prewarmed (37°C) phenol red-free Dulbecco's Modified Eagles Medium/Ham's F-12 Medium (DME/F-12) (Sigma Chemical; St. Louis, MO) to remove residual blood and mucous. The use of human tissues for this study was approved by Vanderbilt University's institutional review board and committee for the protection of human subjects.

Organ cultures of endometrium

Endometrial tissue fragments were divided into multiple groups as required for experimental treatments and suspended as organ cultures within tissue culture inserts (Millipore; Bedford, MA) as previously described. Each culture was maintained under serum-free conditions in DME/F-12 medium supplemented with 1% ITS$^+$ (Collaborative Biomedical; Bedford, MA) and 0.1% Excyte (Miles Scientific; Kankakee, IL), and incubated at 37°C in a humidified chamber with 95% air : 5% CO_2. Treatments included estradiol (10 nM), estradiol plus progesterone (1 nM and 500 nM, respectively) or IL-1α (100 pg/ml) with or without steroids. Organ cultures of human endometrial fragments were maintained for 24 hours before analysis of MMP mRNAs and proteins or use in the nude mouse experimental model as outlined below[19].

Isolation and culture of endometrial stromal cells

Isolation of endometrial stromal cells was accomplished via sequential enzymatic dissociation and sedimentation as previously described[14]. Stromal cells (3×10^5) were cultured on a dry coating of Type I collagen on the bottom surface of tissue culture wells and were allowed to attach 24 hours in DMEM/F-12 with 5% charcoal-stripped, heat-inactivated calf serum before intiation of serum-free experimental conditions. Steroid treatments of isolated stroma included estradiol alone (10 nM), estradiol plus progesterone (1 nM and 500 nM, respectively), estradiol plus IL-1α (100 pg/ml), or estradiol, progesterone plus IL-1α.

Analysis of MMP secretion in endometrial cultures

Secretion of pro-MMP-7 or pro- MMP-3 by endometrial organ cultures was analyzed following ^{35}S-methionine labeling (100μCi) for 18 hours at 37°C in methionine-free medium as previously described[14]. Secreted proteins were quantitated by TCA-precipitation and equivalent TCA-precipitable counts ($0.5 - 1 \times 10^6$ cpm) were selectively immunoprecipitated using antibodies directed against a synthetic peptide corresponding to a deduced sequence in the carboxy terminus of rat prostromelysin-1 (MMP-3)[24] or an internal sequence in human promatrilysin (MMP-7)[25]. The resulting complexes were removed with protein A sepharose and identified by SDS–PAGE and autoradiography.

In situ hybridization

The *in situ* hybridization method using ^{3}H-labeled probes was performed as previously described[13]. Hybridization signal is scored by comparing the silver grain deposition by the anti-sense (messenger RNA) probe with that of the sense (control) probe on serial sections using dark field illumination and 10× magnification.

Interleukin-1α immunohistochemistry

Immunohistochemical studies for IL-1α were performed according to standard methodology. Briefly, formalin fixed, paraffin embedded sections were treated with methanol/peroxide solution and appropriate normal serum in saline to block endogenous peroxidase and nonspecific binding, respectively. Binding of primary antibody to tissue was determined with a streptavidin-peroxidase conjugate to the secondary antibody and visualized with a 3,3'-diaminobenzidine tetrahydrochloride solution, resulting in a brown precipitate. Tissues were counterstained with Gill's hematoxylin. Normal serum was used as a negative control.

Interleukin-1α immunoassay

In vitro secretion of IL-1α activity was measured by ELISA using a commercially available immunoassay kit (Quantikine, R & D Systems). These assays have a sensitivity of 7 pg/ml and a broad working range of 31.2–2000 pg/ml.

Experimental model of endometriosis

Four-week-old athymic (nude), ovariectomized mice were purchased from Taconic Laboratory Animals (Germantown, NY) and housed on site in previously sterilized cages and bedding. The animal room was maintained at 26.7%C with a 12-hour light/12-hour dark cycle and mice were provided with sterile Purina Rodent Chow® and water *ad libitum*. Metafane® (Pittman-Moore, Toledo, OH) was used to anesthetize animals prior to any invasive procedures, which were performed in a laminar flow hood using

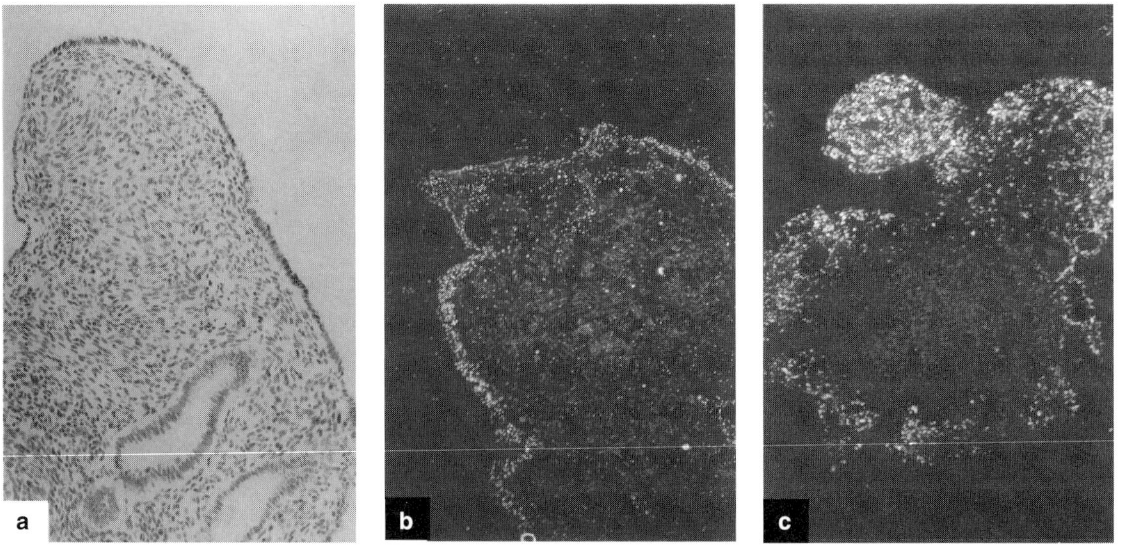

Figure 1 *In situ* hybridization analysis of proliferative phase endometrial organ cultures maintained for 24 hours in the presence of estrogen and progesterone. Under lightfield (a) areas of active re-epithelialization are apparent along the border of this tissue. Darkfield photomicrographs reveal localization of MMP-7 mRNA (b) in epithelial cells actively involved in re-epithelialization and MMP-3 mRNA (c) in stromal cells immediately adjacent to proliferating epithelium. Note a lack of MMP mRNA expression in the interior of the tissue, indicating progesterone suppression of these enzymes. All photomicrographs are at a magnification of 200×

sterile instruments. Mice were randomly divided into groups and sterile 60-day release capsules containing 1.5 mg 17β-estradiol (Innovative Research of America; Sarasota, Florida) were inserted subcutaneously at a site just below the scapula.

Human endometrial tissue, maintained for 24 hours in culture as described above, was washed briefly in PBS before injection into recipient mice. Each animal received a single intraperitoneal injection of 8–10 endometrial tissue fragments in 400 μl sterile PBS using a tuberculin syringe. All animals had received a steroid-releasing capsule 24–96 hours prior to human tissue injections. Ten to twelve days after receiving human tissue injections, mice were killed and necropsied for identification of endometriotic-like lesions. Morphological and immunohistochemical characterization of ectopic lesions by standard methods was done to confirm human endometrial origin.

RESULTS

Interleukin-1α overrides progesterone suppression of MMPs

We have previously demonstrated that progesterone exposure suppresses endometrial secretion of MMP-3 and MMP-7 proteins following 24–48 hours of treatment *in vitro*[14]. However, the time course of suppressing these enzymes *in vitro* suggests that MMP expression may not be uniformly regulated under organ culture conditions. To address this issue in more detail, proliferative phase human endometrial tissues were maintained as organ cultures in the presence of estradiol and progesterone for 24 hours and analyzed for cell-type specific expression of MMP-3 and MMP-7 mRNA. As shown in Figure 1a, under lightfield, areas of active re-epithelialization (ie, proliferation) can be seen along the borders of the tissue. Following *in situ* hybrid-

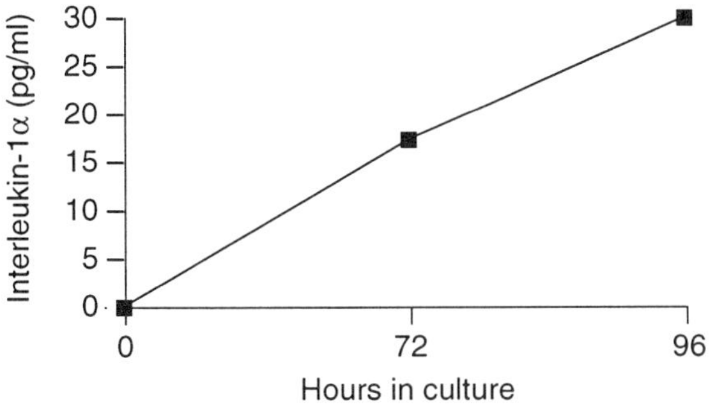

Figure 2 Interleukin-1α secretion by proliferative phase human endometrial epithelial cells cultured on Matrigel and maintained in a steroid-free environment. Cytokine expression was quantified over several days in culture by ELISA

ization localization, darkfield microscopy reveals specific MMP-7 mRNA expression in areas of active re-epithelialization (Figure 1b) as well as MMP-3 mRNA expression in the stromal cells immediately adjacent to the proliferating epithelium (Figure 1c). Reflecting the more generalized suppressive effects of progesterone, MMP mRNAs are not detected in the interior of the tissue, in areas not undergoing repair. These results suggest that the endometrial epithelial cells may act to upregulate local MMP expression during tissue repair, transiently overriding the normally suppressive effects of progesterone on both MMP-7 and MMP-3.

Epithelial-derived interleukin-1α stimulates stromal cell MMP expression

The ability of epithelial cells to mediate repair processes in a variety of tissues is well-established[26]. Our laboratory has previously found that IL-1 is involved in the upregulation of MMP-7 at sites of ectopic pregnancy[22]. Not surprisingly, we also found that IL-1α is released by cultures of human endometrial epithelial cells following cell isolation and serum-free culture (Figure 2). Stimulation of MMP-3 expression in similarly isolated endometrial stromal cells was induced by addition of IL-1α, even in the presence of progesterone (Figure 3). Together with the results of organ culture studies (Figure 1), these results strongly support a role for epithelial-derived IL-1α in opposing progesterone suppression of both stromal-derived MMP-3 and epithelial-derived MMP-7 during re-epithelialization in response to injury.

Effect of interleukin-1α in experimental endometriosis

We have previously demonstrated that progesterone-mediated suppression of endometrial MMPs can prevent the development of endometriotic-like lesions in an experimental model of endometriosis[19]. The above results indicate that IL-1α can oppose the ability of progesterone to suppress endometrial MMPs and thus we investigated whether IL-1α can also inhibit the ability of progesterone to prevent experimental endometriosis. Organ cultures of proliferative phase endometrial tissues were maintained in the presence of estradiol alone, IL-1α alone (IL-1), estradiol plus progesterone, or IL-1α plus estradiol and progesterone. Following 24 hours in culture, tissues were washed with PBS and intraperitoneally injected into ovariectomized nude mice, each previously implanted with an estradiol-releasing pellet. As described in Table 1, a similar percentage of mice receiving IL-1α-treated tissue or estradiol treated tissue developed lesions (87.5% and 90%, respectively) although none of the animals receiving progesterone-treated tissue developed lesions. Co-treatment of

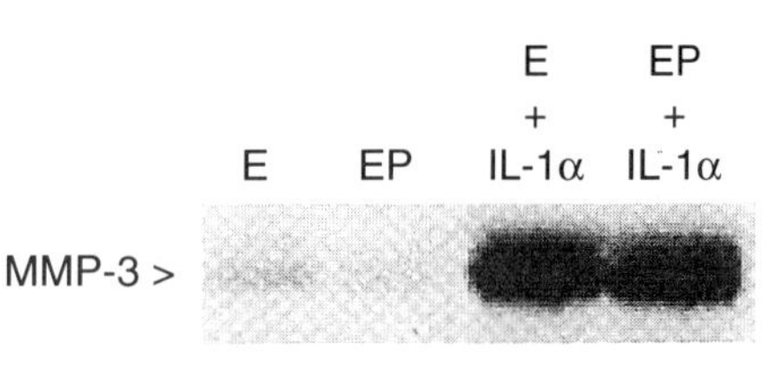

Figure 3 Expression and regulation of MMP-3 in isolated endometrial stromal cells cultured in estradiol (E; 10mM) or estradiol plus progesterone (EP; E=1mM, P=500mM), interleukin-1α (100 pg/ml) or EP + IL-1α

Table 1 Summary of results obtained in the nude mouse model of human endometriosis

Tissue treatment	*Animal treatment*	*Number with lesions*	*Total number*	*Percent with lesions*
E	E	11	12	92
EP	E	0	13	0
IL-1α	E	7	8	87.5
IL-1α + EP	E	8	9	89

E, estradiol; P, progesterone

tissue with IL-1α and progesterone resulted in 89% of mice developing lesions, suggesting that the ability of IL-1α to oppose progesterone suppression of MMPs results in an inability of progesterone to prevent experimental endometriosis.

Expression of interleukin-1α in human endometriosis

Although IL-1α opposition of progesterone suppression of experimental endometriosis is intriguing, it does not directly address whether or not this cytokine plays a role in the human disease. In regard to this question, we have localized by immunohistochemistry IL-1α protein in human endometriosis and in normal endometrium from women without endometriosis. As shown in Figure 4a, normal proliferative endometrium shows little immunolocalization of IL-1α protein. In contrast, an endometriotic lesion surgically removed from a patient during the proliferative phase (Figure 4b) demonstrates abundant expression of IL-1α. Sahakian *et al.*[27] have previously reported the presence of IL-1 receptor antagonist in eutopic, but not ectopic, tissues from women with endometriosis. Taken together, these results support a role for IL-1α action in the pathophysiology of this disease, possibly via induction of MMPs.

SUMMARY

Clinical observations suggest that estrogen plays an important role in the development and maintenance of endometriosis[4, 28] while

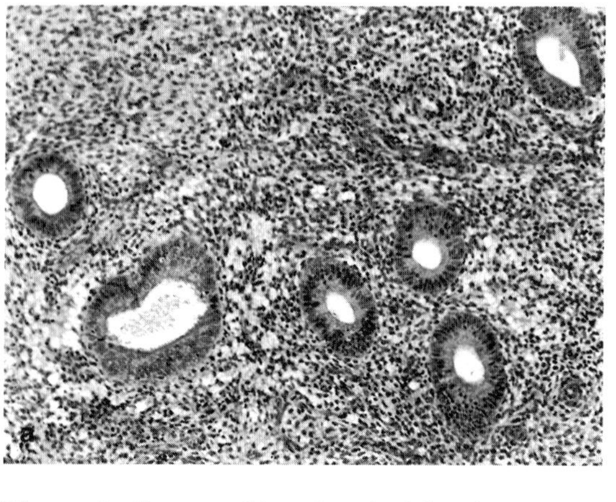

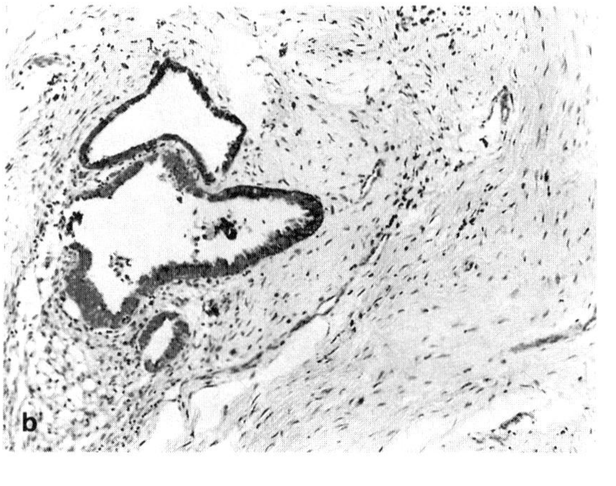

Figure 4 Immunohistochemical localization of IL-1α in formalin-fixed, paraffin-embedded normal proliferative endometrium (a) and in an endometriotic lesion removed from a patient during the proliferative phase (b)

progesterone may prevent or suppress the disease process[5,6]. Unfortunately, many women fail to respond to progesterone therapy, possibly resulting from an insensitivity to this steroid[29,30], or by the exacerbation of local tissue responses which may alter steroid sensitivity. In the normal endometrium, we have previously described both direct and indirect steroid-mediated regulation of the stromelysin family of MMPs, including suppression of these enzymes by progesterone[12–14,16]. In the current study, we demonstrate that endometrial MMPs may be upregulated by IL-1α, secreted locally by epithelial cells during an apparent tissue repair process. One of the most important aspects of stromal-epithelial communication is steroid-driven regulation of MMPs[14,16], and numerous studies have demonstrated that the steroid-sensitive endometrial stromal cell transmits signals to adjacent epithelium in a paracrine fashion[31–33]. In this report, however, we provide evidence that endometrial epithelial cells, via IL-1α secretion, can direct stromal cell MMP expression without regard to the steroid environment. Although this epithelial cell directed pathway may be necessary for normal tissue repair, our study suggests that IL-1α upregulation of MMPs may allow endometrial tissue to more readily establish ectopic sites of growth by opposing progesterone suppression of MMPs. Enhanced expression of IL-1 in the peritoneal fluid of women with endometriosis[23] could further stimulate expression of MMPs, exacerbating disease progression. Developing a better understanding of MMP regulation by both stromal and epithelial cells should provide insight into developing more successful treatment strategies for endometriosis.

References

1. Sampson JA. Peritoneal endometriosis due to menstrual dissemination of endometrial tissue into the peritoneal cavity. *Am J Obstet Gynecol* 1927; 14:422–69
2. Ishimaru T, Masuzaki H. Peritoneal endometriosis: endometrial tissue implantation as a primary etiologic mechanism. *Am J Obstet Gynecol* 1991;165:210–14
3. DiZerga GS, Barber DL, Hodgen GD. Endometriosis: role of steroids in initiation, development, maintenance and suppression. *Fertil Steril* 1980;33:649–53
4. Halme J, Stovall D. Endometriosis and its medical management. In Wallach EE, Zacur HA, eds. *Reproductive Medicine and Surgery*. St Louis, MO: Mosby, 1995:695–710
5. Ramzy, I. Pathology. In Schenken RS, ed. *Endometriosis: Contemporary Concepts and Clinical Management*. Philadelphia: J.B. Lippincott Company, 1989:60
6. Olive DL. Medical treatment: alternatives to danazol. In R.S. Schenken, ed. *Endometriosis: Contempory Concepts and Clinical Management*. Philadelphia: J.B. Lippencott, 1989:192
7. Giudice LC. Growth factors and growth modulators in human uterine endometrium: their potential relevance to reproductive medicine. *Fertil Steril* 1994;61:1–7
8. Tabibzadeh S, Sun X. Cytokine expression in human endometrium throughout the menstrual cycle. *Hum Reprod* 1992;7:1214–21
9. Osteen KG, Bruner KL, Sharpe-Timms, KL. Steroid and growth factor regulation of matrix metalloproteinase expression and endometriosis. *Sem Rep Endocr* 1996;14:247–55
10. Spuijbroek MDEH, Dunselman GAJ, Menheere PPCA, *et al.* Early endometriosis invades the extracellular matrix. *Fertil Steril* 1992;58:929–33
11. Hulboy DL, Rudolph LA, Matrisian LM. Matrix metalloproteinases as mediators of reproductive function. *Mol Hum Reprod* 1997; 3:27–45
12. Rodgers WH, Osteen KG, Matrisian LM, *et al.* Expression and localization of matrilysin, a matrix metalloproteinase, in the human endometrium. *Am J Obstet Gynecol* 1993;168: 253–60
13. Rodgers WH, Matrisian LM, Giudice LC, *et al.* Patterns of matrix metalloproteinase expression in cycling endometrium imply differential functions and regulation by steroids. *J Clin Invest* 1994;94:946–53
14. Osteen KG, Rodgers WH, Gaire M, *et al.* Stromal-epithelial interaction mediates steroidal regulation of matrix metalloproteinase expression in the human endometrium. *Proc Natl Acad Sci USA* 1994;91:10129–33

15. Schatz F, Papp C, Toth-pal E, *et al.* Ovarian-steroid modulation of stromelysin-1 expression in human endometrial stroma and decidual cells. *J Clin Endocrinol Metab* 1994;78:1467–72
16. Bruner KL, Rodgers WH, Korc M, *et al.* Transforming growth factor-β mediates the progesterone suppression of an epithelial metalloproteinase by adjacent stroma in human endometrium. *Proc Natl Acad Sci USA* 1995;92: 7362–6
17. Saito T, Mizumoto H, Kuroki K, *et al.* Expression of MMP-3 and TIMP-1 in endometriosis and the influence of Danazol. *Acta Obstet Gynec Japan* 1995;47:495–6
18. Sharpe-Timms KL, Keisler LW, McIntush EW, *et al.* Tissue inhibitor of metalloproteinase-1 concentrations are attenuated in peritoneal fluid and sera of women with endometriosis and restored in sera by gonadotropin releasing hormone-agonist therapy. *Fertil Steril* 1998; 69:1128–34
19. Bruner KL, Matrisian LM, Rodgers WH, *et al.* Suppression of matrix metalloproteinases inhibits establishment of ectopic lesions by human tissue in nude mice. *J Clin Invest* 1997; 99:2851–7
20. Page RC. The role of inflammatory mediators in the pathogenesis of periodontal disease. *J Peridontal Res* 1991;26:230–42
21. Simon C, Mercader A, Gimeno MJ, *et al.* The interleukin-1 system and human implantation. *Am J Rep Immunol* 1997;37:64–72
22. Osteen KG, Sierra-Rivera E, Keller NR, *et al.* Interleukin-1α opposes progesterone-mediated suppression of MMP-7: a possible role of this cytokine in human implantation. *Ann NY Acad Sci* 1997;828:137–45
23. Fakih H, Bagget B, Holtz G, *et al.* Interleukin-1: possible role in the infertility associated with endometriosis. *Fertil Steril* 1987;47:213–17
24. Matrisian LM, Bowden GT, Kreig P, *et al.* An mRNA coding for the secreted proteinase transin is expressed more abundantly in malignant than benign tumors. *Proc Natl Acad Sci (USA)* 1986; 83:9413–17
25. Busiek DF, Ross FP, McDonnell S, *et al.* The MMP matrilysin (PUMP-1) is expressed in developing human mononuclear phagocytes. *J Biol Chem* 1992;265:9087–92
26. Dignass AU, Podolsky DK. Cytokine modulation of intestinal epithelial cell reconstitution: central role of transforming growth factor-β. *Gastroenterology* 1993;105:1323–32
27. Sahakian V, Anners J, Haskill S, *et al.* Selective localization of interleukin-1 receptor antagonist in eutopic endometrium and endometriotic implants. *Fertil Steril* 1993; 60:276–9
28. Cramer DW, Wilson E, Stillman RJ, *et al.* The relationship of endometriosis to menstrual characteristics, smoking and exercise. *J Am Med Assoc* 1986; 255:1904–8
29. Lessey BA, Metzger DA, Haney AF, *et al.* Immunohistochemical analysis of estrogen and progesterone receptors in endometriosis: comparison with normal endometrium during the menstrual cycle and the effect of medical therapy. *Fertil Steril* 1989; 49:229–35
30. Bergqvist A, Ferno M. Oestrogen and progesterone receptors in endometriotic tissue and endometrium: comparison of different cycle phases and ages. *Hum Rep* 1959;8:2211–17
31. Cunha GR, Bigsby RM, Cooke PS, *et al.* Stromal-epithelial interactions in adult organs. *Cell Differ* 1985;17:137–41
32. Cunha GR, Young P. Role of the stroma in oestrogen induced epithelial proliferation. *Epi Cell Biol* 1992;1:18–31
33. McLachlan JA, Nelson KG, Takahashi T, *et al.* Estrogens and growth factors in the development, growth and function of the female reproductive tract. In Schomberg DW, ed. *Growth Factors in Reproduction.* New York: Springer-Verlag, 1991:197–203

Ovarian steroids and angiogenesis

19

R.N. Taylor, I.P. Ryan, J.F. Tseng, J.L. Shifren, D. Hornung and D.I. Lebovic

INTRODUCTION

Endometriosis is a common gynecologic syndrome associated with infertility, dysmenorrhea and pelvic pain, and characterized by the presence of ectopic endometrial implants. On visualization, these endometriotic lesions are often surrounded by exaggerated vascularity and extrapelvic endometriosis is typically located in well-vascularized tissues[1]. Microscopic studies have confirmed angiogenesis around and within endometriosis implants[2]. Thus, neovascularization of ectopic implants is likely to represent a critical step in the growth and progression of these lesions, and women afflicted with endometriosis may have a greater propensity for peritoneal angiogenesis.

Circulating factors in the peritoneal milieu may be mediators or markers of increased angiogenic activity in women with endometriosis. Oosterlynck *et al.*[3] used chick chorioallantoic membrane assays to demonstrate that 58.3% of pelvic fluid samples from women with endometriosis stimulated positive vascular reactions, whereas only 12.5% of control fluids were positive. Using [^{3}H] thymidine incorporation assays on human endothelial cell cultures *in vitro*[4] we were able to quantify a 1.7-fold increase in peritoneal fluid angiogenic activity in endometriosis cases relative to matched controls ($p < 0.01$, Mann–Whitney test). We observed no relationship between angiogenic activity and severity of endometriosis (Figure 1).

HORMONAL REGULATION OF ENDOMETRIAL VASCULARIZATION

In his classical experiments Markee directly visualized the cyclical changes of primate endometrium transplanted into the eye[5]. Vascularization in this model was observed to occur *pari passu* with tissue growth and differentiation induced by ovarian steroids. Since these hormones are required to

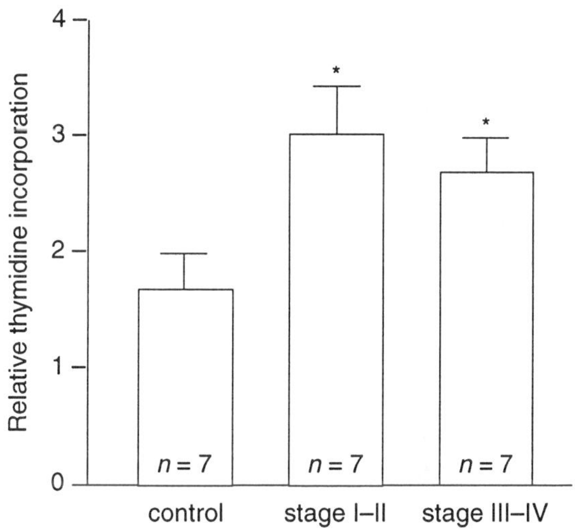

Figure 1 Angiogenic activity in pelvic fluid of endometriosis and control patients. Relative [^{3}H]thymidine incorporation into nascent DNA of quiescent human umbilical vein endothelial (HUVE) cells was used as an indicator of angiogenic activity in peritoneal fluid. Matched endometriosis cases (American Fertility Society classification stages I–II and III–IV) and normal controls were compared. Results were normalized to the amount of thymidine incorporated into HUVE cells exposed to serum-free medium alone and are presented as the mean ± standard error of the mean. The number of specimens analyzed in each group is indicated as '*n*' at the base of each histogram. Asterisks indicate samples that differ significantly from controls by the nonparametric Kruskal–Wallis test and by Mann–Whitney *post hoc* tests with Bonferroni corrections. Data were adapted from Taylor *et al.*[4]

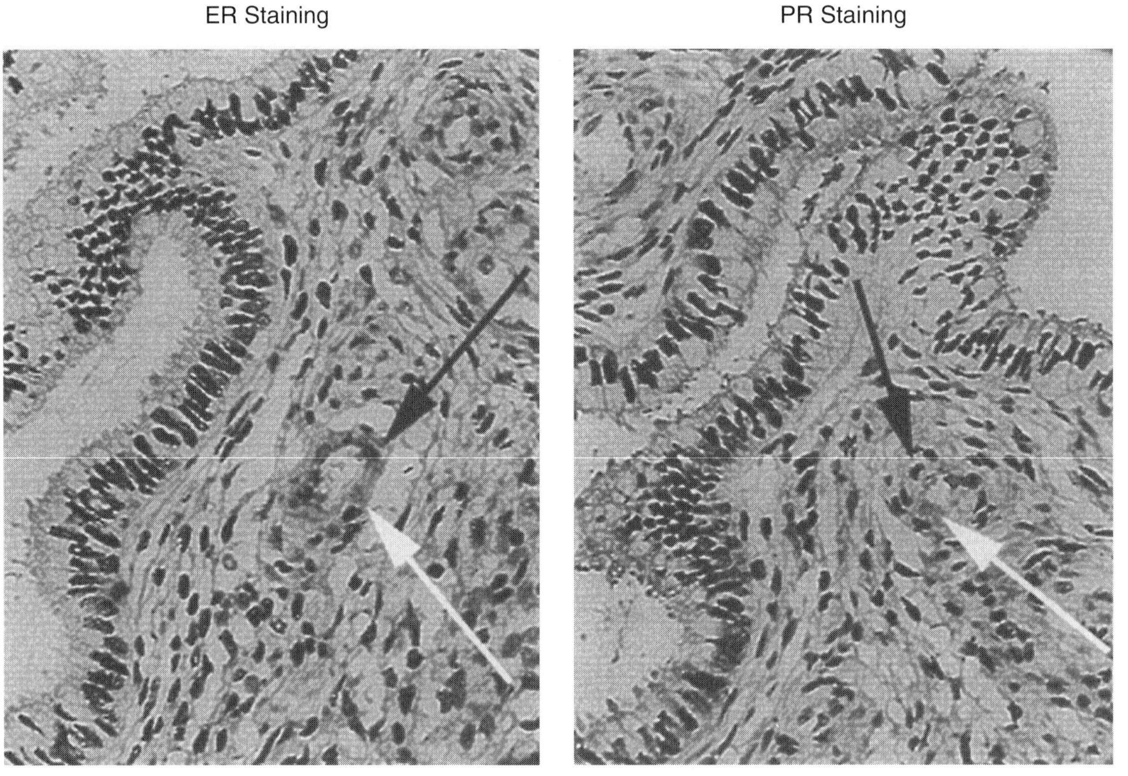

Figure 2 Immunohistochemical localization of estrogen (ER) and progesterone receptors (PR) in secretory phase human endometrium. Note that glandular epithelial and stromal cell nuclei are immunopositive for both receptors. Vascular smooth muscle cells of the spiral arterioles are ER and PR positive (black arrows) but endothelial cells within these vessels are ER and PR negative (white arrows). Original magnification × 400

maintain implants in animal models of endometriosis[6] and the clinical suppression of endogenous ovarian steroid production by GnRH analogs causes lesions to regress[7,8], we postulated that endometriosis implant vascularization also might be hormone dependent.

STEROID HORMONE RECEPTORS IN ENDOMETRIUM AND ENDOMETRIOSIS

Like its normal eutopic counterpart, endometriosis tissue harbors estrogen (ER) and progesterone receptors (PR)[9]. Some authors have suggested that ER and PR concentrations are abnormally regulated in endometriosis implants[10,11], although quantitative studies in isolated endometrial and endometriosis cells indicate that both have similar receptor complements[12].

Morphometric studies of normal human endometrial vascularization indicate that capillary density[13], spiral arteriolar growth and vascular endothelial cell proliferation[14] are most prominent during the secretory phase of the cycle, a time when local estradiol and progesterone concentrations are high. Immunohistochemical evaluation of this tissue reveals expression of estrogen (ER) and progesterone (PR) receptors in the nuclei of glandular epithelial, stromal and vascular smooth muscle cells, but neither receptor was detected in vascular endothelial cells (Figure 2), confirming previous results[15].

PARACRINE EFFECTORS OF ANGIOGENESIS

If endometrial vascular endothelial cell proliferation is not mediated directly by

Table 1 VEGF concentrations in peritoneal fluid from normal controls and women with endometriosis

		Mean (± SD) VEGF concentration (ng/ml)		
Reference	*Normal controls*	*AFS * stage I–II*	*AFS stage III–IV*	*p value*
Shifren *et al.*[20]	0.07 ± 0.02	0.07±0.02	0.11 ± .03	< 0.04**
McLaren *et al.*[23]	13 ± 7	24 ± 15§		< 0.05†

*Laparoscopic staging followed the revised American Fertility Society classification but was applied only to active lesions. **, Data were not normally distributed; nonparametric statistics (Kruskal–Wallis test) were used. §, Endometriosis stage not specified. †, Data were not normally distributed; log transformation and unpaired Student's *t*-test were used.

ovarian steroid receptors, we postulated that ovarian steroids might indirectly stimulate capillary growth via the production of paracrine growth factors. The mitogens responsible for angiogenesis in normal and ectopic endometrium remain incompletely characterized, but in other tissues vascular endothelial growth factor (VEGF), basic fibroblast growth factor (bFGF) and interleukin 8 (IL-8) are known to mediate vascular cell mitogenesis and capillary formation[16]. Our laboratory has investigated several cytokines and growth factors as potential mediators of endometriosis implant neovascularization[4]. This report will focus on the role of VEGF, a 46 kD dimeric glycoprotein that is a specific mitogen for vascular endothelial cells.

Five molecular species of VEGF have been identified to date ($VEGF_{121}$, $VEGF_{145}$, $VEGF_{165}$, $VEGF_{189}$, $VEGF_{206}$) and these are named based on the length of their amino acid sequences. The different proteins are generated by alternate splicing of a single mRNA transcript[17]. VEGF has been found in a variety of normal cells as well as in tumor cells and transformed cell lines, including those of endometrial origin[18]. Using reverse transcription–polymerase chain reaction methods with isoform specific primers, Torry *et al.* determined that the predominant endometrial VEGF isoforms are $VEGF_{121}$ and $VEGF_{165}$[19].

Immunolocalization of VEGF in normal endometrium[19,20] and endometriosis implants[20] revealed two distinct patterns of protein distribution: highly concentrated in secretory granules of glandular epithelial cells and diffusely distributed in the cytoplasm of stromal cells. We postulated that stromal VEGF production, owing to its proximity to the growing endometrial capillary tree, plays a key rolc in endometrial and endometriosis neovascularization. By contrast, epithelial VEGF, which is secreted in an apical, intraluminal direction, may be important in blastocyst apposition and trophoblast proliferation[21]. McLaren and colleagues have shown that peritoneal macrophages can secrete VEGF[22]. Thus, endometriosis implants and peritoneal macrophages both are potential sources of the increased VEGF concentrations detected in peritoneal fluid of patients with endometriosis compared to those without endometriosis[20,23]. It should be emphasized that owing to differences in the VEGF assays the absolute amounts of peritoneal VEGF detected in the two studies differed by ~200-fold (Table 1). In our study we did not detect a correlation between endometriosis stage and peritoneal fluid VEGF concentration[20].

TRANSCRIPTIONAL AND POST-TRANSCRIPTIONAL REGULATION OF VEGF GENE EXPRESSION

The cloned human VEGF gene promoter is 3.4 kb in length and contains a long 5'

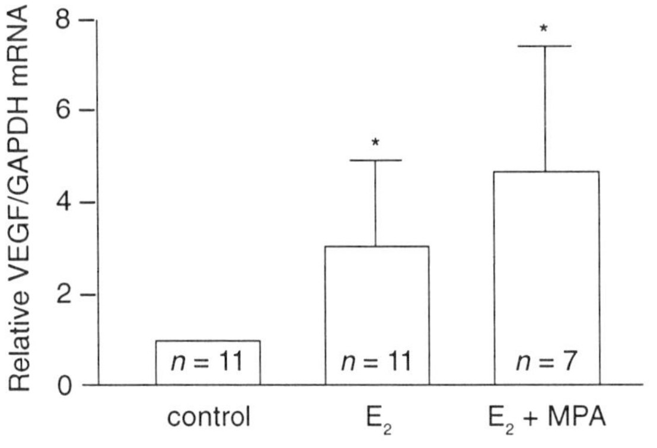

Figure 3 Steady-state VEGF mRNA concentrations in endometrial stromal cell cultures. VEGF mRNA transcripts detected by Northern analyses were quantified by laser densitometry and phosphorimaging and expressed relative to GAPDH mRNA expression in the same blots. The data are presented as the mean ± standard error of the VEGF/GAPDH mRNA densitometry ratios under each of the three hormonal conditions (control, 10 nM estradiol, 10 nM E_2+100 nM MPA). The number of specimens analyzed in each group is indicated as '*n*' at the base of each histogram. Asterisks indicate samples that differ significantly from controls by the nonparametric Kruskal–Wallis test and by Mann–Whitney *post hoc* tests with Bonferroni corrections

untranslated region with a high G + C content upstream from the translation start site[24]. The regulation of VEGF gene expression is modulated by sequence-specific consensus sites that bind various transcription factors as well as by post-transcriptional mechanisms[25]. Analysis of the primary DNA sequence of the VEGF promoter identified several response elements, including AP-1 and AP-2 sites and half-palindromic estrogen and progesterone responsive elements (ERE and PRE, respectively)[24,26].

To test the hypothesis that endometrial VEGF expression is modulated by ovarian steroid hormones, we developed an *in vitro* cell model. Highly purified and well-characterized primary human endometrial stromal cells expressing functional endogenous ER and PR were prepared as described by Ryan *et al.*[12]. Confluent stromal cells grown in 10 cm dishes were incubated in phenol-red free medium containing 2.5% charcoal-stripped fetal calf serum and antibiotics. Cell cultures were treated for 24 h with 0.1% ethanol vehicle (control), 10 nM estradiol or 10 nM estradiol plus 100 nM medroxyprogesterone acetate (E_2+MPA) to mimic proliferative and secretory phase endocrine conditions, respectively. Total RNA was isolated from each culture and subjected to Northern analysis as described[20]. The blots were probed for VEGF mRNA and glyceraldehyde-3-phosphate dehydrogenase (GAPDH) mRNA, a constitutive gene product, to control for sample loading.

VEGF transcripts 4.2–4.4 kb in length were detected in the endometrial stromal cell preparations[20]. Quantification of steady-state VEGF mRNA concentrations, normalized to GAPDH mRNA expression, showed that estradiol and the combination of E_2+MPA resulted in 3.1- and 4.7-fold increases in VEGF gene expression ($p < 0.01$, Kruskal–Wallis test; Figure 3). Despite the absence of a classical palindromic consensus ERE sequence in the 3.4 kb VEGF promoter, estradiol treatment increased the accumulation of VEGF mRNA as rapidly as 1 h following estrogen administration, suggesting a direct effect on VEGF gene transcription[20]. Uterine VEGF gene expression also was shown to be regulated rapidly following *in vivo* administration of estrogen and progesterone to rats[27].

Cell culture supernatants from the human endometrial stromal cells also were analyzed for immunodetectable VEGF protein. An ELISA developed at Genentech, Inc. (South San Francisco, CA), which is linear and sensitive to 30 pg/ml VEGF in conditioned media, was used to quantify VEGF secreted by the stromal cells. The results, reported as pg VEGF secreted/ng cellular DNA, demonstrated that estradiol afforded an 85% and E_2+MPA a 31% increase in VEGF secretion over control cells. Although these effects were small, paired statistical analyses showed them to be significant ($p < 0.04$, Wilcoxon tests with Bonferonni corrections; Figure 4). A discrepancy between VEGF mRNA accumulation and VEGF protein secretion in the E_2+MPA treated samples was observed consistently and

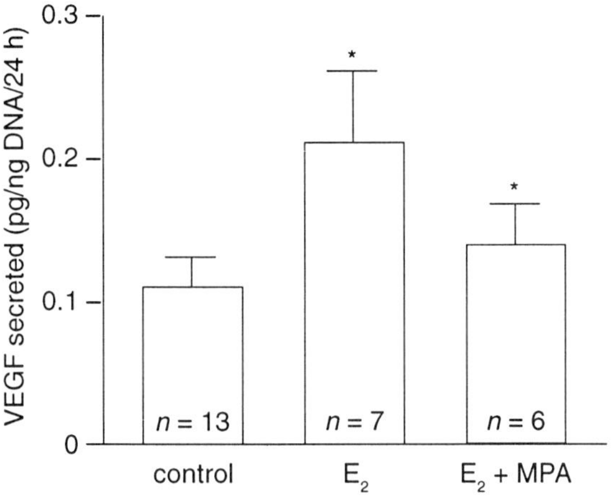

Figure 4 VEGF protein secretion by endometrial stromal cell cultures. Immunodetectable VEGF protein was quantified by ELISA and expressed as pg VEGF secreted/ng cellular DNA/24 h. The data are presented as the mean ± standard error for each of the three hormonal conditions (control, 10 nM estradiol, 10 nM E_2+100 nM MPA). The number of specimens analyzed in each group is indicated as '*n*' at the base of each histogram. Asterisks indicate samples that differ significantly from controls by the nonparametric Wilcoxon paired test with Bonferroni corrections

is not fully understood. We postulate that under the E_2+MPA conditions, translation and/or secretion of VEGF is less efficient than in cells exposed to estradiol alone.

CONCLUSIONS

The recent experiments reviewed above suggest the following model of ovarian steroid hormone action on angiogenesis in human endometrium and endometriosis. Endometrial capillary proliferation is highly correlated with changes in ovarian hormone production, particularly those associated with the luteal phase of the menstrual cycle. The best evidence indicates that endometrial endothelial cells themselves do not express ER or PR, and thus are not direct targets for their cognate hormones. Adjacent endometrial stromal cells, by contrast, express functional ER and PR and synthesize VEGF, a potent paracrine angiogenic protein. Incubation of highly-purified, primary endometrial stromal cell cultures with physiological concentrations of ovarian steroids or their analogs significantly stimulate VEGF mRNA accumulation and protein secretion by these cells. In contrast to what is observed in secretory endometrium *in situ*, acute exposure of endometrial stromal cells by a combination of E_2+MPA does not augment VEGF protein synthesis above that induced by the addition of estradiol alone. Our *in vitro* model may fail to fully simulate secretory phase cellular physiology because endometrial stromal cell decidualization *in vivo* is more complex than acute E_2+MPA treatment. Indeed, a preliminary report from Sharkey *et al.*[28] suggests that long-term decidualization of human endometrial stromal cell cultures results in a dramatic enhancement of VEGF expression, such as that observed *in situ*. Further refinements of the *in vitro* model should improve our understanding of angiogenesis in normal endometrium and endometriosis implants.

ACKNOWLEDGEMENTS

The authors thank Victor Chao, Evelyn Garrett and Drs Eldon Schriock and Carolyn Givens, from the Department of Obstetrics, Gynecology and Reproductive Sciences, UCSF, and Drs Gloria Meng and Napoleone Ferrara from Genentech, Inc., for their generous contributions to the study. This work was supported in part by the following grants and fellowships: NIH grants HD11979, HD33283 (RNT) and HD07263 (DIL), Berlex Scholar Award (IPR), Howard Hughes Medical Student Fellowship (JFT), Deutsche Forschungsgemeinschaft (DH) and American Association of Obstetricians and Gynecologists Fellowship (JLS).

References

1. Ryan IP, Taylor RN. Endometriosis and infertility: new concepts. *Obstet Gynecol Surv* 1997; 52: 365–71
2. Nisolle M, Casanas-Roux F, Anaf V, *et al.* Morphometric study of the stromal vascularization in peritoneal endometriosis. *Fertil Steril* 1993; 59:681–4
3. Oosterlynck DJ, Meuleman C, Sobis H, *et al.* Angiogenic activity of peritoneal fluid from women with endometriosis. *Fertil Steril* 1992; 59:778–82
4. Taylor RN, Ryan IP, Moore ES, *et al.* Angiogenesis and macrophage activation in endometriosis. *Ann NY Acad Sci* 1997; 828:194–207
5. Markee J. Menstruation in intraocular endometrial transplants in the rhesus monkey. *Contr Embryol* 1940;177:219–308
6. DiZerega G, Barber D, Hodgen G. Endometriosis: role of ovarian steroids in initiation, maintenance, and suppression. *Fertil Steril* 1980; 33:649–53
7. Barbieri RL. Hormone treatment of endometriosis: the estrogen threshold hypothesis. *Am J Obstet Gynecol* 1992;166:740–5
8. Henzl MR, Corson SL, Moghissi K, *et al.* Administration of nasal nafarelin as compared with oral danazol for endometriosis. A multicenter double-blind comparative clinical trial. *N Engl J Med* 1988; 318:485–9
9. Jänne O, Kauppila A, Kokko E, *et al.* Estrogen and progestin receptors in endometriosis lesions: comparison with endometrial tissue. *Am J Obstet Gynecol* 1981;141:562–6
10. Lessey BA, Metzger DA, Haney AF, *et al.* Immunohistochemical analysis of estrogen and progesterone receptors in endometriosis: comparison with normal endometrium during the menstrual cycle and the effect of medical therapy. *Fertil Steril* 1989;51:409–15
11. Bergqvist A, Ferno M. Estrogen and progesterone receptors in endometriotic tissue and endometrium: comparison according to localization and recurrence. *Fertil Steril* 1993; 60:63–8
12. Ryan IP, Schriock ED, Taylor RN. Isolation, characterization, and comparison of human endometrial and endometriosis cells *in vitro*. *J Clin Endocrinol Metab* 1994;78:642–9
13. Fanger H, Barker BE. Capillaries and arterioles in normal endometrium. *Obstet Gynecol* 1961; 17:543–50
14. Ferenczy A, Bertrand G, Gelfand MM. Proliferation kinetics of human endometrium during the normal menstrual cycle. *Am J Obstet Gynecol* 1979; 133:859–67
15. Perrot-Applanat M, Groyer-Picard MT, Garcia E, *et al.* Immunocytochemical demonstration of estrogen and progesterone receptors in muscle cells of uterine arteries in rabbits and humans. *Endocrinology* 1988;123:1511–19
16. Folkman J. Angiogenesis in cancer, vascular, rheumatoid and other disease. *Nature Med* 1995; 1:27–31
17. Ferrara N, Houck K, Jakeman L, *et al.* Molecular and biological properties of the vascular endothelial growth factor family of proteins. *Endocrinol Rev* 1992;13:18–32
18. Charnock-Jones DS, Sharkey AM, Rajput-Williams J, *et al.* Identification and localization of alternately spliced mRNAs for vascular endothelial growth factor in human uterus and estrogen regulation in endometrial carcinoma cell lines. *Biol Reprod* 1993;48:1120–8
19. Torry DS, Holt VJ, Keenan JA, *et al.* Vascular endothelial growth factor expression in cycling human endometrium. *Fertil Steril* 1996; 66:72–80
20. Shifren JL, Tseng JF, Zaloudek CJ, *et al.* Ovarian steroid regulation of vascular endothelial growth factor in the human endometrium: implications for angiogenesis during the menstrual cycle and in the pathogenesis of endometriosis. *J Clin Endocrinol Metab* 1996;81:3112–18
21. Hornung D, Lebovic DI, Shifren JL, *et al.* Vectorial secretion of vascular endothelial growth factor by polarized human endometrial epithelial cells. *Fertil Steril* 1998;69:909–15
22. McLaren J, Prentice A, Charnock-Jones DS, *et al.* Vascular endothelial growth factor is produced by peritoneal fluid macrophages in endometriosis and is regulated by ovarian steroids. *J Clin Invest* 1996;98:482–9
23. McLaren J, Prentice A, Charnock-Jones D, *et al.* Vascular endothelial growth factor (VEGF) concentrations are elevated in peritoneal fluid of women with endometriosis. *Hum Reprod* 1996;11:220–3
24. Tischer E, Mitchell R, Harman T, *et al.* The human gene for vascular endothelial growth factor. *J Biol Chem* 1991;266:11947–54
25. Stein I, Itin A, Einat P, *et al.* Translation of vascular endothelial growth factor mRNA by internal ribosome entry: implications for translation under hypoxia. *Mol Cell Biol* 1998; 18:3112–19
26. Garrido C, Saule S, Gospodarowicz D. Transcriptional regulation of vascular endothelial growth factor gene expression in ovarian bovine granulosa cells. *Growth Factors* 1993;8: 109–17
27. Cullinan-Bove K, Koos RD. Vascular endothelial

growth factor/vascular permeability factor expression in the rat uterus: rapid stimulation by estrogen correlates with estrogen-induced increases in uterine capillary permeability and growth. *Endocrinology* 1993; 133:829–37

28. Sharkey AM, Charnock-Jones DS, Day K, *et al.* Regulation of vascular endothelial growth factor expression in human endometrium by steroids and hypoxia: *in vitro* and *in vivo* studies. *J Soc Gynecol Invest* 1998; 5 (Suppl 1):119 (abstract)

Aromatase expression in endometriosis: biology and clinical perspectives

20

S.E. Bulun, K. Zeitoun, K. Takayama, L. Noble, D. Michael, E. Simpson, A. Johns, M. Putman, H. Sasano and B. Carr

INTRODUCTION

Endometriosis is a complex disorder that is characterized by the presence of endometrial tissue in ectopic sites outside the uterus and is linked to pelvic pain and infertility. The prevalence of endometriosis in women of reproductive age is estimated to be as high as 10%[1,2]. Endometriosis is diagnosed in approximately 25% of women who undergo laparoscopy because of pelvic pain and in 20% of infertile women[3–5]. It is a chronic and progressive disease that may give rise to a variety of severe and disabling symptoms including painful menses, painful intercourse, chronic pelvic pain and infertility.

Endometriosis is probably inherited in polygenic manner with an etiology of complex and multifactorial nature[6]. The most widely accepted mechanism for the pelvic disease is implantation of endometrial tissue on the peritoneum through retrograde menstruation, which was first proposed by Sampson[7]. Since retrograde menstruation occurs in at least 90% of all women, the presence of immunological defects in women with endometriosis was hypothesized[6,8–10]. These defects would presumably lead to impaired clearance of the menstrual debris on the peritoneal surfaces. On the other hand, data from other laboratories were suggestive that intrinsic molecular aberrations in the endometrium of women with endometriosis facilitated implantation of the endometrium on the pelvic peritoneum[11]. The proposed intrinsic aberrations that were important in this hypothesis included deficient expression of an integrin[12] and overexpression of complement 3[13] and certain cytokines[14]. Moreover, certain molecules, such as tissue metalloproteinase inhibitor type 1, were shown to be expressed in endometriosis but not in the endometrium[15,16]. We recently demon-strated significant levels of aromatase activity and mRNA in the stromal cell component of endometriosis, whereas aromatase expression was either absent or barely detectable in the eutopic endometrium[17,18]. We would like to clarify the terminology to be used in this manuscript in reference to the tissues and cells that were studied: the terms 'endometriotic tissue' and 'endometriosis' will refer to the pathological ectopic endometrium-like tissues in the pelvic peritoneum or ovaries. Extremely high levels of aromatase expression were found in the stromal cell component of endometriotic tissues. The term 'endometrium' refers to the eutopic or intrauterine endometrial tissue in its normal location. Aromatase expression is absent in the eutopic endometrium of women without endometriosis or any other uterine pathology and is barely detectable (only by RT–PCR) in the eutopic endometrium of women with endometriosis.

Considerable circumstantial and laboratory evidence suggests that endometriosis is an estrogen-dependent disease[19]. For example, the usefulness of gonadatropin releasing hormone (GnRH) agonists to effect suppression of ovarian steroidogenesis and progestins (which act to inhibit estrogen action) in the management of endometriosis is well recognized. Moreover, we recently reported

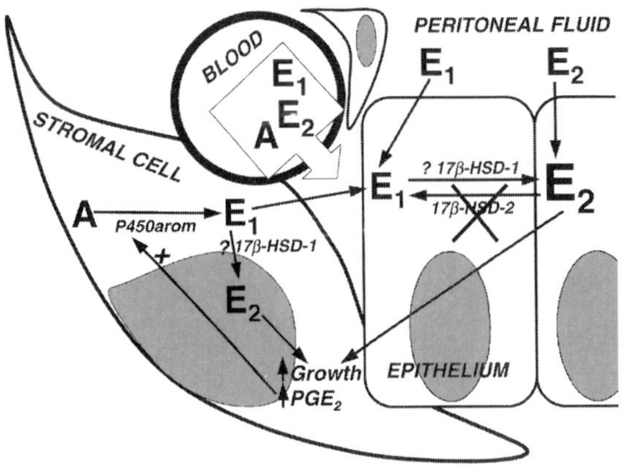

Figure 1 Estrogen biosynthesis and metabolism in endometriotic lesions. Estradiol-17β (E_2) reaches the endometriotic lesion via blood stream (and possibly peritoneal fluid). Aromatase P450 (P450arom) in the stromal cell catalyzes the conversion of androstenedione (A) to estrone (E_1), which is further reduced to E_2 by 17β-HSD type 1 in the endometriotic tissue. (At this time, the cell type that expresses 17β-HSD type 1 in endometriotic lesions is not known). E_2 is normally inactivated by conversion to E_1 by 17β-HSD type 2 in epithelial cells of the eutopic endometrium. In endometriotic tissue, however, E_2 is not metabolized owing to the lack of 17β-HSD type 2 giving rise to increased local concentration of this potent estrogen. Elevated E_2, in turn, will promote the growth of endometriotic tissue and, also, local PGE_2 formation in stromal cells. Since PGE_2 is the most potent known inducer of aromatase in endometriosis, this will complete the positive feedback cycle that favors increased levels of E_2 in endometriosis through enhanced biosynthesis and deficient metabolism

the successful treatment of an unusually aggressive type of recurrent postmenopausal endometriosis using an aromatase inhibitor[20]. The responsiveness of endometriosis to estrogen and progesterone is also evident from hormone-dependent histological changes in this tissue similar to those in eutopic endometrium. Additionally, the expression of estrogen and progesterone receptors has been demonstrated in endometriotic tissue[11,21].

The delivery of estrogen to endometriotic implants has been assumed by many to occur only via the circulating blood in an endocrine fashion. We and others, however, have recently demonstrated markedly high levels of aromatase P450 mRNA and activity in pelvic endometriotic implants[17,22]. Moreover, prostaglandin E_2 (PGE_2), which is produced in very high levels in endometriotic tissues, was found to be the most potent inducer of aromatase activity in endometriosis-derived stromal cells[18,23–25]. The production of PGE_2 in eutopic endometrial stromal cells, in turn, was demonstrated to be greatly stimulated by cytokines and estradiol-17β via enhancement of cyclooxygenase-2 (COX-2) expression[26–28]. Finally, the expression of 17β-hydroxysteroid dehydrogenase (17β-HSD) type 2, the enzyme that is induced by progesterone and inactivates estradiol-17β (by conversion to estrone) in eutopic endometrium, was recently shown to be deficient in endometriotic tissues biopsied during mid-secretory phase of the cycle[29]. Collectively, these data are supportive of the model that alterations in the expression of aromatase, COX-2, and 17β-HSD type 2 in endometriosis may lead to increased local concentrations of estradiol-17β by enhancing its production and diminishing its metabolism (Figure 1). In fact, higher concentrations of estradiol-17β have been detected in the peritoneal fluid of women with endometriosis compared with normal controls[30].

MECHANISMS OF ESTROGEN BIOSYNTHESIS AND METABOLISM IN ENDOMETRIOSIS

Estrogen biosynthesis and metabolism in humans

Aromatase P450 (P450arom) catalyzes the conversion of androstenedione to estrone and testosterone to estradiol-17β in a number of human cells including placental syncytiotrophoblast, ovarian granulosa cells, and adipose and skin fibroblasts[31]. In the human, aromatase expression is regulated by usage of alternative and partially tissue-specific promoters in the placenta (promoter I.1), adipose tissue (promoters I.4, I.3 and II), and ovary (promoter II). Activation of these promoters, and thus aromatase expression, in these tissues is controlled by various hormones. In ovarian granulosa cells FSH stimulates the activation of promoter II via a cAMP-dependent signaling pathway. In adipose fibroblasts, glucocorticoids and members of the IL-6 cytokine family give rise to activation of promoter I.4, whereas treatment with cAMP analogs or PGE_2 switches the promoter use to I.3 and II in these cells. Estrogen biosynthesis in peripheral tissues (adipose tissue, skin, and endometrium) is dependent for substrate on circulating androstenedione, which is produced by the adrenal cortex. Importantly, the product of aromatase activity in these tissues, namely estrone, is of itself only very weakly estrogenic, and must therefore be converted to estradiol-17β in tissue sites of action. Evidence from several laboratories is indicative that 17β-hydroxysteroid dehydrogenase (17β-HSD) type 1, which is present in these peripheral tissues, catalyzes this conversion. We recently demonstrated the expression of 17β-HSD type 1 in endometriotic tissues[29]. Another 17β-HSD isozyme, 17β-HSD type 2, catalyzes the conversions of estradiol-17β to estrone and testosterone to androstenedione in a number of human tissues including the placenta and liver[32]. Additionally, very high levels of 17β-HSD type 2 transcripts have been demonstrated in the glandular epithelial cell fraction of the human endometrium during the secretory phase, suggesting that progesterone stimulates this enzyme[33,34]. In fact, estradiol dehydrogenase activity (oxidation of estradiol-17β to estrone) in endometrial tissues and isolated glandular epithelial component has been shown to be stimulated by progesterone in earlier reports[35–37]. The inactivation of estradiol-17β to estrone by the secretory phase endometrium has been viewed as an important protective mechanism in this estrogen-responsive tissue.

Aromatase expression in Müllerian-derived tissues

Müllerian-derived tissues are targets of estrogen action. Because aromatase is expressed in extraglandular tissues, we have investigated the regulation of expression of this gene in estrogen-dependent neoplasia or disorders that involve Müllerian-derived tissues. Firstly, using a [^{3}H]water assay and quantitative RT–PCR, we were unable to detect aromatase activity or mRNA in disease-free endometrium, myometrium, or endometrial stromal cells in culture (derived from eutopic endometrium of disease-free women)[38]. On the other hand, aromatase expression was demonstrable in the disease states of these tissues. For example, in endometrial cancer, aromatase transcripts are readily demonstrable by RT–PCR, and aromatase expression was found to be regulated by promoter II in this malignant tissue[39]. Next, extremely high levels of aromatase transcripts were found in uterine leiomyoma tissues from 32 of 35 women and in apparently normal myometrial tissues adjacent to leiomyomata (18 of 24 evaluated) but not in normal myometrial tissues from disease-free uteri[40]. In leiomyoma-derived smooth muscle cells maintained in primary culture, treatment with dibutyryl (Bt_2)cAMP acted to increase aromatase activity. Addition of phorbol diacetate potentiated this stimulatory effect of Bt_2cAMP. Again, promoter II was found to be primarily responsible for aromatase expression in leiomyoma tissues and cells. These findings led us to investigate the expression of aromatase in endometriosis, another estrogen-dependent disorder of a Müllerian tissue. In an initial study, we found high levels of P450arom transcripts in all 17 endometriotic tissues from extra-ovarian pelvic sites that were evaluated[17]. The levels of P450arom transcripts (normalized to total RNA) in endometriotic tissues were 3.2 times those in adipose tissue. Eutopic endometrium (obtained by endometrial curettage) from these patients also contained P450arom transcripts, albeit in barely detectable quantities, by RT–PCR[17]. P450arom transcripts could not be detected in the disease-free pelvic peritoneum proximal to endometriotic implants or in the intrauterine endometrial curettings from disease-free

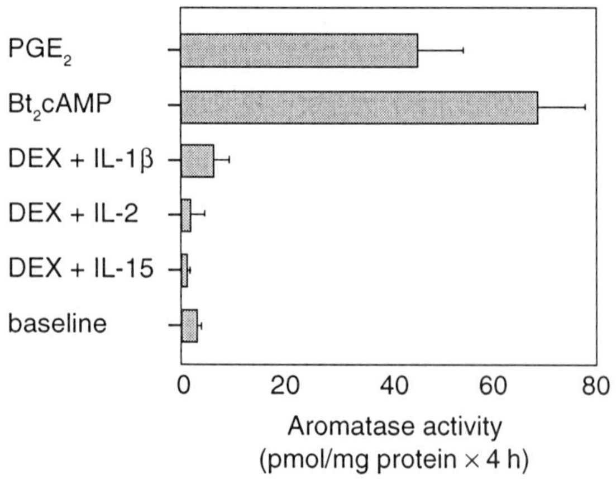

Figure 2 Aromatase activity in endometriosis-derived stromal cells. Confluent stromal cells in primary culture were maintained for 24h in serum-free medium. Treatments consisted of (1) DEX (250 nmol/l) in serum-free medium plus one of the following cytokines: IL-1β (1 ng/ml), IL-1 (2 ng/ml), or IL-15 (2 ng/ml); (2) Bt_2cAMP (0.5 mmol/l) in serum-free medium; and (3) PGE_2 (10^{-8} mol/l). All treatments were continued for 24 h. Please note that Bt_2cAMP or PGE2 treatments gave rise to extremely high activity levels comparable to those in the placental syncytiotrophoblast or ovarian granulosa cells

women. Thus, we hypothesize that estrogen-responsive Müllerian-derived neoplasia and endometriosis are disorders with aberrant aromatase expression that may give rise to an increase in the concentration of bioactive estrogen *in situ*[41] . Moreover, a common cAMP-dependent signaling pathway seems to be responsible for activating P450arom promoter II in these disorders.

Regulation of aromatase expression in endometriotic stromal cells

Upon demonstration of relatively high quantities of P450arom transcripts in endometriosis (much higher than those found in the adipose tissue), we next used endometriotic stromal cells in monolayer culture as a model system to study the regulation of aromatase expression[18]. Glands and stromal cells of ovarian endometriomas and eutopic endometrium were separated by the method of Satyaswaroop *et al.*[35] and the stromal cells were cultured using a previously reported protocol of Ryan *et al.*[42]. These cultured stromal cells were reported to retain estrogen receptors and estrogen responsiveness[42]. The endometriotic stromal cells cultured by this method were also characterized in terms of vimentin and cytokeratin expression[42]. Baseline aromatase activity in endometriotic stromal cells ranged from 0.65 to 6 pmol/mg protein × 4 h. No significant stimulation of aromatase activity was observed by various cytokines (IL-1β, IL-2, IL-6, IL-11, oncostatin M, IL-15, TNFα) or steroids (estradiol-17β, progesterone agonist R5020, dexamethasone). Dibutyryl cAMP induced aromatase activity in these cells by 26- to 60-times the baseline values, whereas the addition of phorbol acetate neither potentiated nor diminished this response. Because of the inflammatory nature of endometriosis, we treated these stromal cells with various prostanoids. Whereas treatments with PGI_2, $PGF_{2\alpha}$ PGJ_2 failed to elicit a response, PGE_2 treatment gave rise to a dose-dependent induction of aromatase activity by up to 19- to 44- fold in endometriosis-derived cells from different patients (Figure 2)[18]. These changes in aromatase activity were accompanied by comparable changes in the levels of P450arom mRNA. A modified rapid amplification of 5'-cDNA ends (5'-RACE)/Southern hybridization of the promoter-specific sequences in P450arom transcripts revealed almost exclusive use of promoter II for aromatase expression in PGE_2- or Bt_2cAMP-treated endometriotic cells.

The summary of our findings thus far is as follows: PGE_2-induction of aromatase activity in endometriotic stromal cells is mediated possibly through increased intracellular levels of cAMP. The basis for markedly high levels of aromatase expression in endometriosis in contrast to absent or barely detectable quantities in the eutopic endometrium may be due to the transformation of endometrial stromal cells after implantation in the pelvic peritoneum and ovary in response to locally produced paracrine factors. The potential aromatization capability of eutopic endometrial cells from women with genetic predisposition to develop endometriosis may facilitate the implantation process and growth in pelvic peritoneum by increasing local estradiol-17β concentrations by the activities of aromatase and 17β-HSD type 1[18,29]. Estradiol-17β, in turn, will induce the activity of COX-2, the rate-limiting enzyme for PGE_2 biosynthesis[27]. The inflammatory process in endometriotic tissues giving rise to increased production of cytokines (e.g., IL-1β, TNFα) by monocytes and macrophages will also promote PGE_2 production in this tissue[43]. Thus a positive feedback cycle is established, whereby local production of estrogen and PGE_2 was enhanced by complex molecular interactions (Figure 3).

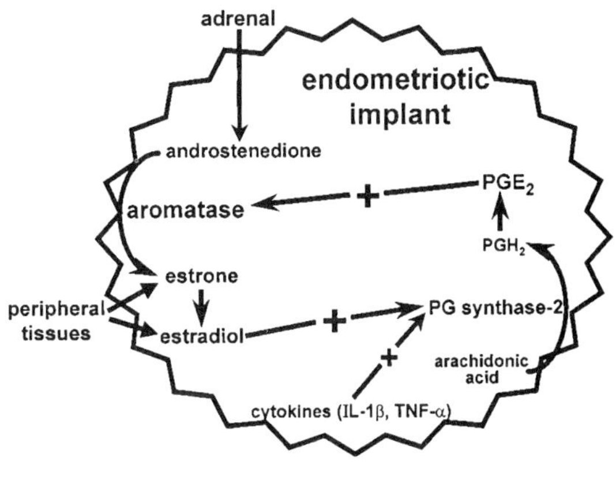

Figure 3 Local estrogen biosynthesis in endometriotic tissue. This model indicates the origin of estradiol-17β in a postmenopausal woman or a woman in her reproductive years who is treated with a GnRH agonist and thus has inactive ovaries. Therefore, the body sites of estrogen biosynthesis are peripheral tissues (adipose and skin) and the endometriotic implant itself. The most important precursor androstenedione of adrenal origin, becomes converted to estrone that is, in turn, reduced to estradiol-17β in the peripheral tissues and endometriotic implants. We demonstrated significant levels of 17β-HSD type 1 expression in endometriosis, which catalyzes the conversion of estrone to estradiol-17β. Estradiol-17β induces prostaglandin synthase-2 (COX-2), which gives rise to elevated concentrations of PGE_2 in endometriotic tissues. PGE_2 in turn, is the most potent known inducer of aromatase in endometriotic stromal cells. Therefore, a positive feedback loop in favor of continuous estrogen formation is established in endometriosis

Stimulation of aromatase P450 promoter (II) activity in endometriosis and its inhibition in endometrium are regulated by competitive binding of SF-1 and COUP-TF to the same kis-acting element[44]

An intriguing observation made during the previous studies was the lack of aromatase expression in eutopic endometrial stromal cells in contrast to significant levels of aromatase mRNA and activity in endometriotic stromal cells, which can be strikingly induced by cAMP analogs. Thus, we sought to determine whether differential binding of transcription factors to the P450arom promoter in response to cAMP is a mechanism involved in this process. First, we demonstrated by 5'-RACE that P450arom expression in pelvic endometriotic lesions is regulated almost exclusively via the alternative promoter II. Then, luciferase reporter plasmids containing deletion mutations of the 5'-flanking region of promoter II were transfected into endometriotic stromal cells. We identified two critical regulatory regions for cAMP induction of promoter II activity: (i) -214/-100 bp proximal region responsible for a 3.7-fold induction, and (ii) -517/-214 distal region responsible for potentiation of cAMP response up to 13-fold. In -214/-100 region, we studied eutopic endometrial and endometriotic nuclear protein binding to a nuclear receptor half-site (NRHS, AGGTCA) and an imperfect cAMP response element (CRE, TGCACGTCA). Using EMSA, CRE-binding activity in nuclear proteins from both endometriotic and eutopic endometrial cells gave rise to formation of identical DNA-protein complexes, which led us to conclude that CRE did not account for differential aromatase expression. The NRHS probe, on the other hand, formed a distinct complex with nuclear proteins from endometriotic cells, which migrated at a much faster rate compared with the complex formed with nuclear proteins from eutopic endometrial cells. Employing recombinant proteins and antibodies against SF-1 and COUP-TF, we demonstrated that COUP-TF but not SF-1 bound to NRHS in eutopic endometrial cells, whereas SF-1 was the primary NRHS-binding protein in endometriotic cells. In fact, COUP-TF transcripts were present in both eutopic endometrial ($n = 12$) and endometriotic tissues ($n = 8$), whereas SF-1 transcripts were detected in all endometriotic tissues ($n = 12$), but in only 3 out of 15 eutopic endometrial tissues. Moreover, we demonstrated a dose-dependent direct competition between SF-1 and COUP-TF for occupancy of the NRHS, to which SF-1 bound with a higher affinity. Finally, overexpression of SF-1 in endometriotic cells strikingly potentiated baseline and cAMP-induced activities of -517 promoter II construct, whereas overexpression of COUP-TF almost completely abolished these activities. In conclusion, COUP-TF is responsible for the inhibition of P450arom expression in eutopic endometrial stromal cells, which lack SF-1 expression in the majority (80%) of the samples; whereas aberrant SF-1 expression in endometriotic stromal cells overrides this inhibition by competing for the same DNA binding site, which is likely to account for high levels of baseline and cAMP-induced aromatase activity (Figure 4).

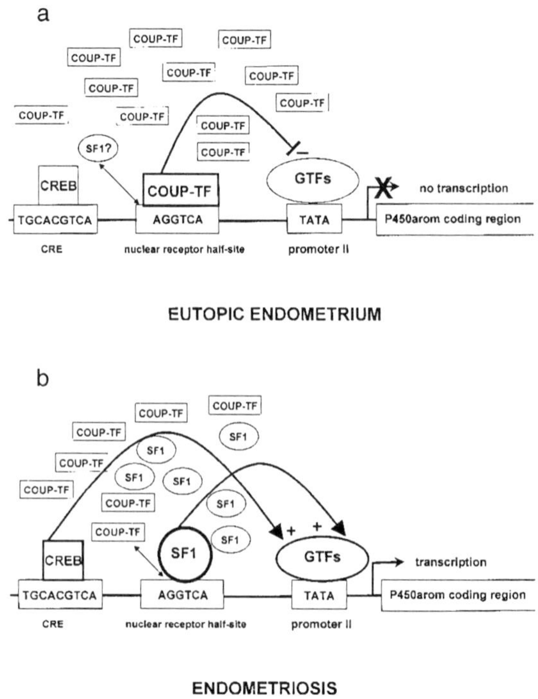

Figure 4 Proposed mechanism for the regulation of aromatase P450 expression by SF-1 and COUP-TF in eutopic endometrium and endometriosis. (a) represents binding of COUP-TF readily to the nuclear receptor half-site in aromatase P450 promoter II in the absence of SF-1 in eutopic endometrial stromal cells. Thus, COUP-TF exerts its inhibitory effect on the complex of general transcription factors (GTFs) that bind to TATA box. (b) In endometriotic stromal cells that contain both SF-1 and COUP-TF, however, SF-1 binds to the nuclear receptor half-site with a higher affinity than that of COUP-TF and synergizes with CREB and other transcription factors to activate the transcription of the *CYP19* (P450arom) gene in response to cAMP

Deficient expression of 17β-HSD type 2 in endometriosis in contrast to eutopic endometrium[29]

Interconversions of estradiol-17β and estrone are catalyzed by two enzymes encoded by two separate genes[45]. 17β-HSD type 1 favors the formation of estradiol-17β, whereas type 2 inactivates estradiol-17β by converting it to estrone. We recently demonstrated by Northern blotting transcripts of 17β-HSD type 1, which catalyzes the conversion of estrone to estradiol-17β, in both eutopic endometrium and endometriosis. Thus, it follows that the product of the aromatase reaction, namely, estrone, that is weakly estrogenic, can be converted to the potent estrogen, estradiol-17β in endometriotic tissues.

It was previously demonstrated that progesterone stimulates the inactivation of estradiol-17β through conversion to estrone in eutopic endometrial epithelial cells. Subsequently, 17β-HSD type 2 was shown to catalyze this reaction, and its transcripts were detected in the epithelial cell component of the eutopic endometrium in secretory phase.

Because estradiol-17β plays a critical role in the development and growth of endometriosis, we studied 17β-HSD type 2 expression in endometriotic tissues and eutopic endometrium. We demonstrated by Northern blotting 17β-HSD type 2 transcripts in all RNA samples of secretory eutopic endometrium ($n = 12$) but not in samples of secretory endometriotic lesions ($n = 10$), including paired samples of secretory eutopic endometrium and endometriosis obtained simultaneously from four patients. These transcripts were not detectable in any paired samples of proliferative eutopic endometrium or endometriosis ($n = 4$), as expected. Next, we confirmed these findings by demonstration of immunoreactive 17β-HSD type 2 in epithelial cells of secretory eutopic endometrium in 11 out of 13 samples employing a monoclonal antibody against 17β-HSD type 2, whereas 17β-HSD type 2 was absent in paired secretory endometriotic tissues ($n = 4$). Proliferative eutopic endometrial ($n = 8$) and endometriotic ($n = 4$) tissues were both negative for immunoreactive 17β-HSD type 2 except for barely detectable levels in one eutopic endometrial sample. Finally, we sought to determine whether deficient 17β-HSD type 2 expression in endometriotic tissues is due to impaired progesterone action in endometriosis. We determined by immunohistochemistry the expression of progesterone and estrogen receptors in these paired samples of secretory ($n = 4$) and proliferative ($n = 4$) eutopic endometrium and endometriosis, and no differences could be demonstrated. In conclusion, inactivation of estradiol-17β is impaired in endometriotic tissues due to deficient expression of 17β-HSD type 2, which is normally expressed in eutopic endometrium in response to progesterone (Figure 1). The lack of 17β-HSD type 2 expression in endometriosis is not due to alterations in the levels of immunoreactive progesterone or estrogen receptors in this tissue and may be related to an inhibitory aberration in the signaling pathway that regulates 17β-HSD type 2 expression.

The first reported use of an aromatase inhibitor to treat endometriosis[20]

Aromatase inhibitors have been widely used to treat breast cancer[46]. We recently evaluated a 57-year-old woman, who presented with recurrent severe endometriosis after hysterectomy and bilateral salpingo-oophorectomy. Two additional laparotomies were performed owing to severe pelvic pain and bilateral ureteral obstruction giving rise to left renal atrophy and right hydronephrosis. Recently, recurrent pelvic endometriosis, evident by a 30-mm vaginal lesion visible on speculum examination, did not respond to an oral megestrol acetate treatment of 4 months. We administered anastrozole (an aromatase inhibitor), orally, 1 mg/day and elemental calcium, 1.5 g/day for 9 months. Alendronate (a non-estrogenic inhibitor of bone resorption), 10 mg/day was added to this regimen. The vaginal lesion was biopsied before and 6 months after the onset of treatment. The circulating levels of estradiol-17β were reduced to approximately 50% of the baseline value after treatment with anastrozole. Pain rapidly decreased and completely disappeared after the second month of treatment. The 30 × 30 × 20 mm bright red polypoid vaginal lesion was reduced to a 3 mm gray tissue by the end of 9 months of treatment. Markedly high pretreatment levels of aromatase P450 mRNA in the endometriotic tissue became undetectable in a rebiopsy specimen after 6 months of treatment. Bone density of lumbar spine decreased by 6.2% after 9 months of treatment. No other side-effects were noted. This was the first description of the use of an aromatase inhibitor in the treatment of endometriosis. The short-term results were extraordinarily successful in elimination of pain and near-complete eradication of implants associated with severe endometriosis not responsive to other therapy. The occurrence of significant bone loss despite the addition of alendronate to the treatment regimen in this particular case should be studied further in large clinical trials. Besides the expected inhibition of aromatase enzyme

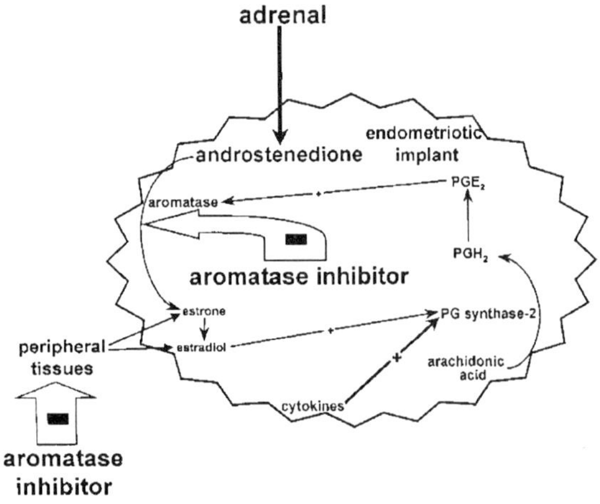

Figure 5 The molecular basis for treatment of endometriosis using an aromatase inhibitor. After administration of a nonsteroidal competitive aromatase inhibitor such as anastrozole, aromatase activity is significantly reduced in the peripheral tissues and in endometriotic implants giving rise to markedly diminished estradiol-17β availability to endometriosis from both sources. Moreover, the positive feedback loop involving PGE_2 stimulation of local aromatase expression is also interrupted. The end result is significantly lower concentrations of estradiol-17β in endometriotic tissues.

activity by anastrozole, the disappearance of aromatase P450 mRNA expression in the lesion may be explicable by denial of estrogen that is known to stimulate local biosynthesis of PGE_2, which in turn, stimulates aromatase ex-pression (Figure 5). We suggest that the recently developed potent aromatase inhibitors are candidate drugs in the treatment of endometriosis that is resistant to standard regimens.

CONCLUSIONS

The development and growth of endometriosis is estrogen-dependent. Several molecular aberrations were found to be present in endometriotic tissues (in contrast to the eutopic endometrium), which favor increased local levels of estradiol-17β. In fact, we uncovered a positive feedback mechanism that is responsible for continuous formation of estradiol-17β and PGE_2 through up-regulation of aromatase and COX-2 in endometriotic stromal cells. Levels of estradiol-17β in endometriotic tissue are further increased by impaired inactivation of this steroid because of deficient 17β-HSD type 2 expression in endometriotic epithelial cells. Aberrant regulation of steroidogenic enzymes in endometriotic tissues giving rise to elevated estradiol-17β levels is possibly one of many metabolic abnormalities that promote the development and growth of this tissue. These studies have already led us to successfully use an aromatase inhibitor to treat endometriosis. We believe that determination of such molecular aberrations in endometriosis will give rise to identification of other molecular targets for potential treatments.

ACKNOWLEDGEMENTS

The authors thank Rosemary Bell for expert editorial assistance. This work was supported in part by an American Association of Obstetricians and Gynecologists Foundation Postdoctoral Fellowship Award to K. Zeitoun.

References

1. Aral SO, Cates W, Jr. The increasing concern with infertility: why now? *J Am Med Assoc* 1983; 250:2327–31
2. Wheeler JM. Epidemiology of endometriosis-associated infertility. *J Reprod Med* 1989; 34: 41–6
3. Hasson HM. Incidence of endometriosis in diagnostic laparoscopy. *J Reprod Med* 1976; 16:135–8
4. Goldstein DP, deCholnoky C, Emans SJ, Leventhal JM. Laparoscopy in the diagnosis and management of pelvic pain in adolescents. *J Reprod Med* 1980;24:251–6
5. Eskenazi B, Warner ML. Epidemiology of

endometriosis. *Obstet Gynecol Clin North Am* 1997; 24:235–58
6. Olive DL, Schwartz LB. Endometriosis. *N Engl J Med* 1993;328:1759–69
7. Sampson JA. Peritoneal endometriosis due to the menstrual dissemination of endometrial tissue into the peritoneal cavity. *Am J Obstet Gynecol* 1927; 14:422
8. Syrop CH, Halme J. Peritoneal fluid environment and infertility. *Fertil Steril* 1987;48:1–9
9. Hill J, Anderson D. Lymphocyte activity in the presence of peritoneal fluid from fertile women and infertile women with and without endometriosis. *Am J Obstet Gynecol* 1989;161: 861–4
10. Hill JA. Immunology and endometriosis. *Fertil Steril* 1992;58:262–4
11. Lessey BA, Metzger DA, Haney AF, McCarty KS, Jr. Immunohistochemical analysis of estrogen and progesterone receptors in endometriosis: comparison with normal endometrium during the menstrual cycle and the effect of medical therapy. *Fertil Steril* 1989;51:409–15
12. Lessey BA, Castelbaum AJ, Sawin SW, *et al.* Aberrant integrin expression in the endometrium of women with endometriosis. *J Clin Endocrinol Metab* 1994;79:643–9
13. Isaacson KB, Galman M, Coutifaris C, Lyttle CR. Endometrial synthesis and secretion of complement component-3 by patients with and without endometriosis. *Fertil Steril* 1990; 53: 836–40
14. Ryan IP, Taylor RN. Endometriosis and infertility: new concepts. *Obstet Gynecol Surv* 1997;52: 365–71
15. Sharpe KL, Zimmer RL, Griffin WT, Penney LL. Polypeptides synthesized and released by human endometriosis differ from those of the uterine endometrium in cell and tissue explant culture. *Fertil Steril* 1993;60:839–51
16. Sharpe-Timms KL, Penney LL, Zimmer RL, Wright JA, Zhang Y, Surewicz K. Partial purification and amino acid sequence analysis of endometriosis protein-II (ENDO-II) reveals homology with tissue inhibitor of metalloproteinase-1 (TIMP-1). *J Clin Endocrinol Metab* 1995;80:3784–7
17. Noble LS, Simpson ER, Johns A, Bulun SE. Aromatase expression in endometriosis. *J Clin Endocrinol Metab* 1996;81:174–9
18. Noble LS, Takayama K, Putman JM, *et al.* Prostaglandin E_2 stimulates aromatase expression in endometriosis-derived stromal cells. *J Clin Endocrinol Metab* 1997;82:600–6
19. Dizerga GS, Barber DL, Hodgen GD. Endometriosis: role of ovarian steroids in initiation, maintenance and suppression. *Fertil Steril* 1980;33:649–53
20. Takayama K, Zeitoun K, Gunby RT, Sasano H, Carr BR, Bulun SE. Treatment of severe postmenopausal endometriosis with an aromatase inhibitor. *Fertil Steril* 1998;69:709–13
21. Lessey BA, Killam AP, Metzger DA, Haney AF, Greene GL, McCarty KS, Jr. Immunohistochemical analysis of human uterine estrogen and progesterone receptors throughout the menstrual cycle. *J Clin Endocrinol Metab* 1988; 67:334–40
22. Kitawaki J, Noguchi T, Amatsu T, *et al.* Expression of aromatase cytochrome P450 protein and messenger ribonucleic acid in human endometriotic and adenomyotic tissues but not in normal endometrium. *Biol Reprod* 1997; 57:514–19
23. Karck U, Reister F, Schafer W, Zahradnik H, Breckwoldt M. PGE_2 and $PGF_{2\alpha}$ release by human peritoneal macrophages in endometriosis. *Prostaglandins* 1996;51:49–60
24. Badawy S, Cuenca V, Marshall L, Munchback R, Rinas A, Coble D. Cellular components in peritoneal fluid in infertile patients with and without endometriosis. *Fertil Steril* 1984; 42: 704–8
25. De Leon FD, Vijayakumar R, Rao CV, Yussman M. Prostaglandin $F_2\alpha$ and E_2 release by peritoneum with and without endometriosis. *Int J Fertil* 1988;33:48–51
26. Ishihara O, Matsuoka K, Kinoshita K, Sullivan M, Elder M. Interleukin-1β-stimulated PGE_2 production from early first trimester human decidual cells is inhibited by dexamethasone and progesterone. *Prostaglandins* 1995;49:15–26
27. Huang JC, Dawood MY, Wu KK. Regulation of cyclooxygenase-2 gene in cultured endo-metrial stromal cells by sex steroids. *Am Soc Reprod Med* 1996;5
28. Kennard E, Zimmerman P, Friedman C, Kniss D. Interleukin-1β induces cyclooxygenase-2 in cultured human decidual cells. *Am J Reprod Immunol* 1995;34:65–71
29. Zeitoun K, Takayama K, Sasano H, *et al.* Deficient 17β-hydroxysteroid dehydrogenase type 2 expression in endometriosis: failure to metabolize estradiol-17β. *J Clin Endocrinol Metab* 1998;83:4474–80
30. DeLeon FD, Vijayakumar R, Brown M, Rao CV, Yussman MA, Schultz G. Peritoneal fluid volume, estrogen, progesterone, prostaglandin, epidermal growth factor concentrations in patients with and without endometriosis. *Obstet Gynecol* 1986;68:189–94
31. Simpson ER, Mahendroo MS, Means GD, *et al.* Aromatase cytochrome P450, the enzyme responsible for estrogen biosynthesis. *Endocr Rev* 1994;15:342–55
32. Andersson S, Moghrabi N. Physiology and molecular genetics of 17β-hydroxysteroid dehydrogenases. *Steroids* 1997;62:143–7

33. Casey ML, MacDonald PC, Andersson S. 17β-Hydroxysteroid dehydrogenase type 2: chromosomal assignment and progestin regulation of gene expression in human endometrium. *J Clin Invest* 1994;94:2135–41
34. Mustonen MVJ, Isomaa VV, Vaskivuo T, *et al.* Human 17β-hydroxysteroid dehydrogenase type 2 messenger ribonucleic acid expression and localization in term placenta and in endometrium during the menstrual cycle. *J Clin Endocrinol Metab* 1998;83:1319–24
35. Satyaswaroop PG, Bressler RS, de la Pena MM, Gurpide E. Isolation and culture of human endometrial glands. *J Clin Endocrinol Metab* 1979; 48:639–41
36. Tseng L, Gurpide E. Estradiol and 20α-dihydroprogesterone dehydrogenase activities in human endometrium during the menstrual cycle. *Endocrinology* 1974;94:419–23
37. Tseng L, Gurpide E. Induction of human endometrial estradiol dehydrogenase by progestins. *Endocrinology* 1975; 97:825–33
38. Bulun SE, Mahendroo MS, Simpson ER. Polymerase chain reaction amplification fails to detect aromatase cytochrome P450 transcripts in normal human endometrium or decidua. *J Clin Endocrinol Metab* 1993;76:1458–63
39. Bulun SE, Economos K, Miller D, Simpson ER. CYP19 (aromatase cytochrome P450) gene expression in human malignant endometrial tumors. *J Clin Endocrinol Metab* 1994; 79:1831–4
40. Bulun SE, Simpson ER, Word RA. Expression of the CYP19 gene and its product aromatase cytochrome P450 in human leiomyoma tissues and cells in culture. *J Clin Endocrinol Metab* 1994; 78:736–43
41. Bulun SE, Noble LS, Takayama K, *et al.* Endocrine disorders associated with inappropriately high aromatase expression. *J Steroid Biochem Mol Biol* 1997;61:133–9
42. Ryan I, Schriock ED, Taylor R. Isolation, characterization, and comparison of human endometrial and endometriosis cells *in vitro*. *J Clin Endocrinol Metab* 1994;78:642–9
43. Guan Z, Baier LD, Morrison AR. p38 Mitogen-activated protein kinase down-regulates nitric oxide and up-regulates prostaglandin E_2 biosynthesis stimulated by interleukin-1β. *J Biol Chem* 1997;272:8083–9
44. Zeitoun K, Takayama K, Michael MD, Bulun SE. Stimulation of aromatase P450 promoter (II) activity in endometriosis and its inhibition in endometrium are regulated by competitive binding of SF-1 and COUP-TF to the same *cis*-acting element. *Mol Endocrinol* 1999;13:239–53
45. Penning TM. Molecular endocrinology of hydroxysteroid dehydrogenases. *Endocr Rev* 1997; 18:281–305
46. Brodie A. Aromatase and its inhibitors – an overview. *J Steroid Biochem Mol Biol* 1991;40:255–61

Excessive angiogenesis: a new theory for endometriosis

21

C. Gargett, J. Tsaltas, P.A.W. Rogers, N. Taylor, M. Lawrence and D.L. Healy

Deposits of endometriosis cannot survive without a blood supply. The establishment of a blood supply and the development of blood vessels between plaques of endometriosis and the underlying tissues involve the process of angiogenesis or new blood vessel formation. This theory is developed in this paper to support a hypothesis that excessive angiogenesis may help explain the development of endometriosis.

ANGIOGENESIS

Angiogenesis is a process by which new capillaries develop from pre-existing vessels. It involves the proliferation of endothelial cells and their migration and formation into rudimentary vascular structures, accompanied by the remodeling of the extracellular matrix[1,2]. There is a complex interplay of basement membrane degradation, extracellular matrix proteolysis and endothelial cell mitosis and migration. Although the precise regulation of these events remains unclear, a number of angiogenic factors and inhibitors have been identified.

Central to the complex changes which occur in the endometrium throughout the menstrual cycle is angiogenesis or new blood vessel growth. Three separate episodes of angiogenesis have been described in the primate endometrium[3]. The rapid cyclical growth of the endometrium necessitates the dynamic remodeling of its vascular supply. A complex process of vascular and glandular proliferation, differentiation, sloughing and regeneration occurs each month. These cyclic changes are controlled primarily by ovarian steroids, with growth factors probably serving as local mediators of endocrine effects. During the proliferative phase, under the influence of estrogen, there is an increase in glandular cells, stromal fibroblasts, and vascular endothelial cells. Straight glands in the endometrium enlarge. With ovulation there is an increase in circulating progesterone, which stimulates the cells of the functional layer of the endometrium to undergo secretory differentiation. As part of this process intracellular glycoproteins accumulate, epithelial cells synthesize secretory proteins, the ratio of glands to the stroma increases and there is also stromal edema and decidualization.

The growth cycle of the endometrium is accompanied by extensive vascular remodeling. The endometrium is supplied by uterine arteries that give rise to arcuate arteries in the myometrium. Radial arteries penetrate the endometrium where basal arteries divide into horizontal branches supplying the basal layer and vertical branches supplying the functional layer[4]. These vessels give rise to spiral arterioles which play a critical role in the regulation of uterine bleeding observed during the menstrual cycle. These vessels, unlike the radial and basal arteries that feed them, are highly sensitive to ovarian steroids. The endometrial vascular architecture changes throughout the menstrual cycle, in parallel with the changes in the intrauterine epithelium and stroma. There is a gradual increase in branching and coiling of spiral arterioles, corresponding to an increase in the length and coiling of endometrial glands. During the late proliferative phase and throughout the luteal phase a complex subepithelial capillary plexus develops[5,6]. At the end of the cycle, particularly from day 25 to 28, there is perivascular and stromal decidualization. In response to progesterone withdrawal vasoconstriction of the distal segments of the spiral arterioles occur and on cycle days 1–4 there is diffuse necrosis, inflammation and vascular thrombosis which occurs with menstruation.

Angiogenesis is a complex process which involves local degradation of the basement membrane of native blood vessels followed by migration and proliferation of endothelial cells to form a new vessel[1,2]. A number of angiogenic factors have been identified in the endometrium. Ovarian steroid hormones regulate a number of changes in the human endometrium during the menstrual cycle but the end response appears to occur through polypeptide growth factors. One of the chief angiogenic factors is probably vascular endothelial growth factor which has been demonstrated both in mouse and human endometrium[7]. It appears that vascular endothelial growth factor plays an important role in the regulation of endometrial angiogenesis throughout the human reproductive cycle.

EXCESSIVE ANGIOGENESIS: A NEW THEORY OF ENDOMETRIOSIS

Surprisingly little attention has been focused on the possible role of the intrauterine endometrium in the pathogenesis of endometriosis. It may actually be that women develop endometriosis because of an abnormality inherent in their eutopic or intrauterine endometrium. The endometrium is unique among adult tissues because it undergoes intense proliferation, secretion, regression and regeneration during each menstrual cycle. It is perfectly plausible to believe that subtle alterations in this complex series of events could lead to proliferation of the endometrial tissue in an environment where it does not normally exist. Our research shows that the endometrium of women with endometriosis has an increased capacity to proliferate and therefore implant and grow in the peritoneal cavity[8].

Our theory is that endometrial angiogenesis is likely to be involved in the pathogenesis of endometriosis. Endometriosis is the engraftment and growth of endometrial implants which require a new vascular supply for the lesion to develop. Endometriotic implants appear to be surrounded by increased vascularity at laparoscopy. It appears also that the peritoneal fluid which is obtained from women with endometriosis has increased angiogenic activity[9]. Other evidence to support an increase in angiogenesis of the endometriotic implant in the development of endometriosis is provided by histological studies in animal experiments which show that endometriotic deposits derived their blood supply from surrounding micro vasculature, that larger deposits grow in areas with a rich blood supply and that the more vascular endometriotic deposits are more active[10].

Two studies at Monash[8,11] have shown that endothelial cell proliferation was significantly greater in the endometrium of patients with endometriosis as opposed to controls (Figures 1 and 2). These studies were undertaken on patients who had proven endometriosis. In particular, in the second study the diagnosis of endometriosis was based on histological as well as visual evidence because all lesions were excised. The endometrium of the patients with endometriosis was compared with the endometrium of women who had a normal pelvis found at the time of tubal ligation. During these studies it was demonstrated that there was an increased number of proliferating endometrial and endothelial cells as well as epithelial and stromal cells in the endometrium of women with endometriosis. This strongly suggests that the endometrium may have an enhanced ability to implant and survive in ectopic locations.

FUTURE DIRECTIONS

Advances in angiogenesis research have important implications for the study of endometriosis. Strategies to develop inhibi-

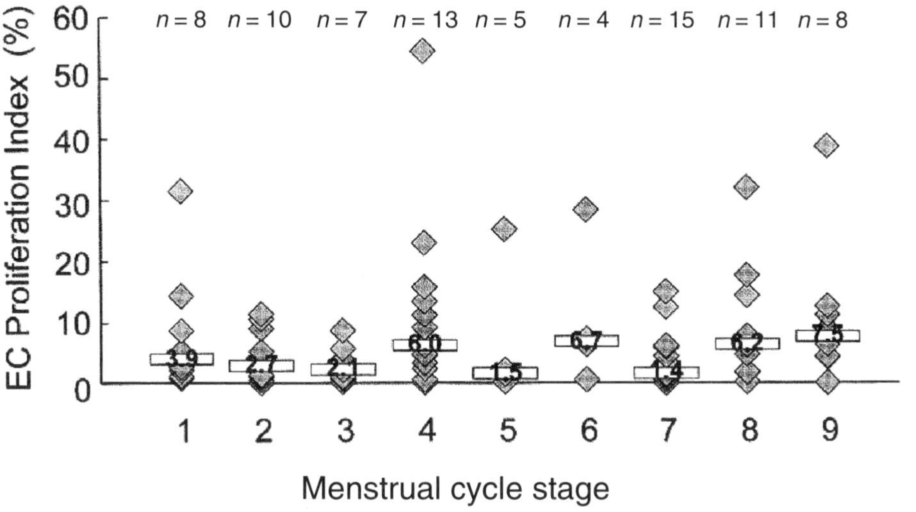

Figure 1 Endothelial cell (EC) proliferation index in nine menstrual cycle stages in normal women without uterine pathology or endometriosis. The numbers and bars represent median values

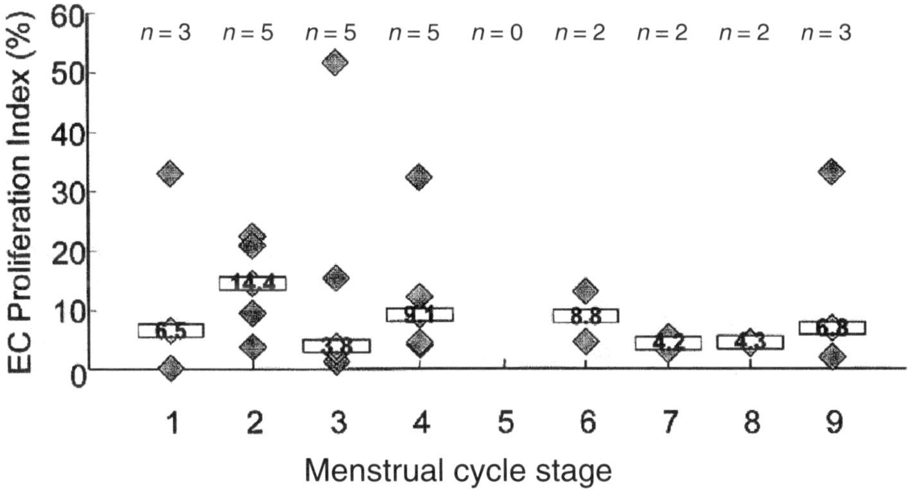

Figure 2 Endothelial cell (EC) proliferation index in nine menstrual cycle stages in endometriosis patients

tors of angiogenesis could be applied to pelvic endometriosis. Local applications of angiogenesis inhibitors, such as via laparoscopy, to deposits of endometriosis may provide an innovative approach to treatment of this disease.

References

1. Risau, W. Mechanisms of angiogenesis. *Nature* 1997;386:671–4
2. Klagsbrun M, D'Amore P. Regulators of angiogenesis. *Ann Rev Physiol* 1991;53:217–39
3. Findlay J K. Angiogenesis in reproductive tissues. *J Endocrinol* 1986;111:357–66
4. Rogers P A W. The endometrial vascular bed. In Cameron I T, Fraser I S, Smith S K, eds. *Clinical Disorders of the Endometrium and Menstrual Cycle.* New York: Oxford University Press, 1998:31–45
5. Kurman R J. Blaustein's pathology of the female genital tract, third ed. New York: Springer, Verlag, 1987
6. Noyes R, Hertig A, Rock J. Dating the endometrial biopsy. *Fertil Steril* 1950;1:3–25
7. Charnock-Jones D, Sharkey A, Rajput-Williams J, *et al.* Identification and localisation of alternatively spliced mRNA's for vascular endothelial growth factor in human uterus and oestrogen regulation in endometrial carcinoma cell lines. *Biol Reprod* 1993;48:1120–8
8. Wingfield M, Macpherson A, Healy DL, Rogers PAW. Cell proliferation is increased in the endometrium of women with endometriosis. *Fertil Steril* 1995;64:340–6
9. Oosterlynck D J, Meuleman C, Sobis H, Vandeputte M, Koninckx P R. Angiogenic activity of peritoneal fluid from women with endometriosis. *Fertil Steril* 1993;59:778–82
10. Vernon M W, Wilson E A. Studies on the surgical induction of endometriosis in the rat. *Fertil Steril* 1985;44:684–94
11. Rogers PAW, Lederman F, Taylor N. Endometrial microvascular growth in normal and dysfunctional states. *Hum Reprod* 1999; in press

Endometriosis management: past, present and future

22

J. Collins

INTRODUCTION

The word endometriosis entered medical terminology over 70 years ago, although the pathological appearance spawned several theories even before Sampson published his convincing observations on retrograde menstruation in the 1920s[1]. Even today endometriosis continues to intrigue theorists and frustrate therapists. Etiological studies have provided insight into potential mechanisms, but the true cause of endometriosis remains unknown. Numerous developments in treatment have helped thousands of women, but we still lack a specific treatment to relieve the pain or infertility associated with endometriosis. This paper reviews the past medical care research evidence on the treatment of endometriosis-associated infertility; considers the value of the present techniques, as published; and offers some inferences for the future based on present-day biological and behavioral research. Although etiological theories, diagnosis and prognosis are also fascinating aspects of endometriosis, the focus is on management. Publications in the latter half of this century are numerous, however, requiring a further concentration on the treatment of infertility associated with mild and minimal endometriosis. A final qualification is needed for the definitions of past, present and future, all of which must necessarily be flexible, given the dynamic nature of biomedical developments.

THE PAST

The early papers

Abnormal growth of endometrial tissue outside the uterus was first described by Rokitansky in 1860[2]. Adeno-myomata or cystadenomata were the original descriptive terms, and involvement of the Fallopian tube and ovary were first described respectively by Cullen in 1896 and Russell in 1899[3, 4]. In all the years prior to Sampson's first paper in 1921 there were less than 20 reported cases and almost as many theories of origin[5].

Sampson's presentation to the American Gynecological Society in May 1922 included 37 cases treated in Albany during the previous year[1]. Color plates of the pathology and excellent drawings of the surgical anatomy illustrate the case reports. Sampson duly acknowledges the earlier theories before developing his concept that these 'implantation adenomas of endometrial type' arise from retrograde menstruation. The paper is also remarkable for the first description of treatment-independent pregnancy in a woman with endometriosis-associated infertility; the 8 week gestation was not discovered, unfortunately, until the uterus was opened in the pathology department. Sampson used the term 'chocolate' in reference to the contents of a cyst which ruptured, but the term endometriosis was not widely used until 1927[3].

The immediate reaction to Sampson's paper was mixed[6]. J. Whitridge Williams led the discussion at the May meeting, noting that Sampson had (1) identified the origin of ovarian hematomata, (2) demonstrated the mechanism by which adenomyomata of the uterus may develop, and (3) proven that uterine epithelium could be transplanted. Another Baltimorean was less convinced: Curtis F. Burnam said he would have to see

Sampson's specimens himself before he would be '. . . convinced that the blood cyst of the ovary is analogous to or the same condition as the adenomyoma of the uterus'. Other participants, including John G. Clark (Philadelphia), Benjamin P. Watson (Toronto) and William C. Danforth (Evanston) were more sympathetic to Sampson's views.

The era of surgery

Sampson's surgical lessons encouraged others to explore hysterectomy and bilateral salpingo-oophorectomy as a treatment for a broader range of presenting problems that were now recognized as endometriosis[7]. Before long, it was reported that conservative surgery with conservation of ovarian tissue appeared to be equally effective in some cases[5]. In a review and aggregate analysis in 1936, improvement in pain and disappearance of lesions occurred in 86 to 100% of cases with 'radical' surgery and in 68 to 96% of cases with 'conservative' surgery. The authors commented that '. . . removal of all ovarian tissue in young women is a very serious matter and we do not feel that it is warranted in this disease where local excision can be performed'.

Hormonal treatment

The use of stilbestrol in the treatment of endometriosis began in 1948, and was adopted readily as it seemed to promise a greater likelihood of conception[8]. Large doses of estrogen inevitably generated concerns about endometrial hyperplasia, however, a side-effect which Scott and Wharton confirmed in an experimental monkey model. Their model also revealed that estrogen had no permanent therapeutic value[9]. By then Meigs had made the recommendation to avoid endometriosis '. . . through early marriage and frequent childbearing . . .' As an alternative, Kistner reported the use of estrogens and progestins to induce a state of 'pseudopregnancy' for 2 to 7 months in 12 patients[10]. The progestins were Delalutin and Enovid, the latter in a dose of 10 mg daily with increases every two weeks up to a total of 40 mg. Only three of the 12 patients had a microscopic diagnosis, but all had cul-de-sac masses and '. . . all subjects were improved during the period of their pseudopregnancy . . . .' Less complex and lower dosage schemes appeared to be similarly effective[11].

The modern era of hormonal therapy began with the description of danazol by Dmowski *et al.* in 1971[12]. By 1987 the aggregate pregnancy rate was 40% in 16 studies involving 511 patients with mild endometriosis[13]. The results of randomized clinical trials suggested, however, that the results were equally good among placebo-treated patients[14]. A pivotal paper from Quebec City in 1984 introduced the concept of downregulation with gonadotropin releasing hormone agonists[15]. The concept would become a key component of ovulation stimulation regimens for *in vitro* fertilization, but with endometriosis-associated infertility, a meta-analysis of studies involving danazol and other ovulation suppression agents showed that the treatments were not effective[16]. By then other authors had concluded without the benefit of meta-analysis that hormonal treatment of mild endometriosis was a failure[17]. Although hormonal treatment continues to be effective for the management of endometriosis-associated pain, it is no longer regarded as an effective or useful treatment for women with minimal or mild endometriosis and infertility.

THE PRESENT

Early reports

Endoscopic treatment of endometriosis-associated infertility is the standard practice. The early reports were promising because the treatment did not delay conception and added very little additional risk over that of a diagnostic laparoscopy. In 1979 Hasson observed more pain relief and better fertility in 19 patients with electrocoagulation compared with six controls[18]. The next year, Sulewski *et al.* found that 40 of 100 consecutive patients treated at laparoscopy conceived, most within 12 months of the operation[19]. Results of coagulation and vaporization studies were similar, as noted in a summary of publications up to 1987[20].

Cohort studies

Comparative studies, including five cohort studies and one alternate assignment study, revealed an aggregate 2.7-fold higher pregnancy rate (95% CI, 2.1–3.5)[16]. The studies showed numerous methodological weaknesses, however, suggesting that clinical practice should not be altered until the results of randomized trials were available.

Randomized clinical trial

There are few well-designed trials of the effectiveness of surgical procedures, but the ENDOCAN study is a superb model for future designs. The study planners resolved numerous issues of enrolment, efficiency, and follow-up, and their hands-on trial management was a key reason for the success of the multi-center study. The study recruited infertile women contemplating laparoscopy, and if endometriosis was seen, the long-distance telephone random allocation system was activated, so that lesion destruction could be initiated within a minute, or the diagnostic laparoscopy could be completed without treatment of the endometriosis. Follow-up was maintained for 36 weeks, and the primary outcome was on-going pregnancy at 20 weeks, a near perfect surrogate for live birth. Women without endometriosis also were followed and all women were encouraged to avoid co-interventions.

The result was a moderate treatment effect with relative benefit increase 1.7 (95% CI, 1.2–2.6). The cumulative 20-week pregnancy rate at 36 weeks was 31% in laparoscopy surgery patients and 18% in diagnostic laparoscopy patients, an absolute difference of 13%, thus implying one would need to do eight laparoscopy surgeries to achieve one more on-going conception than diagnostic laparoscopy alone. Although lesion destruction improved fertility in women with endometriosis, it failed to restore normal fertility; the authors suggest that this may be owing to the continuing effect of additional unknown defects.

THE FUTURE

Reporting on the past and the present is comparatively uncomplicated, although hindsight can mislead even the most conscientious observer. Of course, it goes without saying that predicting the future is downright precarious. This section, therefore, will avoid the uncertainties of prediction and focus on the troubling questions that remain unresolved as yet. Does mild endometriosis cause infertility? What causes endometriosis? And how best can we help patients to make decisions?

DOES MILD ENDOMETRIOSIS CAUSE INFERTILITY?

There is fair agreement that the lesions of endometriosis are more common in women with infertility, and almost as much agreement that the endometriosis implies a worse prognosis for conception[21]. The key question is whether the visible lesions are themselves the cause of the infertility, or a marker for some hidden defect. Thomas and Cooke reported that conception in treated and untreated women was independent of whether the endometriosis lesions had disappeared at the second laparoscopy[22]. Also, lesion destruction or disappearance did not uniformly improve fertility in the early trials[14]. Furthermore, in the ENDOCAN study the impact of lesion destruction was only modest[23], and the untreated prognosis was not significantly impaired in the women with minimal or mild endometriosis, compared with the follow-up group who had unexplained infertility[24]. The question remains open, however: the 36 week probability of conception lasting at least 20 weeks was 23.7% in 263 women with unexplained infertility, 19.4% in 112 women with minimal endometriosis and 15.3% in 56 women with mild endometriosis. The trend was not significant despite the sample size[24].

Thus the best evidence available indicates that the presence of endometriosis lesions has only a small effect on fecundity, and the destruction of the lesions has only a moderate remedial effect. This implies that the visible lesions are either coincidental findings, or if they truly are involved in the etiologic chain, the lesions are only minor participants in the mechanism of impaired fertility.

WHAT IS THE CAUSE OF ENDOMETRIOSIS?

There are at least two options to consider. Endometriosis lesions may be the by-product of a remote primary defect which also causes infertility. Alternatively, the existence of infertility could be an enabling condition for the development of endometriosis. With respect to the former choice, infertility as a by-product of tubal regurgitation at first glance seems unlikely, given that tubal patency is established in most infertile women with minimal or mild endometriosis. Before dismissing Dr Sampson's concept, however, consider that tubal patency testing is far from a sensitive test of tubal motility, and the possibility exists that a subtle disorder of tubal function might coincidentally interfere with embryo tran-sport and cause endometriosis lesions. Similarly, among the theories listed by Schenken[25] other mechanisms of the histogenesis of endometriosis also may be co-existing or pre-existing causes of infertility.

Evidence for the second option is sparse because there are few longitudinal studies that include repeated assessment for the existence of endometriosis. Nevertheless, the existing studies suggest that infertility or childlessness may be an enabling condition for the development of endometriosis. Mahmood and Templeton, for example, found that the frequency of endometriosis was higher after a long pregnancy-free interval either before or after child-bearing[26].

HOW BEST CAN PATIENTS BE GUIDED IN THEIR DECISIONS?

Infertility clinicians have a special understanding of the clinical burden of endometriosis-associated infertility and the needs of affected patients. Medical recommendations will be more effective and more satisfying when they are based on sound evidence, but decisions about management also depend on the patient's wishes, for several reasons. First, the presence of endometriosis does not explain their infertility in a satisfactory manner. Also, the therapy is empiric, because there is no known mechanism to be addressed by specific therapy. Furthermore, the right choice for a given couple will depend on many factors such as the intensity of their feelings with respect to childlessness, their approach to risk-taking and their finances.

Thus, infertility clinicians should adopt a comprehensive approach which aims to help each couple develop a therapy plan that will take into account the lives they are leading at present and provide them, over the long term, with the feeling that they have explored all options that they would consider to be reasonable. Shared decision-making is a new area of study which may be ideally suited to this approach[27]. Infertility clinicians also can be more effective if they help patients to understand the natural prognosis and long-term outcomes that are most likely in each case. Because there is very little guidance from medical care research on the best way to help couples deal with their prognosis, research is needed to explain the factors that facilitate closure and resolution.

References

1. Sampson JA. The life history of ovarian hematomas (hemorrhagic cysts) of endometrial (Mullerian) type. *Am J Obstet Gynecol* 1922;4:451–512
2. Rokitansky C. Ueber die Adenomyome des Uterus und der Tuba. *Zeitschrifte d k -k Gesellsch* 1860;37:577–8
3. Cullen TS. Adeno-myoma of the round ligament. *Bull Johns Hopkins Hosp* 1896;7:112–14
4. Russell WW. Aberrant portions of the Mullerian duct found in an ovary. *Bull Johns Hopkins Hosp* 1899;10:8–13
5. Cattell RB, Swinton NW. Endometriosis. With particular reference to conservative treatment. *N Engl J Med* 1936;214:341–6
6. Sampson J. Society transactions. *Am J Obstet Gynecol* 1922;4:561–3
7. Graves WP. The treatment of obstructing rectovaginal endometriosis. *Am J Obstet Gynecol* 1927;13:728–31
8. Hurxthal LM, Smith AT. Treatment of endometriosis and other gynecologic conditions with large doses of estrogens. *N Engl J Med* 1952; 247:339–43
9. Scott RB, Wharton LR. The effects of excessive amounts of diethylstilbestrol on experimental endometriosis in monkeys. *Am J Obst Gynec* 1955; 69:573–87
10. Kistner RW. The use of newer progestins in the treatment of endometriosis. *Am J Obstet Gynecol* 1958;75:264–78
11. Chalmers JA. Conservative management of endometriosis. *Proc Roy Soc Med* 1968;61:14–16
12. Dmowski WP, Scholer HFL, Mahesh VB, *et al.* Danazol – a synthetic steroid derivative with interesting physiologic properties. *Fertil Steril* 1971;22:9–18
13. Bayer SR, Seibel MM. Medical treatement: danazol. In Schenken RS, ed. *Endometriosis: Contemporary Concepts in Management.* Philadelphia: J.B. Lippincott Company, 1989:169–88
14. Evers JLH. The pregnancy rate of the no-treatment group in randomized clinical trials of endometriosis therapy. *Fertil Steril* 1989;52: 906–7
15. Lemay A, Maheux R, Faure N,*et al.* Reversible hypogonadism induced by a luteinizing hormone-releasing hormone (LH-RH) agonist (Buserelin) as a new therapeutic approach for endometriosis. *Fertil Steril* 1984;41:863–71
16. Hughes E, Fedorkow DM, Collins JA. A quantitative overview of controlled trials in endometriosis-associated infertility. *Fertil Steril* 1993;59:963–70
17. Candiani GB, Vercellini P, Fedele L, *et al.* Medical treatment of mild endometriosis in infertile women: analysis of a failure. *Hum Reprod* 1990; 5:901–5
18. Hasson HM. Electrocoagulation of pelvic endometriotic lesions with laparoscopic control. *Am J Obstet Gynecol* 1979;135:115–21
19. Sulewski JM, Curcio FD, Bronitsky C, *et al.* The treatment of endometriosis at laparoscopy for infertility. *Am J Obstet Gynecol* 1980;138:128–32
20. VanCaille T, Schenken RS. Endoscopic Surgery. In Schenken RS, ed. *Endometriosis:Contemporary Concepts in Clinical Management.* Philadelphia: J.B. Lippincott Company, 1989:249-66
21. Mahmood TA, Templeton A. The impact of treatment on the natural history of endometriosis. *Hum Reprod* 1990;5:965–70
22. Thomas EJ, Cooke ID. Successful treatment of asymptomatic endometriosis: does it benefit infertile women? *Br Med J* 1987;294:1117–19
23. Marcoux S, Maheux R, Berube S, for the The Canadian Collaborative Group on Endometriosis. Laparoscopic surgery in infertile women with minimal or mild endometriosis. *N Engl J Med* 1997;337:217–22
24. Berube S, Marcoux S, Langevin M, *et al.*, for the The Canadian Collaborative Group on Endometriosis. Fecundity of infertile women with minimal or mild endometriosis and women with unexplained infertility. *Fertil Steril* 1998; 69:1034–41
25. Schenken RS. Pathogenesis. In Schenken RS, ed. *Endometriosis:Contemporary Concepts in Clinical Management.* Philadelphia: J.B. Lippincott Company, 1989:1–49
26. Mahmood TA, Templeton A. Prevalence and genesis of endometriosis. *Hum Reprod* 1991;6: 544–9
27. Charles C, Gafni A, Whelan T. Shared decision-making in the medical encounter: what does it mean? (or it takes at least two to tango). *Soc Sci Med* 1997;44:681–92

Three phase therapy is the best treatment for endometriosis with related infertility

23

K.W. Schweppe

INTRODUCTION

Endometriosis is an enigmatic disease with unknown etiology, poorly understood pathogenesis and conflicting results concerning the efficacy of treatment regimens. Endometriosis is probably not one disease – it is a disease name for different entities ranging from deep infiltrating progressive endometriosis to accidental finding of non proliferating implants in the pelvic cavity, which did not cause pain or infertility and are not a disease at all. These facts are not new. As early as 1899 Russell[1] published his work on endometriosis of the ovaries and nine years later Cullen[2] first described deep infiltrating endometriosis. The famous work of Sampson[3] containing the theory of retrograde menstruation describes diffuse peritoneal endometriosis and Vasquez[4] added in 1984 the microscopical form of implants. To systematize these different appearances of endometriosis Donnez and Nissole[5] divided the disease into three groups: (1) deep infiltrating endometriosis (adenomyosis externa); (2) endometrioma and cysts; and (3) peritoneal, superficial endometriosis. This provides an explanation for the conflicting data of the past concerning the effect of different treatment options for endometriosis.

Besides these different types of endometriosis with relation to their localization and macroscopic growing type there is also a wide spectrum of microscopic and electron microscopic differences[4,6] and a wide spectrum of different biochemical characteristics[7] such as steroid receptors and enzyme activity. Thus, no single treatment can be effective in all types and all variations of the enigmatic disease. We have to introduce individual treatment schedules which take into account the different types and the different activity of endometriosis and to prove these individual strategies in prospective randomized studies.

MATERIAL AND METHODS

In 1992 we started a prospective randomized trial to compare the efficacy of surgical therapy alone with surgical therapy followed by 6 months' medical treatment and repeat laparoscopic surgery in patients with peritoneal endometriosis stage I and II according to the revised ASRM classification[8]. Patients with endometriosis related symptoms and/or infertility were included. Pain score, gynecological examination and laparoscopic findings were used to classify the symptoms and the extent of the disease. The following macroscopical[9] and microscopical criteria[10,11] were used to classify the implants in active and inactive endometriosis. Macroscopically active foci are red implants which grow flame like, vesicular or polypoid with hypervascularization of the surrounding tissue. Inactive foci are black or brownish implants from the nodular type with poor vascularization and scars and fibrosis of the surrounding area. The morphological criteria for active disease include extensive, endometrium-like differentiation, cyclic changes, and mitosis of the epithelial cells with edema, good vascularity and inflammatory cells in the stroma. The biopsy is judged inactive if non-endocrine-modulated atrophic glands with little differentiation and little or no mitosis along

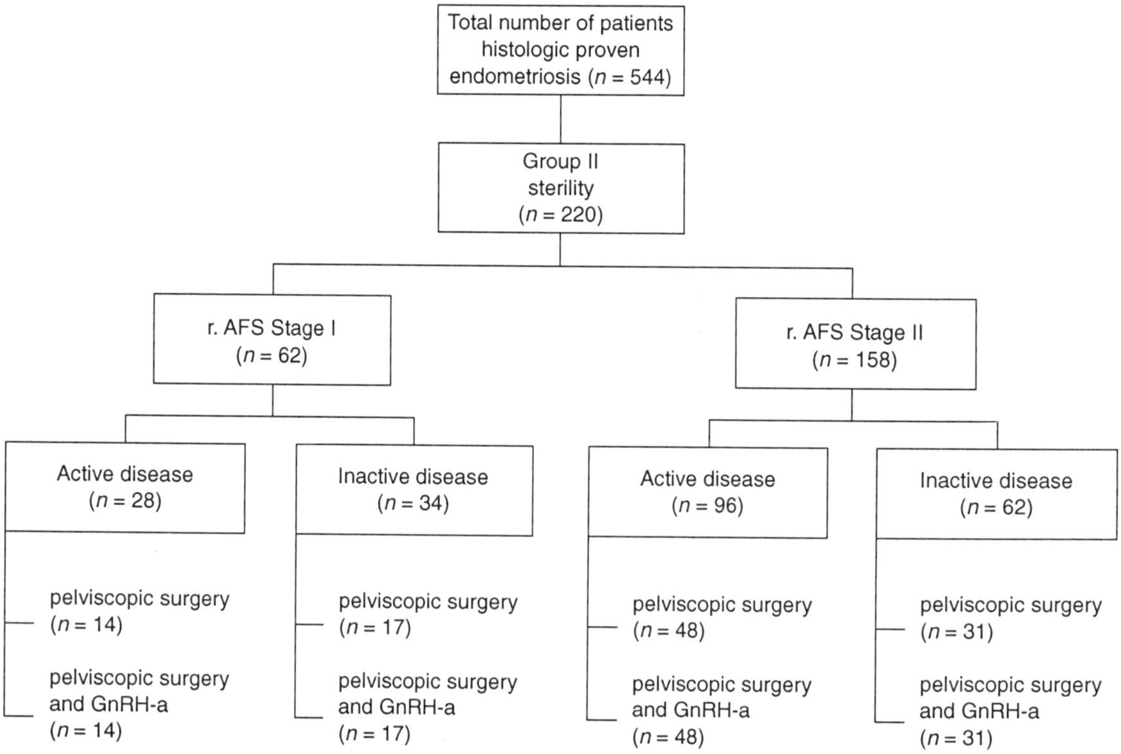

Figure 1 Randomization of patients with infertility with or without pain in relation to the stage and the activity of the disease

with condensed stroma with collagen fibers and siderophages are seen. Cases with mixed appearance of implants are judged active when more than one area of red lesions and microscopically active foci are found.

A total of 544 patients were recruited; 324 treated for pain and 220 treated for endometriosis-associated infertility with or without pain. In infertile patients the pregnancy rate and the time between end of treatment and getting pregnant were the criteria for the effectiveness of treatment. For statistical analysis the SAS-package was used with *t*-test, Wilcoxon Rank test and life table analysis.

The mean age of the study group was 31 years (range 26–40 years) with a mean of 28 years in the pain group and 33 years in the infertile group. The mean duration of infertility was 4.15 years. In the past 72% of the pain patients and 21% of the infertile patients had had treatment for endometriosis before. In the infertile group 268 patients were originally recruited and signed the informed consent for randomization prior to laparoscopy. Only 220 could be enroled with proven endometriosis (82%) because although the other 48 patients had typical or atypical lesions these were not confirmed by morphological examination and thus the patients had to be excluded. During the diagnostic procedure the judgement of active or inactive was made by the above mentioned macroscopic criteria and the microscopic examination of frozen sections. The randomization for the different treatment options is demonstrated in Figure 1. Pelviscopic surgery (PS) was done after representative biopsies and included complete excision, thermocoagulation or vaporization of all visible lesions including fibrosis and sequelae of the disease such as adhesions. Three phase therapy (TPT) as primarily recommended by Riedel and Semm[12] includes biopsies and simple adhesiolysis at the first pelviscopy, followed by 6 months' application of a GnRH-agonist as a depot preparation beginning at the first day of the next menstrual bleeding. Four weeks after the sixth injection the second look pelviscopy was performed with complete surgical removal of residual endometriosis, scars and sequelae. During the follow-up period of two years gynecological examination, pain questionnaire and endocrine parameters were obtained at 3, 6, 9, 12 and 24 months in an endometriosis clinic by one physician only. No other treatment of infertility was allowed (i.e. ovarian stimulation, insemination or other methods of assisted reproduction).

RESULTS

There were no differences in the results and statistics between patients of stage I and stage II endometriosis, therefore the analysis was done in the total study population. This is an indication that the prognostic value of the r-ASRM classification is poor with respect to fecundity. The following data refer to the combined stages.

In the group of sterile patients there were no drop-outs due to side-effects of the medication; three patients did not show up after 12 months and another three decided to try assisted reproduction during the follow-up period. In the pelviscopic surgery alone group we had five losses during the follow-up period and one patient began IVF–ET treatment before the follow-up was completed. In the group of infertile patients with active endometriosis the medical therapy for 6 months using a GnRH agonist followed by laparoscopic eradication of residual endometriosis, fibrosis and adhesions led to a significant higher pregnancy rate and an earlier achievement of pregnancy when compared to laparoscopic surgery alone. Nine months after three phase treatment, 24 out of 62 (38.7%) were pregnant, vs 6 out of 61 (9.8%) in the pelviscopic surgery (PS) only group ($p < 0.001$); 24 months after TPT, 26 of 59 (44.1%) were pregnant, vs 17 of 58 (29.3%) in the PS only group. No significant differences between the treatment schedules were found in patients with inactive endometriosis and infertility. Nine months after TPT, 8 of 48 (16.7%) of the patients were pregnant vs 9 of 47 (19.1%) in the PS only group, and after two years' follow-up the figures were 12 out of 45 (26.7%) in the TPT group vs 14 of 46 (30.4%) ($p > 0.05$) in the PS only group (Figure 2).

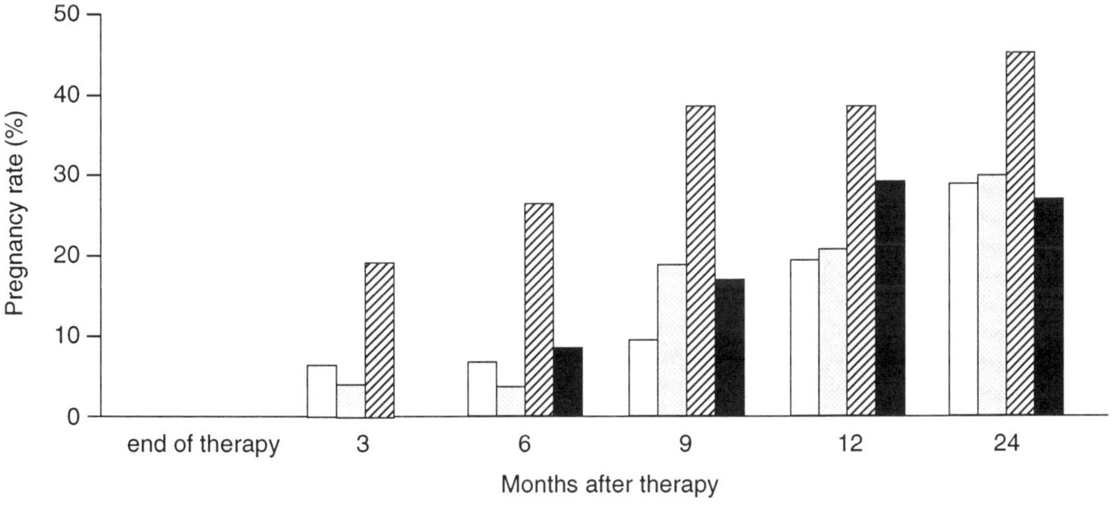

Figure 2 Pregnancy rates (life table analysis) and time taken to become pregnant after treatment in patients with endometriosis-associated infertility. □, active implants treated with pelviscopic surgery alone; □, inactive implants, treated with pelviscopic surgery alone; ▨, active implants treated with three-phase therapy; ■, inactive implants treated with three-phase therapy

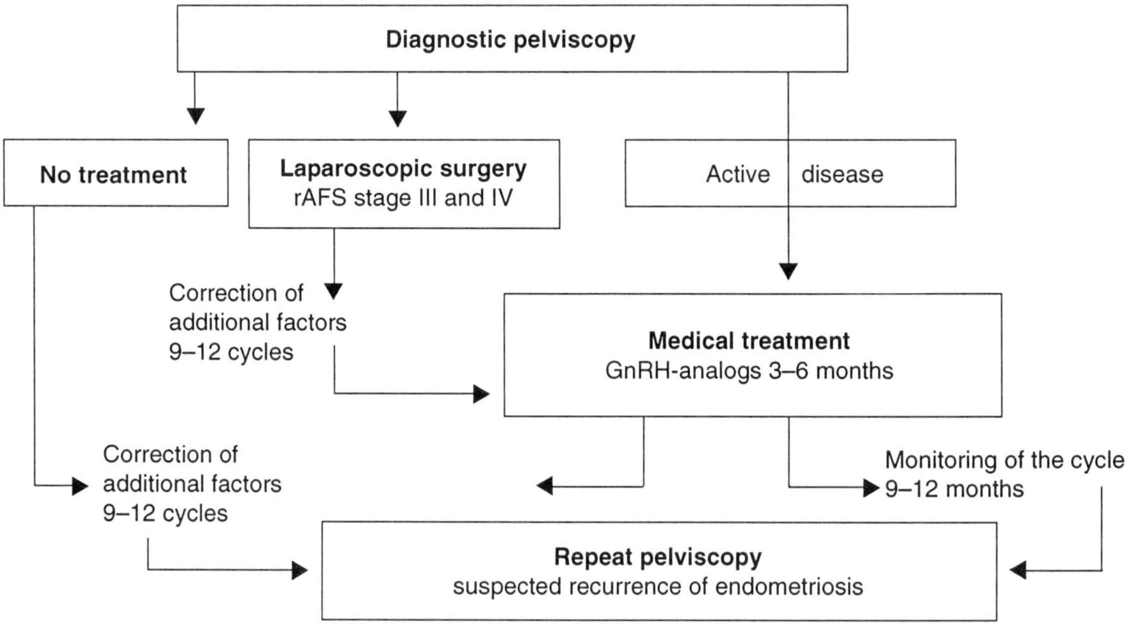

Figure 3 Flow chart for practical procedures in infertile patients with endometriosis for gynecological practice

CONCLUSIONS FOR CLINICAL PRACTICE

The most important decision for the optimal treatment of endometriosis is the diagnostic process. Localization, type, macroscopic and microscopic appearance of endometriotic lesions must be defined, before surgery, medical treatment or a combination of both is recommended. In cases of active peritoneal endometriosis laparoscopic surgery alone is insufficient and medical treatment after surgery will improve the pregnancy rates in infertile patients. In cases of infertility inactive peritoneal disease is probably not a cause of reduced fertility; no medical or surgical therapy is indicated with respect to endometriosis (Figure 3). It is not clear yet whether medical treatment is of similar value in cases of deep infiltrating endometriosis or ovarian endometrioma. Similar prospective, randomized studies are necessary to clarify the unsolved questions of an individual medical and/or surgical approach for the different types of endometriosis.

References

1. Russell WW. Aberrant portions of the Müllerian duct found in an ovary. *Bull Johns Hopkins Hosp* 1899;10:8–10
2. Cullen TS. *Adenomyoma of the uterus*. Philadelphia: W.B. Saunders & Co, 1908
3. Sampson JA. Peritoneal endometriosis due to menstrual dissemination of endometrial tissue into peritoneal cavity. *Am J Obstet Gynecol* 1927; 14:422–69
4. Vasquez G, Cornillie F, Brosens IA. Peritoneal endometriosis: scanning electron microscopy and histology of minimal pelvic endometriotic lesions. *Fertil Steril* 1984;42:696–703
5. Nissole N, Donnez J. Peritoneal endometriosis, ovarian endometriosis, and adenomyotic nodules of the rectovaginal septum are three different entities. *Fertil Steril* 1997;68:585–96
6. Schweppe K-W. *Morphologie und Klinik der*

Endometriose. Stuttgart, New York: Schattauer, 1984:103–76

7. Kauppila A, Rönneberg L, Vihko R. Steroid-rezeptoren in endometriotischem Gewebe. *Endometriose* 1986;4:56–60
8. The American Fertility Society. Revised American Fertility Society classification of endometriosis. *Fertil Steril* 1985;43:351–2
9. Wiegerinck MAHM, Van Dop PA, Brosens IA. The staging of peritoneal endometriosis by the type of active lesion in addition to the revised American Fertility Society classification. *Fertil Steril* 1993;60:461–4
10. Nissole M, Casanas-Roux F, Anaf V, *et al.* Morphometric study of the stromal vascularization in peritoneal endometriosis. *Fertil Steril* 1993;59: 681–4
11. Jansen RP, Russell P. Non pigmented endometriosis: clinical, laparoscopic, and pathologic definition. *Am J Obstet Gynecol* 1986;155:1154–9
12. Riedel HH, Semm K. Extragenital endometriosis and sterility – clinical experiences with a 3-step-therapy. *Proc Clin Biol Res* 1982;112:187–94

Treatment of endometriosis associated with infertility – IVF is the best treatment

24

W.M. Buckett, L.-L. Too and S.L. Tan

INTRODUCTION

Although *in vitro* fertilization (IVF) was initially developed as a treatment for tubal factor infertility[1], it has become a successful treatment for patients with infertility for many indications including male factor infertility and unexplained infertility[2,3]. Patients with moderate or severe endometriosis may have anatomic distortion of the Fallopian tube and ovary which may necessitate the use of IVF. However, even patients with mild or minimal endometriosis, who have failed to become pregnant following expectant management or other treatment for infertility or endometriosis, including surgery, may benefit from IVF, purely because the overall pregnancy rates are higher. This chapter will review the indications for IVF in women with endometriosis, compare the results of IVF for treatment of endometriosis with those for other indications for IVF, compare the outcome of IVF in women with moderate/severe endometriosis with those with minimal/mild endometriosis, discuss the most appropriate ovarian stimulation protocols, and discuss the significance of ovarian endometriomas.

INDICATIONS FOR IVF IN WOMEN WITH ENDOMETRIOSIS

Serum from infertile women with endometriosis has been shown to inhibit fertilization and early embryo development in the murine model when compared with serum from fertile women without endometriosis[4]. The inhibition increased with increasing severity of endometriosis and was improved by laser laparoscopic treatment. When the results of oocytes donation in women with active endometriosis were compared with its use in women without endometriosis, no differences in pregnancy rates or implantation rates were found[5]. Such studies suggest that any putative adverse effect of endometriosis on reproductive outcome is not related to implantation but is probably due to impaired oocyte or embryo quality. These findings also support the appropriateness of IVF for infertility associated with endometriosis, since only cleavage stage embryos are transferred to the uterine cavity.

When expectant treatment was compared with IVF within the first six months following diagnostic laparoscopy, the patients who underwent IVF were noted to conceive earlier (20.6 months *vs.* 27.1 months) and the cumulative conception rate was higher (62% *vs.* 43%)[6]. Nevertheless, IVF is generally indicated only when a couple has failed to conceive one to one and a half years after medical or surgical therapy. The timing of IVF treatment also depends on the age of the woman, the duration of infertility, and the presence or absence of other causes of infertility.

In cases of moderate/severe endometriosis (stages III and IV), where IVF has been compared with women who underwent re-operation (by laparoscopy), the cumulative pregnancy rates 3, 7 and 9 months after laparoscopy were 5.9%, 18.1% and 24.4% respectively compared with 33.3% and 69.6% after one and two cycles of IVF treatment respectively[7]. In this study no significant difference with regard to fertilization, implantation, pregnancy or live birth rates was found between patients with endometriosis and those with tubal infertility.

RESULTS OF IVF IN WOMEN WITH ENDOMETRIOSIS

Several studies have compared the success rates of IVF in women with endometriosis with women who have other indications for IVF. Although initial results suggested that fertilization rates were reduced in women with endometriosis compared with those with tubal or unexplained infertility[8], subsequent larger studies have shown comparable fertilization rates[9,10].

Similarly, there remains some controversy whether endometriosis affects implantation. One retrospective study reporting the results of 35 patients who underwent 89 IVF cycles, suggested that implantation was significantly lower in women with endometriosis (3.9%) compared with those with unexplained infertility (7.2%) or tubal infertility (8.1%)[11]. In another study, there was no difference in the implantation rate between women who had minimal or mild endometriosis and those with tubal infertility, although interestingly, the cleavage rate was lower in the women with endometriosis[12]. The largest study published so far (140 patients who underwent 182 IVF cycles) has shown no difference in the pregnancy rate per embryo transfer in women with all stages of endometriosis (40%) compared to couples with male factor infertility (39%), unexplained infertility (48%) or tubal factor infertility (45%)[10]. This study also reported no increase in the risk of miscarriage.

RESULTS OF IVF ASSOCIATED WITH THE SEVERITY OF ENDOMETRIOSIS

Although some early studies suggested that pregnancy rates following IVF were significantly lower in women with severe endometriosis compared with those with minimal or mild endometriosis (3%/cycle compared with 13%/cycle)[13,14], more recent larger studies have shown no difference in the pregnancy rate following IVF in women with stage III or IV disease compared with stage I or II disease[10,15,16]. This may be because of better ovarian stimulation protocols in the more recent studies (see below).

OVARIAN STIMULATION PROTOCOLS FOR ENDOMETRIOSIS

Some early studies suggested poorer pregnancy rates following IVF in women with endometriosis, however most recent studies show comparable pregnancy rates to women without endometriosis. One reason for this apparent discrepancy may be the increasingly widespread use of GnRH agonists[2]. A retrospective study, involving 145 patients with endometriosis who underwent 174 IVF treatment cycles, compared the use of GnRH agonists for 3 weeks, 3 months or not at all and the study reported significantly higher pregnancy rates in the women who had had the GnRH agonists irrespective of the duration of use[17].

Two prospective studies have compared prolonged pituitary suppression with GnRH agonists before IVF with IVF alone (without GnRH agonists)[18] or with the short or ultrashort GnRH agonist protocols[19] and reported significantly better pregnancy rates in the groups who received prolonged GnRH agonists.

Whether prolonged treatment with GnRH agonists in women with endometriosis is significantly better than the long protocol for IVF is unclear and further studies are needed in this area.

ENDOMETRIOMAS AND IVF

The presence of endometriomata does not generally impair the results of IVF but it increases the risk of infection. There have been several case reports of ovarian abscess after puncture of endometriomata during ultrasound guided oocyte retrieval[20,21]. A recent case series reported that there remains a significant risk of pelvic abscess even with the prophylactic use of broad spectrum antibiotics[22].

These findings would suggest that avoidance of endometriomata during oocyte retrieval is essential if it is possible. In some cases puncture of endometriomata may be unavoidable, and, for these patients, intra-operative and post-operative antibiotics should be given although they will remain at increased risk of developing infection. These patients should be advised to seek early treatment if symptoms of infection arise and intravenous antibiotics, given as an in-patient admission, would then be necessary.

CONCLUSIONS

In vitro fertilization is an effective treatment of infertility associated with endometriosis but it is generally used only when the woman has failed to conceive 1–1½ years after medical or surgical therapy. The timing of IVF treatment also depends on the age of the woman, the duration of the infertility, and the presence or absence of other causes of infertility. In women with endometriosis who have failed to conceive after surgery, IVF should offer higher pregnancy rates than repeat surgery. Results following IVF in women with endometriosis are comparable to those for women without endometriosis and they do not seem to be affected by the severity of the disease. The use of GnRH agonists in a long-protocol of ovarian stimulation leads to the highest pregnancy rates, although the role of prolonged pituitary suppression remains unclear. The presence of endometriomata does not generally impair the results of IVF but it increases the risk of infection. If possible, transvaginal drainage of endometriomata at oocyte collection is best avoided, but if this is not possible, prophylactic antibiotics must be given.

References

1. Steptoe PC, Edwards RG. Birth after re-implantation of a human embryo. *Lancet* 1978;ii:366
2. Tan SL, Royston P, Campbell S, *et al.* Cumulative conception and live birth rates after *in vitro* fertilisation. *Lancet* 1992;339:1390–4
3. Martin JS, Nisker JA, Parker JI, *et al.* The pregnancy rates of cohorts of idiopathic infertility couples give insights into the underlying mechanism of infertility. *Fertil Steril* 1995;64:98–102
4. Miller KA, Pittaway DE, Deatin JL. The effect of serum from infertile women with endometriosis on fertilization and early embryonic development in a murine *in vitro* model. *Fertil Steril* 1995;64:623–6
5. Sung L, Mukherjee T, Takeshige T, *et al.* Endometriosis is not detrimental to embryo implantation in oocyte recipients. *J Assist Reprod Genet* 1997;14:152–6
6. Kodama H, Fukuda J, Karube H, *et al.* Benefit of *in vitro* fertilization treatment for endometriosis-associated infertility. *Fertil Steril* 1996;66:974–9
7. Pagidas K, Falcone T, Hemmings R, *et al.* Comparison of reoperation for moderate (stage III) and severe (stage IV) endometriosis-related infertility with *in vitro* fertilization–embryo transfer. *Fertil Steril* 1996;65:791–5
8. Wardle PG, Mitchell JD, McLaughlin EA, *et al.* Endometriosis and ovulatory disorder: reduced fertilization *in vitro* compared with tubal and unexplained infertility. *Lancet* 1985;ii:236–9
9. Matson PL, Yovich JL. The treatment of infertility associated with endometriosis by *in vitro* fertilization. *Fertil Steril* 1986;46:432–4
10. Geber S, Paraschos T, Atkinson G, *et al.* Results of IVF in patients with endometriosis: the severity of the disease does not affect outcome, or the incidence of miscarriage. *Hum Reprod* 1995;10:1507–11
11. Arici A, Oral E, Bukulmez O, *et al.* The effect of endometriosis on implantation: results from the Yale University *in vitro* fertilization program. *Fertil Steril* 1996;65:603–7
12. Tanbo T, Omland A, Dale PO, *et al.* *In vitro* fertilization/embryo transfer in unexplained

infertility and minimal peritoneal endometriosis. *Acta Obstet Gynecol Scand* 1995;74:539–43
13. Yovich JL, Matson PL. The influence of infertility etiology on the outcome of IVF–ET and GIFT treatments. *Int J Fertil* 1990;35:26–33
14. Chillick CF, Acosta AA, Garcia JE, *et al.* The role of *in vitro* fertilization in infertile patients with endometriosis. *Fertil Steril* 1985;44:56–61
15. Dmowski WP, Rana N, Michalowska J, *et al.* The effect of endometriosis, its stage and activity, and of auto antibodies on *in vitro* fertilization and embryo transfer success rates. *Fertil Steril* 1995; 63:555–62
16. Olivennes F, Feldberg D, Liu HC, *et al.* Endometriosis: a stage by stage analysis – the role of *in vitro* fertilization. *Fertil Steril* 1995;64:392–8
17. Chedid S, Camus M, Smitz J, *et al.* Comparison among different ovarian stimulation regimens for assisted procreation procedures in patients with endometriosis. *Hum Reprod* 1995;10:2406–11
18. Dicker D, Goldman GA, Ashkenazi J, *et al.* The value of pre-treatment with gonadotrophin-releasing hormone (GnRH) analogue in IVF–ET therapy for severe endometriosis. *Hum Reprod* 1990;5:418–20
19. Marcus SF, Edwards RG. High rates of pregnancy after long-term down-regulation of women with severe endometriosis. *Am J Obstet Gynecol* 1994; 171:812–17
20. Padilla SL. Ovarian abscess following puncture of an endometrioma during ultrasound guided oocyte retrieval. *Hum Reprod* 1993;8:1282–3
21. Yaron Y, Peyser MR, Samuel D, *et al.* Infected endometriotic cysts secondary to oocyte aspiration for *in vitro* fertilization. *Hum Reprod* 1994;9:1759–60
22. Younis JS, Ezra Y, Laufer N, *et al.* Late manifestation of pelvic abscess following oocyte retrieval, for *in vitro* fertilization, in patients with severe endometriosis and ovarian endometriomata. *J Assist Reprod Genet* 1997;14:343–6

Endometriosis: arguments against proposed therapeutic options

25

A.H. DeCherney and S. Daneshmand

The optimal management of endometriosis remains controversial. Over the years, endometriosis has been the target of countless attempts at therapeutic interventions including ovarian suppression therapy, surgical treatment or a combination of these therapies. Controversy also still exists regarding the cause of endometriosis-associated infertility. Although the association between endometriosis and subfertility is well documented, causality is poorly understood[1]. The very few prospective and randomized studies which have been performed on endometriotic patients indicate that monthly fecundity rates in patients with endometriosis are about half those without endometriosis[1]. Several theories have been proposed to explain the decreased fecundity. These include ovulatory dysfunction, altered folliculogenesis, sperm phagocytosis, impaired fertilization, defective implantation, luteal phase defect, inhibition of early embryo development and immunological alterations[2]. Fertility can also be compromised by mechanical factors if there is distortion of pelvic structures, particularly if the Fallopian tube and ovarian relationship is disrupted.

New research developments have focused on the immunological sequelae of pelvic endometriosis as a factor leading to infertility. Halme *et al.* have identified peritoneal macrophage activation as a central contributor to the pathogenesis of endometriosis[3]. These macrophages can be actively recruited to the sites of inflammation by chemokines and induced to undergo activation by cytokine stimulation or in response to foreign antigens. The macrophages themselves can also secrete a variety of cytokines which can contribute to a feed forward loop exacerbating local inflammation[4]. Certain cytokines may be toxic to sperm or embryos and in this way can directly interfere with fertilization and implantation[4].

The endometrium may also provide another clue in the etiology of endometriosis-associated infertility. Certain investigators have found that while retrograde menstruation occurs in about 90% of cycling women, only 10–15% of women are actually diagnosed with endometriosis. This discrepancy raises the question about certain features of reflux endometrium in patients with endometriosis which may allow for greater adherence and proliferation of implants on peritoneal surfaces. Integrins, which are a family of adhesion molecules, have been implicated in endometriosis-associated infertility[4]. Integrins bond various extracellular matrix components and mediate cell matrix interactions during cell adhesion and migration. These proteins are important to the process of endometrial proliferation and shedding as well as embryo recognition and implantation. In the human endometrium, β_3 integrin is selectively upregulated during the window of implantation from cycle days 20–24[4]. This particular integrin seems to be the most sensitive and specific marker of implantation. Infertile patients with endometriosis lack expression of the β_3 integrin, whereas fertile patients with endometriosis as well as fertile controls have normal expression of this integrin during the luteal phase[4]. This β_3 integrin may be a marker of endometriosis-associated infertility. Some investigators have postulated that a reduced β_3 integrin expression in patients with endometriosis may account for abnormal endometrial/embryo interactions resulting in reduced pregnancy rates. Further research on integrins in endometriosis is needed to clarify their role as adhesion molecules in the pathogenesis of endometriosis.

TREATMENT OPTIONS

The options for treatment of endometriosis include expectant management, ovarian suppression with medical treatment, surgical treatment by laparoscopy, ovarian stimulation with or without intrauterine insemination and assisted reproductive technologies.

A significant number of studies have addressed these treatments for important, however, many of them have significant limitations because they are retrospective or lack controls. It has been even more difficult to ascertain whether surgical treatment is the optimal treatment for endometriosis since prospective randomized trials are rarely performed in surgical studies. Even prospective studies done with controls have limitations because of differences among the treatment groups. It is important to assess the data from these studies in terms of monthly fecundity rate (MFR) and not overall pregnancy rate. This paper will discuss the efficacy of different treatment options in the light of the available information.

Ovulation suppression

Figure 1 summarizes the results of six controlled studies comparing ovulation suppression versus no treatment in patients with endometriosis-associated infertility[5–10]. In these studies, ovulation suppression agents, danazol, medroxyprogesterone acetate (MPA) or gestrinone, were compared with either placebo or no treatment. Three of the studies were randomized clinical trials and none used a crossover design. In these studies, treatment was generally allocated on the basis of disease severity. The odds ratios for individual studies ranged from 0.4 to 1.33, all with 95% confidence intervals including unity.

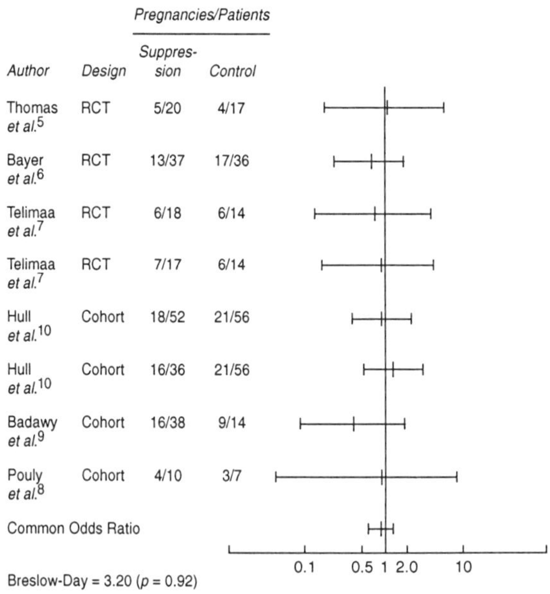

Figure 1 Controlled studies comparing ovarian suppression *vs.* no treatment in women with endometriosis-associated infertility (reproduced with permission from Hughes *et al.*[22])

Figure2 summarizes the results of six randomized controlled trials comparing ovulation suppression versus danazol in women with endometriosis-associated infertility[11–15]. Common odds ratios for pregnancy for these ovulation suppression agents compared with danazol was 1.07 (95% CI, 0.71–1.61). Analysis of this combined data from trials comparing danazol, gestrinone or medroxyprogesterone acetate with placebo or no treatment failed to show any significant treatment benefit. Furthermore, trials comparing gestrinone, GnRH agonists or an oral contraceptive pill with an active control, danazol, demonstrated no difference in subsequent fecundity between groups[11–15].

Fedele performed a randomized clinical trial to compare the efficacy of an intranasal GnRH agonist with expectant management in the treatment of endometriosis-associated infertility (Stage I and II of revised AFS classification)[16]. In this study the median follow-up was 17 months in the buserelin

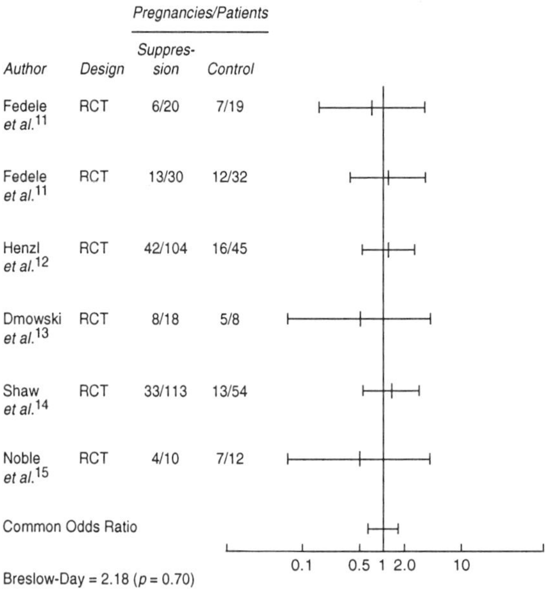

Figure 2 Randomized controlled trials comparing ovulation suppression *vs.* danazol in women with endometriosis-associated infertility (reproduced with permission from Hughes *et al.*[22])

group and 18 months in the women who underwent expectant management. A total of 17 pregnancies were observed both in the GnRH agonist treated patients and in the expectant management group and the authors concluded that treatment with gonadotropin releasing hormone agonist is unlikely to have a marked influence on the reproductive outcome of infertile women with minimal or mild endometriosis[16].

Adamson *et al.* performed a meta-analysis on all the papers in the English language literature since 1977 (Figure 3)[17]. In this meta-analysis, interventions consisted of no treatment, medical treatment or surgical treatment by laparoscopy or laparotomy. The main out-come measures were pregnancy rates. The authors of this study concluded from their meta-analysis that either no treatment or surgery was superior to medical treatment for minimal and mild endometriosis associated with infertility. The authors of this study also confirmed that medical treatment of endometriosis-associated infertility is inappropriate whether alone or after surgery because pregnancy rates are not improved and the duration of time in treatment, treatment costs and medication side-effects represent losses to the patient.

Thus, there is no evidence in the literature that shows any treatment benefit for ovarian suppression. Further research is needed to ascertain the role for presurgical ovarian suppression in the treatment of endometriosis-associated infertility.

Laparoscopic surgery

Adamson *et al.* conducted a study comparing pregnancy rates in 579 infertility patients diagnosed with endometriosis at laparoscopy[18]. This study compared pregnancy rates among patients in four endometriosis treatment groups: diagnostic laparoscopy followed by no treatment, diagnostic laparoscopy followed by medical treatment, operative laparoscopy performed at the time

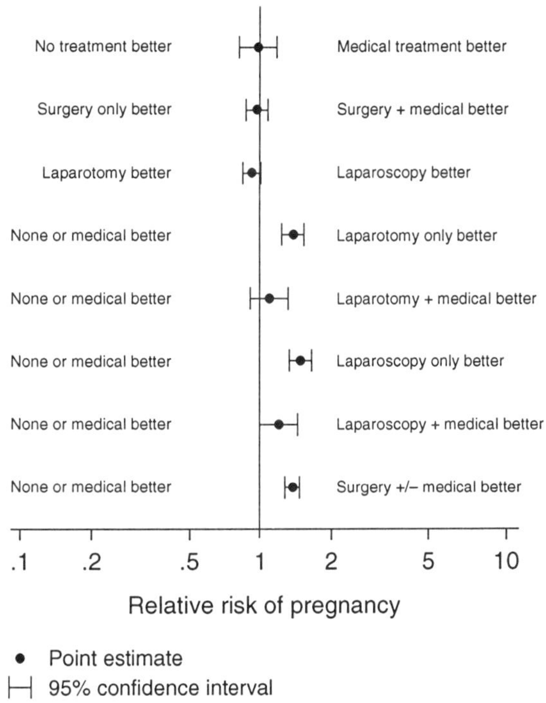

Figure 3 Summary of meta-analysis estimates for endometriosis-associated infertility (reproduced with permission from Adamson[2])

Table 1 Estimated cumulative pregnancy rates by treatment group (reproduced with permission from Adamson[2])

	Entire patient population					*Endometriosis-only subset*				
			Pregnant					*Pregnant*		
Minimal/Mild	*No.*	*No. pregnant in 3 years*	*1 year %*	*2 years %*	*3 years %*	*No.*	*No. pregnant in 3 years*	*1 year %*	*2 years %*	*3 years %*
No treatment	15	10	53.3 ± 12.9*	66.7 ± 12.2	66.7 ± 12.2	13	9	61.5 ± 13.5	69.2 ± 12.8	69.2 ± 12.8
Medical treatment	44	20	26.5 ± 7.2	53.0 ± 8.9	62.3 ± 9.3	32	13	25.6 8.4	47.7 ± 10.2	55.2 ± 11.2
Laparoscopy	241	122	43.6 ± 3.5	59.6 ± 3.8	67.8 ± 4.1	134	70	45.5 ± 4.7	60.4 ± 5.1	70.3 ± 5.4
Laparotomy	46	28	55.7 ± 7.9	65.6 ± 7.9	74.3 ± 8.1	13	6	38.0 ± 15.1	50.4 ± 16.4	64.5 ± 16.8

*Values are estimates ± SE

Table 2 Comparison of treatments for endometriosis-associated infertility controlling for significant variables using survival analysis with fixed covariates (reproduced with permission from Adamson[2]).

	*Entire patient population**			
	Number of patients in each treatment arm	*Estimate*† (%)	χ^2	*p value*
Laparoscopy vs. no treatment	361/20	7	0.05	0.83
Laparoscopy vs. medical treatment	361/50	42	2.92	0.087
Laparoscopy vs. laparotomy	361/148	29	2.27	0.13
No treatment vs. medical treatment	20/50	33	0.64	0.43
No treatment vs. laparotomy	20/148	20	0.30	0.58
Laparotomy vs. medical treatment	148/50	11	0.15	0.70

*Controlled for years infertile, revised AFS total score, ovulation treatment, fimbria score, tubes score
†Percentage by which first treatment pregnancy rate is greater than second treatment rate

of diagnostic laparoscopy, and laparotomy. In this study no significant differences were found in pregnancy rates achieved after three years comparing no treatment versus laparoscopy. Table 1 shows the cumulative life table pregnancy rates by treatment group for different stages of endometriosis. Table 2 shows the pairwise comparison of treatment groups controlling for significant variables using survival analysis with fixed covarieties. In the entire population there were no significant differences in cumulative pregnancy rate[4] among treatment groups. There were also no significant differences when treatment groups were compared among the entire patient population.

In a separate study, Adamson *et al.* compared 64 patients who had endometriosis and adhesions vaporized with a CO_2 laser with a control group of 44 patients who had laparoscopy[19]. In this study the monthly fecundity rates were not significantly different in the laparoscopic CO_2 laser vaporization group as compared to the controls.

It is important to note that the majority of surgical studies performed on infertile endometriosis patients suffer from a lack of prospective design, standardized surgical approaches, documentation of completeness of disease resection and awareness of atypical forms of endometriosis, especially in earlier studies. The ENDOCAN study performed by Marcoux *et al.* in 1997 was the first large scale prospective randomized trial on the effect of stage I–II disease ablation on fertility[20]. In this study 341 patients with endometriosis-associated infertility were studied with a 17% drop-out rate and a 36-week follow-up. The authors in this study reported a significant increase in live birth rate, 29% versus 17%, $p < 0.03$ and time to conception with ablation versus diagnostic laparoscopy only. However, there was only a marginal increase in the monthly fecundity rates in the patients treated with ablation (4.7 vs. 2.4, $p < 0.05$).

Expectant management

Table 1 shows the estimated cumulative life table pregnancy rates in one of the largest prospective controlled trials in the literature[18]. These data show that expectant management or no treatments and surgery have success rates that are no different and both of which are higher than ovarian suppression for minimal or mild disease.

It is important to note that this paper suffered from the absence of randomized controls and insufficient power to differentiate no treatment from surgical success rates. The meta-analysis performed by Adamson in patients with minimal and mild endometriosis comparing no treatment, laparoscopy and laparotomy had equivalent three-year estimated cumulative live pregnancy rates that were also higher than medical treatment pregnancy rates (Figure 3). Based on the results of these studies there seems to be no improvement in reproductive outcome when infertile patients with endometriosis are treated expectantly.

Assisted reproductive technologies

Assisted reproductive technologies (ART) refers to procedures such as *in vitro* fertilization (IVF), gamete intrafallopian transfer (GIFT), tubal embryo transfer (TET) and intracytoplasmic sperm injection (ICSI). When assessing outcome according to diagnosis, patients with endometriosis have lower pregnancy rates compared with patients with tubal factor infertility. It is difficult to assess the role of IVF and ART in the treatment of endometriosis-associated infertility as there are too few well designed trials evaluating this treatment regimen. Also, endometriosis-associated infertility is often confounded by additional factors or variables that affect the choice of treatments including age, duration of infertility, prior pregnancy history, number of previous IVF cycles and cost. Earlier studies showed the success of IVF with more advanced stages of endometriosis which may have been a function of ovarian accessibility at laparoscopy[2]. More recent data show similar rates to other non-male factor patients.

Given these confounding factors, treatment of endometriosis-associated infertility will depend on each couple's unique situation and can include *in vitro* fertilization. However, at this time there are no well designed studies revealing that IVF is a treatment of choice in endometriosis-associated infertility. What is known is that pregnancy outcome in patients with endometriosis is not different from that in those with tubal infertility and thus ART may potentially bypass the deleterious effects of endometriosis on infertility[21].

CONCLUSION

There is considerable controversy regarding the treatment of endometriosis-associated infertility because of a paucity of data on which to base decisions. Clearly, ovarian suppression has almost no role except for its possible use before *in vitro* fertilization in patients with severe or extensive disease. In regards to laparoscopic surgery, with the exception of the ENDOCAN study there is little evidence to support this mode of therapy for endometriosis-associated infertility. Given the role of peritoneal macrophages and cytokines in endometriosis-associated infertility, one approach which can potentially be used for treatment is to inhibit cytokine production or action. There are therapeutic trials under way using this cytokine-targeted approach[4]. Rheumatoid arthritis patients who have been treated experimentally with antibodies against interleukin-6 and TNF-α have shown some response and this therapy might be of benefit to patients with endometriosis. Identification of those cytokines that play pivotal roles in the pathogenesis and sequelae of endometriosis will provide targets for cytokine blockade which may offer targeted therapy early in the disease process.

References

1. Olive D, Haney A. Endometriosis – associated infertility: a critical review of therapeutic approaches. *Obstet Gynecol Surv* 1986;41:538–55
2. Adamson GD. Treatment of endometriosis-associated infertility. *Sem Reprod Endocrinol* 1997;15(3):263–71
3. Halme J, Becker S, Wihg, R. Accentuated cyclic activation of peritoneal macrophages in patients with endometriosis. *Am J Obstet Gynecol* 1981;148:83
4. Ryan IP, Taylor RN. Endometriosis and infertility: new concepts. *Ob-Gyn Survey* 1997;52:365–70
5. Thomas EJ, Cooke I. Successful treatment of asymptomatic endometriosis: does it benefit infertile women? *Br Med J* 1987;294:1117–19
6. Bayer SR, Seibel M, Saffan DS, *et al.* Efficacy of danazol treatment for minimal endometriosis in infertile women. *J Reprod Med* 1988;33:179–83
7. Telimaa S. Danazol and medroxyprogesterone acetate inefficacious in the treatment of infertility in endometriosis. *Fertil Steril* 1988;60:872–5
8. Pouly JL, Manhea H, Mage G, *et al.* Laparoscopic treatment of endometriosis (laser excluded). *Contrib Gynecol Obstet* 1987;16:280–5
9. Badawy SZA, Elbakry MM, Samuel F, Dize M. Cumulative pregnancy rates in infertile women with endometriosis. *J Reprod Med* 1988;33:757–80
10. Hull ME, Moghissi K, Magyar DF, *et al.* Comparison of different treatment modalities of endometriosis in infertile women. *Fertil Steril* 1987;47:40–4
11. Fedele L, Bianchi S, Viezzoli T, *et al.* Gestrinone versus danazol in the treatment of endometriosis. *Fertil Steril* 1989;51:781–5
12. Henzl MR, Corson SL, Moghissi K, *et al.* Administration of nasal nafarelin as compared with oral danazol for endometriosis. *N Engl J Med* 1988;318:485–9
13. Dmowski WP, Radwanska E, *et al.* Ovarian suppression induced with buserelin or danazol in the management of endometriosis: a randomized, comparative study. *Fertil Steril* 1989;51:395–400
14. Shaw RW. An open randomized comparative study of the effect of goserelin depot and danazol in the treatment of endometriosis. *Fertil Steril* 1992;58:265–72
15. Noble AD, Letchworth AT. Medical treatment of endometriosis: a comparative trial. *Postgrad Med J* 1979;55:37–9
16. Fedele L, Bianchi S, Arcaini L, *et al.* Buserelin versus danazol in the treatment of endometriosis-associated infertility. *Am J Obstet Gynec* 1989;161:871–6
17. Adamson GD, Campbell J, Pasta DJ. Surgical treatment of endometriosis-associated infertility: meta-analysis compared with survival analysis. *Am J Obstet Gynecol* 1994;171:1488–505
18. Adamson GD, Hurd SJ, Pasta DJ, *et al.* Laparoscopic endometriosis treatment: is it better? *Fertil Steril* 1993;59:35–44
19. Adamson GD, Lu J, Subak LL. Laparoscopic CO_2 laser vaporization of endometriosis compared with traditional treatments. *Fertil Steril* 1988;50:704–10
20. Marcoux S, Maheux R, Berhle S, *et al.* Canadian Collaborative Group in Endometriosis. Laparoscopic surgery in infertile women with minimal or mild endometriosis. *New Eng J Med* 1997;377:212
21. Oliveness F, Feldberg D, *et al.* Endometriosis: a stage by stage analysis – the role of IVF. *Fertil Steril* 1995;64:342
22. Hughes EG, Fedorkow DM, Collins JA. A quantitative overview of controlled trials in endometriosis-associated infertility. *Fertil Steril* 1993;59:963–70

Endometriosis and pelvic pain: the evidence in favor of surgery

26

G.L. Schattman

Endometriosis may not be a disease, but a natural result of retrograde menstruation. In the majority of women, normal defense mechanisms are able to remove these foreign cells from this extraneous environment. In some, the bodies, defenses are not as competent, allowing lesions of endometriotic disease to grow and cause the symptoms of pain or other pertubations of bodily functions. It is this subset of women, those with documented endometriosis and pain, who suffer for many years before being properly diagnosed and aggressively treated for their disease[1]. Since definitive diagnosis requires operative interventions which are not without risk (i.e. laparoscopy or laparotomy) and histologic confirmation of ectopic endometrial glands and stroma, many patients suffer needlessly while we attempt to do everything possible to avoid surgery, including repeating courses of therapy that have previously failed.

The main question we need to pose to begin this discussion is whether or not surgery can 'cure' endometriosis. If not, how long does surgery palliate the symptoms and in which situations does it work? To actually cure the disease, we need to be able to complete four tasks. They are:

(1) identify all the lesions wherever they may be;

(2) remove all the disease;

(3) restore normal anatomy;

(4) prevent recurrences.

If we are not able to complete all these tasks, then surgery will not be curative, rather it can only be considered cytoreductive or palliative.

Are we able to identify all the lesions? To do so, we rely on the resolution of our video system and our eyes. Our eyes are only as good as our experience and it has been clearly demonstrated that with increasing experience, our ability to detect lesions of endometriosis other than the classic black powder-burn lesions improves dramatically[2,3]. Even now, with all our abilities and experience, we are realizing that it may not be possible to identify all endometriotic disease, and some lesions may only be identified after the use of flourescent dyes[4] or other methods. Additionally, it is unlikely that we will have removed all disease even if we think we have based on its macroscopic appearance. This was well demonstrated by Cornillie[5] who realized that even after complete excision of deep lesions, when they evaluated their specimens histologically, they found evidence of endometriotic disease extending into the margins of their resection, indicating that the excision was incomplete. Microscopic disease as well may predispose these patients to experience a recurrence of their symptoms despite aggressive surgical excision of all visible lesions.

With these thoughts in mind, let us look at the available data with regard to the relief of symptoms in those patients with pelvic pain who have endometriosis. There are a number of retrospective studies looking at patients who have endometriosis. Unfortunately, most of these studies have looked at results of a heterogeneous population of patients with pain, infertility, pelvic masses or a number of other problems. These data, unfortunately, do not allow us to make any interpretable conclusions about our specific patient population[6–12]. Most of the prospective studies are similarly flawed and not randomized; however, they are of some benefit to look at. Hornstein *et al.*[13] studied a homogeneous group of 44 patients with pelvic pain who were found to have endometriosis at laparoscopy, and ablated their lesions with laser or cautery and followed them for 24 months. They randomized the patients after surgery to receive either postoperative GnRH-a treatment or placebo. Forty-seven percent of patients did not complete the study because of treatment failure. In those patients receiving postoperative placebo, 57% required additional medical therapies within the two years because the surgery failed to provide adequate relief of pain. Interestingly, when postoperative GnRH-a was combined to augment the surgical procedure, only 31% of patients required additional medical therapies secondary to persistent or recurrence of pain. Winkel *et al.*[14] presented very interesting data at last year's world congress where patients underwent surgical therapy either by ablation or excision and were followed up prospectively for 24 months. Only 23% of patients undergoing ablative therapies were improved at 24 months compared with 60% improvement in patients who had their visible implants excised.

There is only one randomized, double-blind, placebo-controlled trial that I am aware of in the literature evaluating the effectiveness of surgical therapy in patients with pelvic pain who are found to have endometriosis. This wonderful paper by Sutton *et al.*[9] randomized patients with pelvic pain who were found to have stages I, II or III endometriosis at laparoscopy. Patients with stage IV disease were excluded by the institute's IRB because they felt it was 'unethical to withold treatment from patients in severe pain due to stage IV disease'. Unfortunately, their IRB, as well as many patients and physicians were unaware of the fact that AFS staging and pain scores are unrelated. Patients with 'minimal' disease may indeed have severe pain. Patients who have pain tend to have deeper, more invasive lesions as a possible cause for their pain, despite having only a small area of visible disease[15]. What Sutton and his colleagues did was to randomize patients with stage I, II or III disease to have either a diagnostic laparoscopy with removal of any peritoneal fluid to fully evaluate the pelvis or laser ablation of all visible lesions and utero-sacral nerve ablation (LUNA). Patients, as well as the nurse following up the patients at 3 and 6 months, were blinded as to which procedure they had done and at 6 months the code was broken. What was found was surprising. At 3 months, there was no difference in relief of pain between the two groups! At 6 months, 63% of those patients who had laser ablation and LUNA experienced relief of their symptom while only 23% of those patients who had a diagnostic procedure only were better. Even more interesting was the fact that patients with 'less severe' forms of the disease did not gain as much benefit from the surgery as did patients with more advanced disease. Only 38% of patients with stage I disease were improved after operative intervention, whereas 69% and 100% of patients with stage II and stage III disease respectively were better. When these patients were followed up at one year, 56% of patients still had some relief of their initial symptoms. This means that 44% of patients were still suffering despite aggressive surgical intervention. When five patients were re-operated on at 6 months because of a recurrence of pain, two of them were found to have evidence of endometriosis in areas that were previously lasered and in new areas. This means that the initial surgical procedure resulted in incomplete destruction of endometriotic disease despite being performed by an accomplished and experienced surgeon. Three other patients who had persistent pain had no evidence of endometriosis at their repeat laparoscopy, possibly demonstrating a re-growth of normal peritoneum over an area of deep endometriosis incompletely treated at the initial procedure.

Despite all this aggressive surgical intervention, what we begin to realize from these data is that there is still approximately a 40 to

60% chance that a woman is going to experience a recurrence of pelvic pain after surgery alone. Because we are unable to identify and destroy or resect all endometriotic disease, and the failure rate of surgery alone is significant (> 40%), surgery must be considered cytoreductive and only palliative. Other treatment modalities or adjuvant medical therapies must be utilized to allow these patients who have been suffering for many years to get some relief. In patients for whom oral contraceptives or progestational therapy fail prior to surgery, there is no evidence that these agents will be any more effective postoperatively. GnRH-a appear to be our best option currently and should probably be used to augment our surgical debulking in all patients regardless of 'stage'.

References

1. Dmowski WP, Lesniewicz R, Rana N, *et al.* Changing trends in the diagnosis of endometriosis: a comparative study of women with pelvic endometriosis presenting with chronic pelvic pain or infertility. *Fertil Steril* 1997;67: 238–43
2. Martin DC, Hubert GD, Vander Zwaag R, *et al.* Laparoscopic appearance of peritoneal endometriosis. *Fertil Steril* 1989;51:63
3. Stripling MC, Martin DC, Chatmon DL, *et al.* Subtle appearance of pelvic endometriosis. *Fertil Steril* 1988;49:427
4. Malik E, Trutenau D, Berg C, *et al.* Photodynamic diagnosis of endometriosis, Abstract, VI World Congress on Endometriosis, July 1998, Quebec City, Canada
5. Cornillie FJ, Oosterlynck D, Lauweryns JM, *et al.* Deeply infiltrating endometriosis: histology and clinical significance. *Fertil Steril* 1990;53:978–83
6. Puolakka J, Kauppila A, Ronnberg L. Results in the operative treatment of pelvic endometriosis. *Acta Obstet Gynecol Scand* 1980;59:429–31
7. Hasson HM. Electrocoagulation of pelvic endometriotic lesions with laparoscopic control. *Am J Obstet Gynecol* 1979;135:115–21
8. Keye WR, Hansen LW, Astin M, *et al.* Argon laser therapy of endometriosis: a review of 92 consecutive patients. *Fertil Steril* 1987;47:208–12
9. Sutton CJG, Ewen S, Whitelaw N, *et al.* Prospective, randomized, double-blind controlled trial of laser laparoscopy in the treatment of pelvic pain associated with minimal, mild or moderate endometriosis. *Fertil Steril* 1994;62:696–700
10. Howard FM. The role of laparoscopy in chronic pelvic pain: promise and pitfalls. *Obstet Gynecol Surv* 1993;48:357–87
11. Howard FM. Laparoscopic evaluation and treatment of women with chronic pelvic pain. *J Am Assoc Gynecol Laparosc* 1994;1:325–31
12. Redwine DB. Conservative laparoscopic excision of endometriosis by sharp dissection: life table analysis of reoperation and persistent or recurrent disease. *Fertil Steril* 1991; 56:628–34
13. Hornstein MD, Hemmings R, Yuzpe AA, *et al.* Use of nafarelin versus placebo after reductive laparoscopic surgery for endometriosis. *Fertil Steril* 1997; 68:860–4
14. Winkel C, Bray M. Treatment of women with endometriosis using excision alone, ablation alone or ablation with a combination with Leuprolide acetate. Presented at Vth World Congress on Endometriosis, 1997, Yokohama, P55
15. Konickx PR, Neulemon C, Demeyere S, *et al.* Long term evaluation that pelvic endometriosis is a progressive disease whereas deeply infiltrating endometriosis is associated with pelvic pain. *Fertil Steril* 1991;55:759–65

Laparoscopic excision of endometriosis 27

D.B. Redwine

INTRODUCTION

The most common and most specific symptom of endometriosis is pain. Since no medicine eradicates endometriosis, most physicians treat it surgically. Since 1980 the author has treated almost 1300 patients by laparoscopic excision. In this referral practice, only 18% of patients have had no previous therapy for endometriosis. Most patients have had multiple medical and surgical treatments (including removal of the uterus, tubes and ovaries) and are still bothered by pain symptoms thought to be due to endometriosis. They have had everything done to them and to their disease except one thing: the disease has not been removed from their body. Laparoscopic excision of endometriosis is the only form of treatment which can treat any manifestation of endometriosis with any depth of invasion anywhere in the body.

CLINICAL FINDINGS

Patients with endometriosis frequently begin having pain associated with menses early in their menstrual life. Careful questioning reveals that this is not always uterine cramping, but can be a menstrual aggravation of pain which may have had its onset around ovulation. Some patients may experience uterine cramping in addition to menstrual aggravation of pre-existing pain. When the cul-de-sac or uterosacral ligaments are involved, deep dyspareunia and pain with bowel movements during menses are common. When obliteration of the cul-de-sac and a rectal nodule of endometriosis are present, some patients will have painful bowel movements throughout the month. Ovarian endometriomas may produce lateral pain. On examination, tenderness of the uterosacral liga-ments, with or without nodularity, is usually due to endometriosis. Ultrasonography, X-rays, and other imaging tests are of limited value in the preoperative diagnosis of endometriosis, and tests do not relieve pain or eliminate the need for diagnostic and therapeutic surgery.

SURGERY FOR ENDOMETRIOSIS

Patient positioning for surgery

The patient is placed in the low lithotomy position with a retention catheter in the bladder. Because operative endoscopy can be a lengthy procedure, positioning of the legs is particularly important. If knee stirrups are used, extra thick padding is needed to avoid peroneal nerve paresis. To avoid patient hypothermia, a warming blanket can be placed under the patient, and blankets are placed around the upper torso, head and arms. The arms are ideally tucked along the side of the patient to allow full mobility by the surgeon and the assistant. Irrigation fluid can be passed through a blood warming coil. An intrauterine manipulator is placed for intraoperative manipulation, and the table is placed in steep Trendelenburg position.

After placing a Hulka intrauterine manipulator, a 10 mm umbilical sheath is inserted directly. There is no reason to place a Verress needle blindly first, since this increases the risk of intra-abdominal injury resulting from blind insertion by 100% over simply placing the umbilical trocar directly (1 blind insertion vs 2 blind insertions). A 10 mm operating laparoscope with a 3 mm operating channel accepting a 3 mm scissors is placed through this 10 mm umbilical sheath. Laser laparoscopes are to be avoided, since they have a 5 mm air channel which reduces optical resolution and allows bothersome play in the shaft of the 3 mm scissors during surgery. Two 5.5 mm trocars are placed lateral to the inferior epigastric vessels near the top of the pubic hair line with a suction-irrigator passing through the right lower quadrant sheath. A 5 mm grasper with fine teeth is passed through the left lower quadrant sheath. A high flow insufflator is helpful, but a video camera and monitor are unnecessary and in fact will reduce surgical speed. Ninety to 110 watts of pure cutting current or 50 watts of coagulation current are passed through the scissors tips, depending on the tissue situation encountered.

Superficial peritoneal resection

The peritoneum adjacent to the lesion is grasped and elevated, a touch cut created with 90 W of pure cutting current, and the peritoneum is bluntly dissected away from the underlying vital structures, then removed.

Deep peritoneal resection

When a lesion is larger, has fibrosis, or retroperitoneal invasion is suspected because vessels or the ureter cannot be seen, the peritoneum adjacent to the lesion should be opened with a touch cut, and the hole grasped and elevated medially so the scissors can bluntly dissect the lesion away from underlying structures. Then, grasping either the lesion or the adjacent normal peritoneum as required, slide cuts can extend the line of incision around the lesion, with retroperitoneal dissection working toward the center of the bottom of the lesion. It is only during retroperitoneal dissection that the invasiveness of endometriosis will be appreciated. Coagulation cutting beneath the peritoneum is useful for severing tendrils of tissue left from blunt dissection. At any given power setting on the electrosurgical generator, coagulation current has a higher voltage than cutting current, which means it has more power for cutting into parenchymal or fatty tissue. This is important when dealing with endometriosis of the cul-de-sac[1].

Resection of the uterosacral ligament

Either uterosacral ligament can be involved in invasive endometriosis with the volume of a man's thumb, with fibrotic extension down to the sacrum. This depth of disease will be impossible to treat with laser vaporization or electrocoagulation. Resection of the entire uterosacral ligament is the only treatment that will ensure complete removal. To resect the uterosacral ligament, incise the peritoneum lateral and parallel to it using touch and slide cutting. This incision over the adjacent broad ligament results in automatic retraction of the peritoneum with resultant visualization of the retroperitoneal structures. The ureter and uterine vessels can now be dissected bluntly laterally to ensure that they are not near the uterosacral ligament. The ligament can actually be partially undermined along its length, and this will define much of the ensuing dissection. With bulky invasive disease, fibrosis will extend laterally to involve the ureter or branches of the uterine vessels descending along the lateral vaginal wall. In this case the dissection must begin in uninvolved peritoneum more posteriorly along the broad ligament with the dissection working around the ureter toward the uterosacral ligament. Just medial to the point where the uterine vessels cross the ureter are the inferior branches of the uterine vessels. Blunt dissection alternating with meticulous use of monopolar current is necessary to separate the uterosacral ligament from these vessels. If bleeding is encountered, it can be safely controlled with unipolar coagulation because the dissection at this point is well medial to the previously identified ureter. Once the lateral margin of the uterosacral ligament has been dissected away from these branches of the uterine vessels, a peritoneal incision is made medial and parallel to the ligament. Next, the insertion of the uterosacral ligament into the posterior cervix is divided with coagulation cutting. The uterosacral ligament is grasped and dissected off the pelvic floor using a combination of sharp, blunt and electro dissection. As the dissection retreats from the area of the cervix and the endometriotic invasion is completely undermined, it will be seen that the utero-sacral ligament becomes less dense and spreads out into the surrounding perirectal connective tissue. At this distal point the ligament is transected with coagulation cutting and removed.

Ureterolysis and angiolysis

Retroperitoneal fibrosis associated with invasive endometriosis will commonly invest the ureters and occasionally the internal iliac vessels and their branches. The ureters can be involved by fibrosis extending from invasive endometriosis of the uterosacral ligaments. In these situations, gentle mechanical dissection is required in order to ensure complete removal of disease. An uninvolved area of normal peritoneum is chosen adjacent to the lesion, then grasped and elevated. The 3 mm graspers allow just the outer layers of peritoneum to be grasped so the ureter will not tent up into the area of surgery. The elevated peritoneum is then touch cut with the scissors. The scissors are inserted retro-peritoneally and undermine the peritoneum, bluntly separating it from the underlying vital structures. The peritoneal incision can then be extended with slide cuts along the lesion. This further exposes the retroperitoneal space, and the ureter must be identified. In thin patients, the peristalsis may be quite obvious, while further gentle blunt dissection may be required to identify the ureter in other patients. Although it is taught at laparotomy that the ureter is commonly found attached to the peritoneum that is dissected medially off the pelvic sidewall, the laparoscopic perspective is different. With laparoscopic surgery, the peritoneum directly over the ureter is more commonly incised first, and the ureter will often be seen to lie directly beneath the area of dissection in the visual axis of observation. The graspers can now alternately grasp either the peritoneum or the ureter as the scissors bluntly dissect the ureter out of the fibrosis. Occasional short bursts of mono-polar coagulating current will bloodlessly transect peritoneal vessels. It is occasionally necessary to lay the ureter completely bare from the pelvic brim to the uterine vessels. In rare instances the uterine vessels must be sacrificed with bipolar coagulation or endoloops in order to dissect the ureter completely out of investing fibrosis, which may extend toward the base of the bladder.

Retroperitoneal fibrosis resulting from invasive endometriosis can pass the ureter to involve the large pelvic blood vessels, most commonly the branches of the internal iliac artery. The thinner-walled veins fortunately lie deeper along the pelvic sidewall and it is rarely necessary to operate around them. The rigidity of the arteries and the fact that they are less commonly involved with severe fibrosis than is the ureter make the dissection easier, since an artery is a more stable structure than the ureter. Nevertheless, it is necessary to proceed with caution in this area. The use of monopolar coagulation current along the sidewall will occasionally result in stimulation of the muscles controlled by the unseen obturator or femoral nerves. While this does not seem to result in any deficit whatsoever, it is prudent to switch to bipolar coagulation if this recurs often.

Obliteration of the cul-de-sac

Many clinicians view obliteration of the cul-de-sac as an adhesive process only: the colon is stuck to the back of the cervix and it must be unstuck. While this is partly true, the question must be asked 'What is the significance of the rectosigmoid adhering to the back of the cervix and to the uterosacral ligaments in patients with endometriosis?' The answer to this question has two parts. First, since the cul-de-sac and uterosacral ligaments are among the pelvic areas most frequently involved in endometriosis[2], it must be assumed that they are involved by invasive disease. Second, it must be recognized that invasive disease may exist in the wall of the adherent bowel. When these points are recognized, the clinician will realize that laparoscopic surgical treatment must be expanded to accomplish complete excision of disease in all of these areas, otherwise most patients will have persistent disease[3].

The standard laparoscopic technique which will[4] ensure comprehensive treatment of the obliterated cul-de-sac is reproducible and straightforward. Pure cutting current at 90 to 110 watts is used to create lines of incision in normal peritoneum lateral and parallel to the uterosacral ligaments along the length of the ligament to be resected. This will expose the venous structures of the broad ligaments and isolate the pathology into the center of the pelvis. By moving the scissors continuously and using high current density, there is very little lateral thermal spread, making it safe to operate on or around the bowel with electrosurgery. A blunt probe can be used to dissect behind the ligaments just below their insertion into the posterior cervix, isolating the ligaments away from the ureter and uterine vessels. The line of incision in normal peritoneum then leads around the base of each ligament toward the bowel wall, then up and over the bowel wall adjacent to the nodule, meeting the incision from the opposite side. A transverse incision is made across the cervix above the point of adherence of the bowel, then a slightly intrafascial dissection is carried down the posterior cervix toward the rectovaginal septum. Once the cervix is passed, the surgeon will encounter a thin layer of reddish areolar tissue. The yellow fat of the rectovaginal septum will be encountered just beyond this layer of reddish tissue. Once the rectovaginal septum has been dissected bluntly, the uterosacral ligaments now stand isolated on each side of the rectum. They can be transected at their insertions into the posterior cervix using monopolar scissors. The uterosacral ligaments are then dissected off the pelvic floor, working from the cervix posteriorly toward the line of peritoneal incision around the base of the ligaments. The now-exposed fibrous attachments of the rectum to the lateral pelvic walls are progressively severed until sufficient mobility of the bowel has been achieved. All nodular disease of the cul-de-sac, uterosacral ligaments and rectal wall is now isolated in the center of the pelvis attached to the anterior wall of the rectum. The cul-de-sac remains obliterated! The fatty tissue of the rectovaginal septum is stripped off the bowel to expose the longitudinal layer of outer muscularis distal to the mass. At this point, the decision is made either to perform a partial or full thickness disc resection as discussed above, or to perform a segmental resection with end to end anastomosis. With full thickness resections, the surgical specimen can be retrieved transanally.

RESULTS

Excision of endometriosis results in long lasting relief of pain due to endometriosis[5] and a 19% chance of finding new disease in the pelvis five years after surgery[6]. Complications are rare[6] and there have been no significant complications from the use of monopolar electroexcision. Most patients are discharged after an overnight stay, while those undergoing bowel surgery stay until adequate intestinal function has returned. In summary, most cases of endometriosis, including most cases of intestinal endometriosis, can be treated completely by excision, but not by laser vaporization, electrocoagulation, or medical therapy.

References

1. Redwine DB. Treatment of endometriosis of the cul-de-sac. In Nezhat CR, Buttram VB, Berger GS, Nezhat FR, eds. *Modern Surgical Management of Endometriosis*. New York: Springer-Verlag, 1995:105–15
2. Redwine DB. The distribution of endometriosis in the pelvis by age groups and fertility. *Fertil Steril* 1987;47:173–5
3. Reich H, McGlynn F, Salvat J. Laparoscopic treatment of cul-de-sac obliteration secondary to retrocervical deep fibrotic endometriosis. *J Reprod Med* 1991;36:516–22
4. Redwine DB. Laparoscopic en bloc resection for treatment of the obliterated cul de sac in endometriosis. *J Reprod Med*, 1992;37:695–8
5. Redwine DB. Treatment of endometriosis-associated pain. In Olive DL, ed. *Endometriosis: Infertility and Reproductive Medicine Clinics of North America*. Philadelphia: WB Saunders, 1992: 697–720
6. Redwine DB. Conservative laparoscopic excision of endometriosis by sharp dissection: life table analysis of reoperation and persistent or recurrent disease. *Fertil Steril* 1991;56:628–34

Hysterectomy without bilateral salpingo-oophorectomy for endometriosis

28

A.J.M. Audebert and F. Dubecq-Princeteau

INTRODUCTION

For many years certain technical aspects of hysterectomy have generated many debates and controversial opinions concerning the route of choice (including laparoscopy), and whether or not the cervix and the ovaries should be removed.

In cases of severe endometriosis, when a definitive therapy is required, total abdominal hysterectomy (TAH) with bilateral salpingo-oophorectomy (BSO) is usually the recommended procedure[1].

However, opinion is still divided about the value of oophorectomy; in the light of recent data, we intend to critically reassess the benefits and drawbacks of ovarian preservation in cases of surgically treated endometriosis.

GENERAL CONSIDERATIONS ON HYSTERECTOMY

Before discussing the issue of ovarian preservation, a review of some general considerations on hysterectomy appears useful in trying to clarify various relevant aspects which are not specifically related to endometriosis but which may interfere with some issues.

Hysterectomy for endometriosis

As a definitive therapy, TAH with or without BSO is usually indicated in patients with:

(1) severe endometriosis;

(2) intractable and refractory pain;

(3) failure of other treatments;

(4) no desire of further childbearing; and

(5) desire of permanent cure.

In the USA 600 000 hysterectomies are performed each year with 17% of them because of chronic pelvic pain.

In a general gynecological center, 6% of hysterectomies are performed because of endometriosis[2]. In patients with stages III or IV of the disease a radical definitive therapy is required in 10–15% of them.

In a large series of 832 hysterectomies, BSO was performed in 63.5% of 419 patients with endometriosis and in 59.8% of 413 patients without endometriosis[3]. In a more recent series of 138 hysterectomies with the diagnosis of endometriosis BSO was performed in 79% of the patients[4]. These two series indicate that BSO is not performed in 21 to 36.5% of hysterectomies for endometriosis and that there has been a trend during recent years to perform BSO more frequently.

Hormonal consequences of castration

The usual consequences of surgical castration have been assumed to be similar to those of natural menopause. This assumption must, however, be reassessed.

With natural menopause circulating estradiol levels fall progressively and when ovarian production is completely arrested the only remaining source of estrogen is aromatization of adrenocortical androgens in the peripheral adipose tissue[5]. The post-menopausal ovary is still an active endocrine organ with its stroma producing 50% of the testosterone and 30% of the androstenedione available in the circulation[6].

On the other hand BSO induces not only a major decline of circulating estradiol within 24 hours, but also a significant decline of circulating testosterone level. As a consequence, vasomotor symptoms are more acute and more intense and bone loss is more rapid and more profound; within 5 months bone loss is expected to be similar to that measured after 6 months of GnRH agonist therapy. Therefore, estrogen replacement therapy (ERT) should preferably be prescribed as early as possible, and testosterone replacement has to be considered[7].

Table 1 Causes of pain after hysterectomy for endometriosis

Recurrence of endometriosis
Functional disorders
Other causes:
intrinsic vaginal apex pain
post-operative adhesions
residual ovary syndrome
ovarian remnant syndrome

Post-hysterectomy syndrome

This syndrome was first described in 1973[8]. Its determining characteristics as initially described include: pelvic pain, urinary tract symptoms (incontinence and urgency), hormonal changes (in a minority of patients and transient, because of alteration of ovarian blood supply), psychologic abnormalities (e.g. depression), and vasomotor symptoms (even present without BSO).

Subsequent pain following hysterectomy is indeed the most challenging drawback, especially when hysterectomy is indicated to cure intractable pain suspected to be of uterine origin. In a prospective cohort study of 308 women who had hysterectomy for chronic pelvic pain, at one year follow-up 74% of them were cured, 21 % had some improvement, but 5% had either no change or complained of worsened pain[9]. The difficulty when facing such continuous pain is to distinguish between recurrence of pre-operative disease (i.e. endometriosis) and the occurrence of functional disorders[10].

In addition to endometriosis, which will be discussed later, there are several potential causes of recurrent chronic pain, including intrinsic vaginal apex pain, post-operative adhesions, residual ovary and ovarian remnant syndrome (Table 1)[10].

Post-operative adhesions occur in approximately 60 to 90% of women who have had a previous laparotomy[11]. In a prospective cohort study of 590 women undergoing a laparoscopy, visualization of the umbilical area with a microlaparoscope placed at the Palmer's point revealed the presence of adhesions in 48% of those with a midline incision[12]; if adhesions present at other sites are added, a high proportion of patients do have *de novo* formation or re-formation of adhesions. The real cause–effect relationship of adhesions for the origin of pelvic pain is always debatable and pain mapping appears to be a very helpful tool in evaluating this problem.

Pain due to residual ovarian tissue is attributed to adhesions and functional cyst formation, being in this latter case intermittent and responsive to medical treatment by hormonal suppression. Even a normal looking ovary can cause pain; pain mapping is very helpful in deciding whether or not to perform an oophorectomy[10].

Ovarian remnant syndrome[13] is a major concern when BSO is performed for extensive pelvic inflammatory disease or severe endometriosis; careful and often difficult complete ovarian excision is mandatory in order to avoid this secondary complication which may also arise after laparoscopic oophorectomy[14]. This syndrome has been increasingly reported in recent years[15] probably because of more care in its identification. Multiple surgical procedures often stand out as landmarks in the past history of these patients. Despite some alternative modalities such as GnRH agonists or radiotherapy[16], the conventional therapeutic approach is surgical (by laparotomy or laparoscopy) with a risk of recurrence varying from 10% to 20%, as reported in the literature.

Ovarian cancer risk

Ovarian cancer affects approximately 1.2% of women according to epidemiologic evaluation.

In a theoretical calculation, analyzing the past history of patients with ovarian cancer it has been calculated that systematic oophorectomy at the time of hysterectomy for women 40 years old or more would have prevented 5.2% of all potential new cases of ovarian cancer[17].

Another approach is to evaluate ovarian cancers occurring subsequently to hysterectomy without BSO. A meta-analysis of 24 254 hysterectomies without BSO recorded 66 cases of subsequent ovarian cancer. According to the series included in the meta-analysis, rates varied from 0% to 1.2%[18], suggesting that the frequency of ovarian cancer after hysterectomy may indeed be reduced. It is thus estimated that to prevent one ovarian cancer, 500 to 700 BSO should be performed, indicating the magnitude of the problem.

BENEFITS OF OVARIAN PRESERVATION

Ovarian preservation at the time of hysterectomy is associated with multiple alleged protective effects on women's health.

Morbidity and mortality

Any adjunct procedure performed during hysterectomy may theoretically increase morbidity and mortality rates. Morbidity due to BSO has not been accurately evaluated for abdominal hysterectomy; when dealing with severe endometriosis involving both adnexa, it may be difficult to achieve BSO as well as the removal of all endometriotic lesions; when ovaries are free of abnormality, BSO should not significantly increase the morbidity rate.

In cases of abdominal hysterectomy, it has been calculated that BSO increases the mortality rate from 6 to 9 in 10 000 cases[19].

Maintenance of endocrine ovarian activity

In premenopausal women, preservation of ovarian tissue maintains their endocrine function thus preventing short and long term effects of hormonal deficiency. Indeed, after oophorectomy ERT should be considered for all women after definite surgical treatment for endometriosis.

If addition of progestin appears unnecessary then, as previously mentioned, testosterone therapy should be considered at least in some women. The weight of evidence suggests that testosterone may act at the level of the central nervous system, containing in some areas androgen receptors, and in association with estrogen appears to increase bone mass by 2 to 4%[20]. Androgens are effective in women complaining of low energy level, fatigue, loss of well-being, and decreased libido[20].

Timing of ERT is a matter of debate: acute hormonal effects following castration are indicative of immediate replacement therapy. A recent study suggests that patients who begin ERT immediately after TAH with BSO are not at greater risk of recurrent pain than those who delay ERT for more than 6 weeks[21].

The major drawback of ERT is its variable patient compliance. If compliance to replacement therapy seems better in women after hysterectomy and BSO in comparison with women after natural menopause, long-term compliance rates have been usually reported to be poor[22]. Thirty-one percent to 98% of women do not begin the prescribed replacement therapy[23]. If appropriate patient education is used, this improves compliance as reported in more recent studies. For current users aged 50 or above, median compliance rates with HRT have increased from 24 months in 1991 to 60 months in 1995[24]. For women ovariectomized at a young age, an ERT duration of 5 years leaves many years with an unfavorable hormonal milieu before reaching the usual age of natural menopause.

Risk of ovarian cancer

The risk of malignant transformation of endometriosis is rare (1%), with the ovary being the more commonly affected site. Extragonadal sites may also occur accounting for approximately 25% of all cases of malignant transformation; some cases have been reported after TAH with BSO and unopposed estrogen therapy.

A decreased relative risk (RR) for cancer in preserved ovaries has been demonstrated, depending upon the age when hysterectomy was performed. The RR are respectively 0.58 and 0.52 for women less than 40 years old and those older at the time of hysterectomy with a follow-up of 10 years[25]. In a case control study the RR for ovarian cancer was 0.50 when hysterectomy had been performed at least 15 years before[26].

Psychological impact

Patients' attitudes to hysterectomy and oophorectomy are variable. Removal of the ovaries may induce secondary psychological disturbances with alterations of orgasmic capacity, femininity perception and sexual life[27]. A survey on the attitude to oophorectomy of 109 women at the time of hysterectomy indicates that 62.6% of them had expressed regret at undergoing BSO[28].

DISADVANTAGES OF OVARIAN PRESERVATION

Recurrence of the symptoms or of the disease and potential reoperation are the main issues in patients who undergo an intended definitive surgical therapy, usually after a long past history of severe pain and multiple failed treatments, both medical and/or surgical.

The analysis of published reports on recurrences is very confusing for the following reasons:

(1) the definition of recurrences is variable (i.e. symptoms, pain, endometriotic lesions or reoperation);

(2) all studies are usually retrospective and non-randomized;

(3) the length of follow-up is variable; and

(4) there is unavoidable center selection bias in some series.

Recurrent symptoms

For practical reasons I will concentrate on the recurrence of pain, since it is the most common of all symptoms in the large series reviewed.

We have seen that not only recurrent endometriosis may cause pain but also other reasons are frequently responsible for the discomfort (e.g. adhesions, residual ovary syndrome, ovarian remnant syndrome . . .); it has been assumed that 90% of women with postoperative pain have adhesions present and no evidence of recurrent disease[10]. However, if recurrent endometriosis is present, it is not necessarily the cause of the pelvic pain[29].

A review of published series indicates a trend for earlier reports to support ovarian preservation, and in contrast a tendency for advising oophorectomy in more recent articles (Table 2).

In 1988 Wilson quoted a 3% recurrence rate for persistent symptoms after TAH without BSO[30]. In a review of published data with a total number of 1300 patients, the rate of recurrent symptoms or reoperation after hysterectomy with ovarian conservation was 7%[31]; in the same review, 373 patients with ERT after hysterectomy and BSO had a recurrence rate of 8%[29].

Table 2 Symptom recurrences and reoperation rates reported in the literature

Author	*Year*	*Recurrences of symptoms* (%)	*Reoperations* (%)
TH without BSO			
Sheets *et al.*[35]; Ranney[36];	1963, 1970	–	1–3
Andrews & Larsen[37]	1974		
Hammond *et al.*[39]	1976	–	85
Wilson[30]	1988	3	–
Walters[31]	1989	7	–
Henderson & Studd[28]	1991	–	25
Namnoum *et al.*[4]	1995	62	31
TH with BSO			
Henderson & Studd[28]	1991	–	1.1
Walters[31]	1988	8	–
Namnoum *et al.*[4]	1995	10	3.7

More recently, a prospective study of 109 women who underwent hysterectomy with the diagnosis of endometriosis compares the recurrence rate of pain. While 10% of oophorectomized women had some type of recurrent symptoms, the frequency was 62% in those in whom some ovarian tissue was preserved[4]. The calculated relative risk for recurrence of pain in women not having undergone BSO has been estimated as 6.1[4].

Replacement therapy does not seem to affect notably the recurrence of pain, even if it is well known that reactivation of endometriotic lesions can occur[4]. On the other hand, progression of endometriosis after definitive therapy including ovarian removal, has been reported even in the absence of estrogen therapy[32].

Reoperation

Reoperation as another indicator of the outcome of hysterectomy with or without BSO, may be more reliable since its definition is clear.

Depending on the real cause and the severity of recurrent pain, a medical treatment should always be recommended before proceeding to surgery. If hormonal therapy is not always effective for the treatment of endometriosis occurring after oophorectomy[33], in the future new modalities such as aromatase inhibitors may prove to be more efficient[34].

Again, reported reoperative rates are extremely variable. Earlier studies reported that very few women require reoperation (1% to 3%) following TAH with ovarian conservation[35–38]. However, other studies report higher rates of reoperation, ranging from 25% to 85% when the ovaries have been retained at the time of hysterectomy[28,39].

In a study previously quoted[4], reoperation rates for women having undergone hysterectomy were respectively 3.7% after BSO and 31% without BSO; the calculated relative risk for reoperation was 8.1 when ovaries were retained[4].

CONCLUSIONS

Complete ablation of endometriosis is claimed to be 90% effective in relieving symptoms of pain[40] and definitive surgery therapy is required in 12 to 15% of the women with severe forms of the disease.

The decision to perform the removal of the ovaries at the time of hysterectomy cannot be made on evidence-based medicine: present data on the frequency of symptoms recurrence and reoperation when some ovarian tissue has been retained, are very controversial and no randomized control studies have been published. It does seem, however, that ovarian preservation may expose the patient to more symptom recurrence and reoperations. Furthermore, pain persistence following hysterectomy is related, in a great number of cases, to causes other than recurrent endometriosis.

The consequences of ovarian castration can be prevented by hormonal replacement therapy, but in general routine practice the patient's compliance appears to be still far from what is desirable; proper counseling may improve the compliance as indicated by a few recent studies.

Thus, the decision whether or not to perform bilateral oophorectomy at the time of hysterectomy should be individualized, weighing the risks and benefits of both alternatives.

TAH without BSO appears reasonable in younger women, with less severe damage and preferably without bowel or urinary involvement, wishing to preserve their ovaries providing they are willing to accept a greater risk of recurrent symptoms and a possible increased need for reoperation.

References

1. Lu PY, Ory SJ. Endometriosis: current management. *Mayo Clin Proc* 1995;70:453–63
2. DeMeeus JB, Magnin G. Indications of laparoscopic hysterectomy. *Eur J Obstet Gynecol Reprod Biol* 1997;74:49–52
3. Williams TJ, Pratt JH. Endometriosis in 1,000 consecutives celiotomies: incidence and management. *Am J Obstet Gynecol* 1977;129:245–50
4. Namnoum AB, Gehlbach DL, Hickman TN, *et al.* Incidence of symptoms recurrence after hysterectomy for endometriosis. *Fertil Steril* 1995;64:898–902
5. Vermeulen A. The hormonal activity of the postmenopausal ovary. *J Clin Endocrinol Med* 1976; 42:247–53
6. Adashi EY. The climacteric ovary as a functional gonadotropin driven androgen producing gland. *Fertil Steril* 1994;62:2027
7. Studd J, Khastgir G. Hormone replacement therapy after hysterectomy. In Studd J, ed. *The Management of the Menopause. Annual Review 1998.* New York: Parthenon Publishing,1998:257–70
8. Richars DS. A post hysterectomy syndrome. *Lancet* 1973;11:430
9. Hillis SD, Marchbanks PA, Peterson HB. The effectiveness of hysterectomy for chronic pelvic pain. *Obstet Gynecol* 1995;86:941–5
10. Steege JF. Pain after hysterectomy. In Steege JF , Metzger DA, Levt BS, eds. *Chronic Pelvic Pain.* Philadelphia: W.B. Saunders Co., 1998:135–44
11. Monk BJ, Berman ML , Montz FI. Adhesions after extensive gynecologic surgery: clinical significance, etiology and prevention. *Am J Obstet Gynecol* 1994;170:1396–401
12. Audebert AJM. The role of microlaparoscopy for safer wall entry: incidence of umbilical adhesions according to past-surgical history. *Fertil Steril* 1999; in press
13. Shemwell RE, Weed JC. Ovarian Remnant Syndrome. *Obstet Gynecol* 1970;36:299–303
14. Nezhat F, Nezhat C. Operative laparoscopy for treatment of ovarian remnant syndrome. *Fertil Steril* 1992;57:1003–7
15. Lafferty HW, Angioli RJ, Rudolph J, *et al.* Ovarian remnant syndrome: experience at Jackson Memorial Hospital, University of Miami, 1985 through 1993. *Am J Obstet Gynecol* 1996;174: 641–5
16. Thoms WW, Hughes LL, Rock J. Palliation of recurrent endometriosis with radiotherapeutic ablation of ovarian remnants. *Fertil Steril* 1997; 68:938–40
17. Slighter S, Boike G, Estape R , *et al.* Ovarian cancer in women with prior hysterectomy: a 14 year experience at the university of Miami. *Obstet Gynecol* 1991;78:681–5
18. Kazadi Buanga J, Rira Montane J, Laparte ES, *et al.* L'ovaire restant après hystérectomie. *Rev Fr Gynécol Obstét* 1994;89:14–20
19. Cole P, Berlin J. Elective hysterectomy. *Am J Obstet Gynecol* 1977;129:117–23
20. Sherwin BB. Efficacy of combined estrogen-androgen preparations in the menopause. In Studd J, ed. *The Management of the Menopause. Annual Review 1998.* New York: Parthenon Publishing, 1998:271–7
21. Hickman TN , Namnoum AB, Hinton EL, *et al.* Timing of estrogen replacement therapy

following hysterectomy with oophorectomy for endometriosis. *Obstet Gynecol* 1998;91:673–7
22. Hammond CB. Women's concerns with hormone replacement therapy. *Fertil Steril* 1994; 62:157S–160S
23. Speroff T, Dawson N, Speroff L, *et al.* A risk benefit analysis of elective bilateral oophorectomy: effect of changes in compliance with estrogen therapy on outcome. *Am J Obstet Gynecol* 1991;164:165–74
24. Mac Lemman AM, Wilson DH, Taylor AW. Hormone replacement therapy: prevalence, compliance and the 'healthy woman' notion. *Climacteric* 1998;1:42–9
25. Whittemore A, Harris R, Itnyre J. Characteristics relating to ovarian cancer risk: collaborative analysis of 12 US case control studies. *Am J Epidemiol* 1992;136:1184–203
26. Parazinni F, Negri E, Lavechia C, *et al.* Hysterectomy, oophorectomy and subsequent ovarian cancer risk. *Obstet Gynecol* 1993; 81: 363–6
27. Nathorst-Boos J, Von Schoultz B. Psychological reactions and sexual life after hysterectomy with and without oophorectomy. *Gynecol Obstet Invest* 1992;34:97–102
28. Henderson AF, Studd JWW. The role of definitive surgery and hormone replacement therapy in the treatment of endometriosis. In Thomas E, Rock J, eds. *Modern Approaches to Endometriosis.* Dordrecht: Kluwer Academic Publishers, 1991:275–90
29. Stout AL, Steege JF, Dodson WC, *et al.* Relationship of laparoscopic findings to self-report of pelvic pain. *Am J Obstet Gynecol* 1991;164:73–9
30. Wilson EA. Surgical therapy for endometriosis. *Clin Obstet Gynecol* 1988;31:857–65
31. Walters MD. Definitive surgery. In Schenken RS, ed. *Endometriosis. Contemporary Concepts in Clinical Management.* Philadelphia: JB Lippincott Company, 1989:267–78
32. Redwine DB. Endometriosis persisting after castration: clinical characteristics and results of surgical management. *Obstet Gynecol* 1994;83: 405–9
33. Metzger DA, Lessey BA, Soper JT, *et al.* Hormone-resistant endometriosis following total abdominal hysterectomy and bilateral salpingo-oophorectomy: correlation with histology and steroid receptor content. *Obstet Gynecol* 1977;78: 946–50
34. Takamaya K, Zeitoun K, Gunby RT, *et al.* Treatment of severe postmenopausal endometriosis with an aromatase inhibitor. *Fertil Steril* 1998;69:709–13
35. Sheets JL, Symmonds RE, Banner EA. Conservative surgical management of endometriosis. *Obstet Gynecol* 1963;23:625–8
36. Ranney B. Endometriosis I. Conservative operations. *Am J Obstet Gynecol* 1970;107:743–53
37. Andrews WC, Larsen GD. Endometriosis treatment with hormonal pseudopregnancy and/or operation. *Am J Obstet Gynecol* 1974; 118:643–51
38. Wheeler JH, Malinak LR. Recurrent endometriosis: incidence, management and prognosis. *Am J Obstet Gynecol* 1983;146:247–53
39. Hammond CB, Rock JA, Parker RT. Conservative treatment of endometriosis: the effects of limited surgery and hormonal pseudopregnancy. *Fertil Steril* 1976;27:756–66
40. Olive DL, Schwartz LB. Endometriosis. *N Engl J Med* 1993;328:1759–69

Laparoscopic treatment of extensive endometriosis of the bowel, bladder, ureter and diaphragm

29

C.H. Nezhat, F. Nezhat and C. Nezhat

Severe pelvic endometriosis frequently involves the lower rectosigmoid colon, rectum, ureter, bladder and occasionally the small bowel and diaphragm. In this presentation we describe our approach for the treatment of severe endometriosis involved with these organs.

PREOPERATIVE EVALUATION

Preoperative evaluation includes thorough clinical and laboratory evaluation, imaging techniques such as pelvic ultrasound for the evaluation of the uterus and ovaries and IVP, barium enema or sigmoidoscopy in selected cases. Mechanical and antibiotic out-patient bowel preparation is performed the day before the procedure. Preoperative and intraoperative consultations with a colorectal surgeon and/or urologist, and in the case of diaphragmatic endometriosis a thoracic surgeon, is necessary. Informed consent is obtained.

SURGICAL TECHNIQUE

Under general endotracheal anesthesia, the patient is placed in the modified dorsolithotomy position. Multiple puncture videolaseroscopy begins with the placement of the intra-umbilical operative laparoscope and three suprapubic portals. The suction irrigation probe, bipolar electrodesiccating forceps and the grasping forceps are introduced. Needle holders, laparoscopic endostapler or scissors are substituted as necessary. Superpulse or UltraPulse high power CO_2 laser is used through the operative channel of the laparoscope for the purpose of excision and vaporization. The abdominal and pelvic cavity is explored and the lesions are identified and any associated procedures are performed.

URINARY TRACT ENDOMETRIOSIS

Urinary tract involvement is estimated to occur in 1% to 16% of patients with endometriosis. Fewer than 1% are reported to have obstruction or infiltrative disease. We define urinary tract involvement as full thickness or deep infiltration of the muscularis layer in the bladder and partial or complete obstruction of the ureter. Of the 28 patients in our series, 7 (25%) had vesical and 21 (75%) had ureteral disease. Involvement of the urinary tract with endometriosis is relatively uncommon, but it can be clinically significant. It can involve the bladder or completely obstruct the ureter resulting in loss of kidney function.

BLADDER ENDOMETRIOSIS

Using hydrodissection, the peritoneum over the bladder is opened and a bladder flap is created. After dissecting the bladder from the surrounding tissue, the bladder is entered via cystotomy and the involved area is resected using the CO_2 laser or scissors. Simultaneous cystoscopy is performed to improve observation of the ureteral orifices and for retrograde catheterization. The defect is closed in one layer using the extra or intracorporeal knot tying technique with 4-0 polydioxanone or 0 polyglactin suture and cystoscopy is performed at the end of the procedure to ensure water tight closure. Bladder drainage is continued for 7–14 days based on the size of the defect postoperatively. Before discontinuing bladder drainage, cystogram is performed to confirm that the bladder has healed and there is no leakage.

URETERAL ENDOMETRIOSIS

Extensive enterolysis is required, i.e. mobilization of the ureter adhered to the pelvic wall. The retroperitoneal space is entered at the level of the pelvic brim. The overlying peritoneum is opened with the CO_2 laser and elevated by injecting irrigation fluid. The opening is enlarged and an irrigation probe is inserted with more fluid introduced into the retroperitoneal space along the course of the ureter. The fluid surrounding the ureter moves it posteriorly, and allows safe superficial laser desiccation or vaporization. If the endometrial implant is imbedded and deeply scarred, the ureter is freed from surrounding tissue using hydrodissection and CO_2 laser, avoiding damage to the major pelvic wall and blood vessels. Any bleeding that is not controlled by the laser is managed with bipolar electrodesiccation.

After ureterolysis is completed, endometriosis and fibrosis are vaporized or excised until the ureter is dissected completely and free of disease. At this point, if the ureter is obstructed partially or completely, requiring resection, a retrograde ureteral catheter is placed via cystoscopy with laparoscopic guidance. Partial wall resection is done over the catheter. Pinpoint entries to the lumen are not repaired.

When the lumen is invaded, the ureter is repaired in one layer using 4-0 polydioxanone sutures. If the lumen was occluded completely and retrograde catheter placement was unsuccessful, we transect the ureter at that point using the laser or sharp scissors and excise the obstructed section. Indigo carmine is injected antegrade to verify patency of the proximal lumen. Anastomosis is performed over the ureteral catheter with four interrupted through-and-through, 4-0 polydioxanone sutures at 3,6,9 and 12 o'clock to approximate the proximal and distal ureteral segments or to rejoin the ureter and bladder using intracorporeal or extra-corporeal knot tying. The ureteral stent is removed 2 to 8 weeks postoperatively after the integrity of the repair is confirmed by IV pyelogram.

BOWEL ENDOMETRIOSIS

The incidence of intestinal endometriosis is hard to define because patient selection biases most reports. Accordingly, estimates have a wide range, from 3 to 37%. It has been estimated that 50% of patients with severe endometriosis have some degree of bowel involvement. The most common sites of bowel endometriosis are the rectum, rectosigmoid colon, appendix and ileocecum. We have defined bowel endometriosis as a disease that has invaded the muscularis of the intestine.

The treatment of intestinal endometriosis has evolved considerably over the last decade. The traditional management has been ovarian ablation, either medical or surgical, with most surgeons reluctant to resect the colon or rectum for fear of complications. However, currently many surgeons support a more aggressive approach that includes resecting all visible and detectable endometriosis, and preserving fertility whenever feasible and desired by the patient.

Advocates of radical bowel resection note that large endometriotic bowel lesions may be fibrotic and unresponsive to hormonal manipulation. This is consistent with the observation that bowel endometriosis can occur even in postmenopausal women. In addition, large implants of the bowel may scar, and ultimately lead to obstruction. Complete resection of all endometriotic bowel lesions may also prevent local recurrence and the need for subsequent surgery, and avoid possible, though rare, malignant degeneration of colorectal endometriomas.

Some authorities still reserve bowel resection for near-obstructing lesions and those suspected of malignancy. One of the major arguments against colorectal resection for endometriosis is the potential morbidity of the resection and anastomosis. A second concern is the increased incidence of adhesions, and consequently potential decrease in fertility, as most patients with endometriosis are young and interested in future childbearing. Thus, it is apparent that when an aggressive surgical approach is chosen for benign, non life-threatening disease, a low associated operative morbidity is essential to warrant the operation. Our laparoscopic and/or laparoscopically-assisted surgical techniques, aimed at achieving minimal morbidity without compromising the complete resection of the endometriotic bowel lesion will be described. This goal is accomplished by carefully devising the extent of laparoscopic operation according to the degree of endometriosis bowel infiltration. We have used several techniques for the treatment of bowel endometriosis, based on the location and degree of involvement.

Shaving technique

This technique is used when the lesion is infiltrative to the muscularis layers, but does not involve the full thickness of the bowel. Several centimeters of the rectosigmoid colon can be involved with the disease, including the fibrofatty tissue surrounding the rectum and rectosigmoid. A combination of excision and vaporization is used to remove the lesion. Constant irrigation and suction are performed to remove the plume and tissue debris. If an enterotomy occurs, or if the muscularis is completely denuded and the mucosa reached, this is repaired in one layer, through-and-through, using 3-0 silk, 4-0 PDS, or vicryl sutures.

Disk excision

Disk excision can be performed completely laparoscopically, transvaginally, or transrectally, based on the location of the lesion. Full-thickness excision begins above the area of visible disease. For a complete laparoscopic approach, after mobilization of the bowel and identifying normal tissue, the lesion is held at its proximal end with grasping forceps. An incision is made through the bowel serosa, muscularis and mucosa, and the lumen is entered. The lesion is completely excised from the anterior rectal wall. Following complete excision of the lesion, the pelvic cavity is thoroughly irrigated and suctioned. Two traction sutures are applied to each side of the bowel defect, transforming it into a transverse opening. The bowel is then repaired by placing several interrupted through-and-through sutures spaced 0.3 to 0.6 cm apart using 3-0 silk, 0-polyglactin, or 4-0 PDS laparoscopic sutures and a straight or curved needle with extracorporeal or intracorporeal knot tying.

Anterior rectosigmoid resection with transanal or transvaginal prolapse

When there are multiple lesions or a larger portion of the bowel is involved, an entire segment of bowel is resected. The technique used depends on the location of the lesion. If the lesion is in the rectum or lower rectosigmoid colon, the bowel is mobilized by entering the pararectal area, rectovaginal septum, and posterior rectosigmoid colon from the presacral space to the levator muscles, as is done via laparotomy. The branches of the inferior mesenteric vessels are electrodesiccated and cut if necessary. The involved segment is prolapsed either transvaginally or transrectally.

The lesion is transected. The anal (distal) portion of the transected rectum is replaced into the pelvic cavity. The resected segment is sent for pathologic diagnosis, and a 2-0 polypropylene pursestring suture is placed around the circumference of the proximal limb of the bowel. The anvil of an ILS 29 or 33 stapler (Ethicon) is placed through the pursestring into the proximal bowel, and the proximal limb of the bowel is replaced into the pelvis. Using Babcock clamps, the distal rectal segment is prolapsed through the anal canal, closed with an RL60 (when the initial resection is not being performed by stapler), and replaced through the anal or vaginal canal into the pelvis. In a modification of this technique, after the bowel is mobilized, it is divided intra abdominally using the CO_2 laser or a 60 mm Endostapler (Ethicon®, Cincinatti, USA) above or below the lesion. The proximal portion is then exteriorized transanally or transvaginally.

The ILS circular stapler is then placed into the rectum, and the anvil trocar within the proximal bowel is inserted into the stapling device using the laparoscope and a laparoscopic anvil holder. The device is fired, creating an end-to-end anastomosis. A proctoscope is used to examine the anastomosis for structural integrity and bleeding.

Segmental resection through a minilaparotomy

When the lesion is on the upper portion of the sigmoid, ileocecum, or small bowel, this technique is utilized. The portion of bowel to be resected is mobilized using the CO_2 laser or scissors for cutting and bipolar, surgical clips, or laparoscopic stapler (EZ35W, Ethicon, Inc.) to desiccate or clip the mesocolon attachment and vasculature. The location and size of the ancillary incision are modified on the basis of the area of the involved bowel. A minilaparotomy is performed in the mid-suprapubic, left, or right-lower quadrant by extending the corresponding ancillary incision. The bowel is guided to the minilaparotomy with grasping forceps. Resection and anastomosis are performed in a routine manner and the bowel is returned to the abdominal cavity.

Before termination of the procedure and at the end of all surgical techniques the pelvis is filled with lactated Ringer's solution and observed with the laparoscope as the rectum is insufflated with air to check for leakage.

DIAPHRAGMATIC ENDOMETRIOSIS

Diaphragmatic endometriosis has been the subject of incidental case reports. It may be asymptomatic, produce pain in the right or left upper quadrant of the abdomen, or refer to pain of the left shoulder. When there has been penetration of the diaphragm with extension into the pleural space pneumothorax or hemothorax, then hemoptysis may result. This rare condition raises several diagnostic and treatment challenges. We have treated a series of patients diagnosed with diaphragmatic endometriosis with good results.

Laparoscopy is performed through an umbilical site in the manner previously described. If endometriosis infiltrating the muscularis of the diaphragm is unexpectedly encountered, treatment should not begin until it has been verified that a cardiothoracic surgeon is immediately available, if needed.

All procedures are performed under general endotracheal anesthesia with the patients in a modified dorsolithotomy position. The diaphragm is examined as part of the routine abdominal exploration completed during the initial phase of every laparoscopic procedure. If better visualization of the diaphragm is required, patients are placed in a steep reverse Trendelenburg position. When endometriosis involving the diaphragm is highly suspected, or if surgical treatment is needed after making the diagnosis, additional trocars are placed in the upper quadrant, right or left according to the implant location, similar to the arrangement for laparoscopic cholecystectomy or splenectomy. An atraumatic grasping forceps or suction irrigator probe is used to push down the liver from the operative field and enable better exposure of the diaphragm. When the lesions are superficial (only serosal surface involvement without penetration to the muscularis), they are vaporized using a combination of hydrodissection and a carbon dioxide (CO_2) laser (15–25 watts) or cavitational ultrasonographic surgical aspirator (CUSA). Hemostasis is achieved with bipolar electrocoagulation.

Deep endometriotic lesions infiltrating the diaphragm muscularis are removed using hydrodissection and sharp dissection with the aid of the CO_2 laser set at 20–25 watts. A laparoscopic aspirating needle is inserted through one of the ancillary ports and used to inject 5–10 cc lactated Ringer's under the lesion. The lesion is grasped with a grasping forceps and the CO_2 laser is used to make an incision around the lesion. While the suction irrigator probe is used for traction, evacuation of smoke, and as a backstop for the CO_2 laser, the lesion is excised. Any remaining lesions are vaporized. Biopsies are not routinely performed because of technical difficulty and danger of perforating the diaphragm.

CONCLUSION

Involvement of the extragenital organs with endometriosis is not uncommon. Careful preoperative evaluation can guide the surgeon towards the involvement. Appropriate preparation and consultation along with other disciplines, such as the colorectal, urological and thoracic surgeons should be performed. In the hands of a skilled laparoscopist, familiar with endometriosis and its natural course, most of these procedures can be safely and effectively carried out laparoscopically.

References

1. Andrews WC. Medical versus surgical management of endometriosis. *Clin Obstet Gynecol* 1980; 23:917–24
2. Fianu S, Ingelman-Sundberg A, Nasiell K, *et al.* Surgical treatment of post abortum endometriosis of the bladder and postoperative bladder function. *Scand J Urol Nephrol* 1980; 14:151–5
3. Neto WA, Lopes, RN, Cury M, *et al.* Vesical endometriosis. *Urology* 1984;24:271–4
4. Nezhat CR, Nezhat FR, Luciano AA, *et al.* *Operative Gynecologic Laparoscopy: Principles and Techniques.* New York, NY: McGraw Hill, 1995
5. Nezhat C, Berger S, Nezhat F, *et al. Endometriosis: Advanced Management and Surgical Techniques.* New York, NY: Springer Verlag, 1995
6. Smith MS. Cystotomy and vesicostomy. In Glenn JF, ed. *Urologic Surgery*, 4th edn. Philadelphia: J.B. Lippincott, 1995: 1042
7. Nezhat C, Nezhat F. In Gomel V, Taylor P, eds. *Diagnostic and Operative Gynecologic Laparoscopy.* New York: Mosby-Year Book, Inc., 1995:201–18
8. Nezhat C, Nezhat F, Nezhat CH, *et al.* Urinary tract endometriosis treated by laparoscopy. *Fertil Steril* 1996;66:920–4
9. Gray LA. Endometriosis of the bowel; role of bowel resection, superficial excision and oophorectomy. *Ann Surg* 1973;177:580–7
10. Bailey HR. Colorectal endometriosis. *Perspect Colon Rectal Surg* 1992;5:251–9
11. Weed JC, Ray JE. Endometriosis of the bowel. *Obstet Gynecol* 1987;69:727–30
12. Coronado C, Franklin RR, Lotze EC, *et al.* Surgical treatment of symptomatic colorectal endometriosis. *Fertil Steril* 1990;53:411–16
13. Nezhat F, Nezhat C, Pennington E. Laparoscopic proctectomy for infiltrating endometriosis of the rectum. *Fertil Steril* 1992;57:1129–32
14. Nezhat F, Nezhat C, Pennington E, *et al.* Laparoscopic segmental resection for infiltrating endometriosis of the rectosigmoid colon: a preliminary report. *Surg Laparosc Endos* 1992;2: 212–16
15. Nezhat CH, Seidman D, Nezhat F, *et al.* Laparoscopic surgical management of diaphragmatic endometriosis. *Fertil Steril* 1998

Differential effects of GnRH agonist therapies: implications regarding the estrogen threshold hypothesis

30

S.K. Agarwal

Over the last two decades, GnRH agonists have been widely used for a number of gynecologic indications. Apart from endometriosis, which is probably the main use for these drugs by the general gynecologist, other uses for women's health include the medical management of fibroids, polycystic ovary syndrome, premenstrual syndrome, central precocious puberty, breast cancer, assisted reproduction and via pulsatile administration for ovulation induction in situations such as Kallman's syndrome.

DIFFERENTIAL EFFECTS OF GNRH AGONISTS

A number of chemically distinct agents are now available within this class of drug. They are administered by a variety of routes and in various doses. However, for the treatment of endometriosis, conventional thought has been that their biological actions with regard to efficacy and adverse event profiles are indistinguishable. Thus the choice of drug used is dependent solely upon cost and physician and patient convenience, the main determining factors being cost and route of administration.

Figure 1 shows the amino acid sequences of a number of currently available GnRH agonists. The synthetic analogs, as well as endogenous GnRH, are all decapeptides. Gonadorelin is a synthetic replica of endogenous GnRH, while others all have substitutions at either the sixth or the tenth amino acid position. The reason for these substitutions is that GnRH and the analogs are lysed by blood borne peptidases at the sixth and tenth positions, which leads to their inactivation. Amino acid substitution at these sites confers a degree of protection from this degradation. Since GnRH and the analogs circulate within the hypophyseal portal system almost totally unbound to carrier proteins, any protection from the circulating proteases enhances half-life and thus the potency of the drugs. For example, endogenous GnRH and Gonadorelin have half-lives of between two and four minutes. In contrast, nafarelin and leuprolide have half-lives of approximately three hours. Another factor that influences the half-life of these drugs is the actual amino acid composition. Substitutions of amino acids for more hydrophobic ones confers further protection from degradation and hence translates into a further extension in half-life.

The route of administration also has the potential to impact on the clinical profile of these drugs. Currently used GnRH agonists can be administered subcutaneously, by intramuscular injection, intranasally, or as implants. In addition, it is possible that inhalation may also one day be a viable route of administration for this class of drug. The degree of absorption varies with the route of administration and bioavailability of the agents is thereby affected.

The administered dose varies by agent and route such that studies of nafarelin have ranged from 125 to 800 μg/d, leuprolide from 1.0 to 11.25 mg in the form of daily, monthly or three monthly preparations, goserelin has

	Peptide position									
AGENT	1	2	3	4	5	6	7	8	9	10
GnRH	Pyrog	His	Trp	Ser	Tyr	Gly	Leu	Arg	Pro	Gly
Gonadorelin	Pyrog	His	Trp	Ser	Tyr	Gly	Leu	Arg	Pro	Gly
Leuprolide*	Pyrog	His	Trp	Ser	Tyr	**Leu**	Leu	Arg	Pro	**Ethylamide**
Nafarelin*	Pyrog	His	Trp	Ser	Tyr	**Nap**	Leu	Arg	Pro	Gly
Goserelin*	Pyrog	His	Trp	Ser	Tyr	**Ser**	Leu	Arg	Pro	**Aza-Gly**
Buserelin	Pyrog	His	Trp	Ser	Tyr	**Ser**	Leu	Arg	Pro	**Ethylamide**
Tryptorelin	Pyrog	His	Trp	Ser	Tyr	**Trp**	Leu	Arg	Pro	Gly

Major sites of cleavage (between positions 5 and 6, and between positions 9 and 10)

*FDA approved for the treatment of endometriosis

Figure 1 Peptide sequences of endogenous gonadotropin-releasing hormone (GnRH) and synthetic analogs. The half-life of a GnRH agonist is increased by incorporation of hydrophobic amino acids. Adapted from Agarwal, 1998[11]

uniformly been studied at 3.6 mg implants dosage and buserelin has been evaluated at doses from 200–1200 µg.

Although chemical structure, route of administration and dose can independently influence the therapeutic profile of GnRH agonists, it is the collective effect of the therapeutic regimen that is of clinical importance. Given the wide variability in possible therapeutic regimens, it would not be surprising if differences in efficacy or side-effect profile were to exist.

Clearly, the ideal manner in which to compare the clinical profiles of the various GnRH agonists would be via a direct comparison in the form of a well designed, randomized clinical trial. Because many of the parameters of drug efficacy including dyspareunia, dysmenorrhea and pelvic pain and of adverse events such as hot flushes are subjective, blinding and placebo control are critical components in any study design. In addition, the study should have the power to detect small differences in any of the important points. A major side-effect of these drugs is a decrease in trabecular bone mineral density and hence, when assessing this, a sensitive technique such as dual energy X-ray absorptiometry (DEXA) should be employed and the bone mineral density (BMD) should be measured at a site that is sensitive to the effects of hypoestrogenemia such as the vertebrae.

Only two studies are available that directly compare the effects of different GnRH agonists. The first concentrated on the effects of these drugs on BMD[1]. It was a randomized study with eight women receiving leuprolide 1.6 mg intranasally per day, eight women randomized to goserelin 1.2 mg intranasally per day while the third arm had nine women who received subcutaneous buserelin 200 µg/day. There was a six month treatment phase and all subjects received one gram of calcium per day. Bone mineral density was measured at the lumbar site by dual photon absorptiometry (DPA). The design employed a single blind (observer) and no placebo was used. No changes in bone mineral density were observed. This is not surprising, since the study was small with just eight or nine subjects per arm and DPA was used to measure BMD, a technique which lacks sensitivity. The chances of detecting any differences in BMD were remote. A second, larger and more recent study compared the efficacy and side-effect profiles of nafarelin and leuprolide[2]. This was a randomized study with over 90 subjects per arm, randomized to receive either nafarelin 400 µg intranasal per day or leuprolide 3.75 mg intramuscularly per month. These were the lowest FDA approved doses for the treatment of endometriosis and treatment was administered for six months, with a subsequent six-month post treatment observation phase. Bone mineral density was

Table 1 The effect of 6 months, GnRHa treatment on vertebral BMD as measured by QCT

Study	*n*	*GnRHa*	*Dose*	*% BMD loss*
Cann *et al.*[3]	19	Nafarelin	400 μg/d	7.2
	18	Nafarelin	800 μg/d	6.7
Whitehouse *et al.*[6]	15	Nafarelin	400 μg/d	5.9
Matta *et al.*[7]	11	Buserelin	1200 μg/d	5.9
Dawood *et al.*[8]	18	Buserelin	1200 μg/d	7.4
Wheeler *et al.*[9]	8	Leuprolide	3.75 mg/m	15.1
Dlugi *et al.*[10]	8	Leuprolide	3.75 mg/m	11.8

Reproduced, by permission, from Agarwal, 1998[11]

measured at the lumbar site by DEXA. A double-blind and double-placebo study design was incorporated. The efficacy end points recorded were pelvic pain, dysmenorrhea, dyspareunia, pelvic tenderness and pelvic induration. The findings with respect to efficacy were not surprising in that both treatment regimens were equally efficacious. However, with regard to the side-effect profiles, surprisingly, significant differences were detected. Subjects receiving leuprolide were noted to experience a higher number of days with hot flushes and there was a tendency for these flushes to be more severe. In addition, the BMD loss at the end of six months treatment was significantly greater ($p = 0.002$) in the subjects receiving leuprolide. Analysis of serum estradiol levels indicated that women on leuprolide tended to have a greater suppression of ovarian function with lower circulating levels of estradiol than those receiving nafarelin. It is possible that the differences in circulating estradiol concentrations help to explain why the hypo-estrogenic side-effects were worse in those receiving leuprolide. In view of the difference in side-effect profiles, it is interesting that the efficacy of the two therapeutic regimens was comparable.

For further evaluation of the comparative effects of GnRH agonists, one has to resort to comparing studies. Since most are small, employing a variety of patient profiles, measuring BMD using a number of different technologies and techniques, very little can be conclusively derived from such an analysis. However, a couple of observations can be made. Table 1 shows the adverse effects of GnRH agonist treatments for endometriosis on BMD from a number of studies. These have been selected because they measured bone mineral density loss at the vertebrae as measured by quantitative computerized tomography (QCT) after six months of treatment. QCT is a highly sensitive technique for measuring trabecular BMD, but is not used clinically because of the excessive radiation exposures. One can see that the study by Cann in 1987[3] evaluating two doses of nafarelin found a similar decrease in bone mineral density after six months of treatment, was despite a two-fold increase in dose in one arm. The other observation is that the regimens employing nafarelin or buserelin (both of which are administered on a daily basis) produce less BMD loss than those studies employing leuprolide which, in these studies, was administered on a monthly basis.

Table 2 shows the efficacy of GnRH agonists for the treatment of symptomatic endometriosis in a number of studies. It can be seen that the depot preparations leuprolide and goserelin as well as the higher dose of nafarelin 400 μg bid produce a greater suppression of estradiol – in the range of 13–15 pg/ml. The studies evaluating intranasal buserelin 300 μg tid and intranasal nafarelin 200 μg bid produced less estradiol

Table 2 The efficacy of 6 months' GnRHa administration in the treatment of endometriosis

Study	*n*	*GnRHa*	*Dose*	*Estradiol concentration* (pg/ml)	*% Decrease in AFS score*	*Pain relief % women*
Henzl *et al.*[12]	77	Nafarelin	200 μg bid IN	28	43	73
	79	Nafarelin	400 μg bid IN	15	42	77
Cirkel *et al.*[13]	40	Buserelin	300 μg tid IN	28	51	–
Dlugi *et al.*[10]	52	Leuprolide	3.75 μg/m IM*	15	–	89
Shaw[14]	40	Goserelin	3.6 mg implant	13	50	70

*20 week treatment; reproduced with permission from Agarwal, 1998[11]

suppression – in the range of approximately 28 pg/ml. However, this differential suppression of estradiol did not appear to result in differences in the degree of pain relief experienced by the women.

The implication of these studies is that a decrease in circulating estradiol level to the range of 30–40 pg/ml as has been observed with nafarelin and buserelin regimens is therapeutically as effective as suppression of estradiol to levels of 15 pg/ml or less that is commonly encountered with depot preparations of leuprolide or goserelin. This differential suppression of estradiol does, however, seem to result in a greater loss of BMD in those receiving the depot prepa-rations.

THE SIGNIFICANCE OF BMD LOSS DUE TO GNRH AGONIST THERAPY

Although there is an increase in BMD once GnRH agonist therapy is stopped, I have concerns about therapies that may lead to some overall loss in BMD. It is unknown as to whether such therapy leads to an overall increased risk of fracture in later years. Any loss of BMD with therapy is particularly important since we cannot predict whether the patient will receive further GnRH agonist treatment in years to come; therapy that may further impact on her BMD. Lifestyle factors such as smoking or alcohol and caffeine intake may further lead to an accelerated loss of BMD or failure to reach peak BMD. It has been documented that a slight decrease in BMD at menopause can translate into several additional years with a BMD below the fracture threshold (Figure 2). This is of considerable concern given that women are now living longer and more women-years are being spent at an age vulnerable to osteoporotic fractures. Since the correlation between BMD and fracture risk is strong and, in fact, better than that between serum lipids and risk of cardiovascular event, the extra time

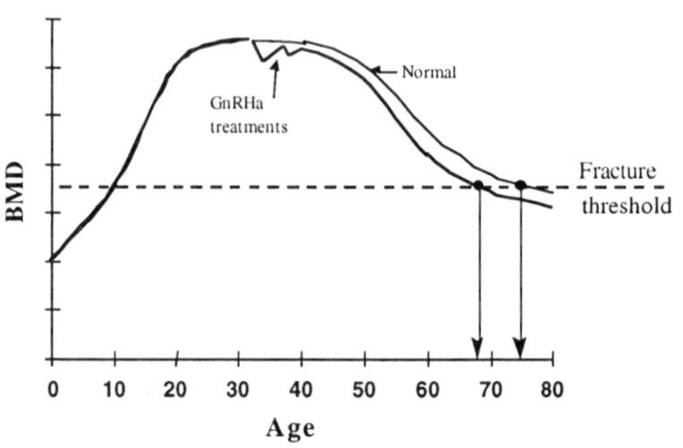

Figure 2 Potential long-term effects of gonadotropin-releasing hormone (GnRH) agonist therapy on bone mineral density (BMD). It is possible that with repeated or prolonged GnRH agonist therapy, a woman will reach menopause with less than her optimal BMD. A small decrease in BMD at this time of accelerated loss can translate into the woman spending an additional several years with a BMD below the fracture threshold – several years at significant risk for osteoporotic fractures

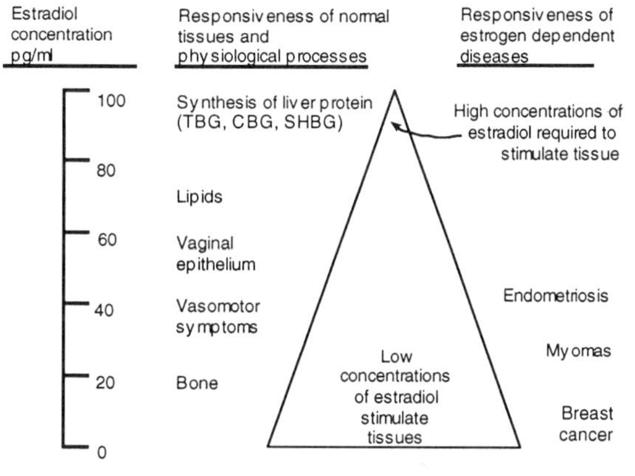

Figure 3 Variation in sensitivity to estradiol of normal and disease processes. TBG, thyroxine-binding globulin; CBG, corticosteroid-binding globulin; SHBG, sex-hormone binding globulin. Adapted with permission from Barbieri, 1992[4]

spent with a BMD below the fracture threshold represents a very real time at significant risk of fracture. Although post-menopausal estrogen replacement can be used to prevent osteoporosis, most women do not take this hormonal therapy for long enough for it to prevent osteoporosis.

THE ESTROGEN THRESHOLD HYPOTHESIS

The above information has some bearing on the estrogen threshold hypothesis that was published in 1992[4]. The basis for this hypothesis was that tissues vary in their sensitivity to estradiol[5]. The hypothesis highlighted the observation that although decreasing estradiol produced changes in bone mineral density, lipids, vaginal epithelium, vasomotor symptoms and endometrium, the magnitude of alteration varied between these tissue systems. Figure 3 shows the responsiveness of normal tissues to changes in circulating estradiol levels. A significant loss in BMD does not occur until the estradiol level is below approximately 20 pg/ml, vasomotor symptoms begin at a higher estradiol level of about 40 pg/ml, vaginal epithelium starts to become atrophic just below about 60 pg/ml and so on. The figure also outlines the responsiveness of various disease processes to estradiol level. For the treatment of breast cancer suppression of estradiol has to be below 10 pg/ml. For the treatment of myomas one has to achieve an estradiol level of below about 25 pg/ml and for the treatment of symptomatic endometriosis, an estradiol level of below approximately 40 pg/ml is required. Therefore, one can see with regard to the treatment of endometriosis, that there is what has been termed a 'therapeutic window' with an estradiol concentration of between 30 and 50 pg/ml. If a decrease in circulating estradiol concentration to this range is achieved, it would be expected that the loss of BMD will be minimized without compromising the treatment of endometriosis. Clearly, the exact therapeutic window will vary from woman to woman but a circulating estradiol level of between 30 and 50 pg/ml should, in general, be the target.

Other supporting data

Further evidence supporting the estrogen threshold hypothesis comes from the observation that after bilateral oophorectomy for endometriosis, low dose estrogen replacement therapy decreases menopausal symptoms without a dramatic increase in the recurrence of endometriosis lesions. Three studies have evaluated the impact of estrogen replacement therapy in women after bilateral oophorectomy for endometriosis. Table 3 shows the results from these studies and it can

Table 3 Estrogen replacement and symptom recurrence

Investigator	*No. studied*	*No. (%) with pain recurrence after ERT*
Ranney[15]	46	0 (0)
Gray[16]	119	21 (18)
Hammond *et al.*[17]	96	5 (5)
Total	261	26 (10)

Adapted from Barbieri, 1998[18]

be seen that on average there is a 10% recurrence rate for pain, presumably due to reactivation of endometriosis. These data suggest that low circulating levels of estrogen, as occurs with hormone replacement therapy, are sufficiently high to alleviate vasomotor symptoms but are generally insufficient to reactivate symptomatic endometriosis.

In conclusion, increasing evidence is available validating the estrogen threshold hypothesis. The data suggest that, in accordance with this hypothesis, it may be possible to modify current GnRH agonist therapies for the treatment of endometriosis so as to reduce hypoestrogenic side-effects while maintaining efficacy.

References

1. Tummon IS, Ali A, Pepping ME, *et al.* Bone mineral density in women with endometriosis before and during ovarian suppression with gonadotropin-releasing hormone agonists or danazol. *Fertil Steril* 1988;49:792–6
2. Agarwal SK, Hamrang C, Henzl MR, *et al.* Nafarelin vs. Leuprolide acetate depot for endometriosis: changes in bone mineral density and vasomotor symptoms. *J Reprod Med* 1997; 42:413–23
3. Cann CE, Henzl MR, Burry KA, *et al.* Reversible bone loss is produced by the GnRH agonist nafarelin. In Cohn DV, Martin TJ, Meunier PJ, eds. *Calcium regulation and bone metabolism: Basic and clinical aspects.* Amsterdam: Excerpta Medica 1987:123–7
4. Barbieri RL. Hormone treatment of endometriosis: the estrogen threshold hypothesis. *Am J Obstet Gynecol* 1992;166:740–5
5. Chetkowski RJ, Meldrum DR, Steingold KA, *et al.* Biologic effects of transdermal estradiol. *N Eng J Med* 1986;314:1615–20
6. Whitehouse RW, Adams JE, Bancroft K, *et al.* The effects of nafarelin and danazol on vertebral trabecular bone mass in patients with endometriosis. *Clin Endocrinol* 1990;33:365–73
7. Matta WH, Shaw RW, Hesp R, *et al.* Reversible trabecular bone density loss following induced hypo-oestrogenism with the GnRH analogue buserelin in premenopausal women. *Clin Endocrinol* 1988;29:45–51
8. Dawood MY, Lewis V, Ramos J. Cortical and trabecular bone mineral content in women with endometriosis: effect of gonadotropin-releasing hormone agonist and danazol. *Fertil Steril* 1989;52:21–6
9. Wheeler JM, Knittle JD, Miller JD. Depot leuprolide acetate versus danazol in the treatment of women with symptomatic endometriosis: a multicenter, double-blind randomized clinical trial. II. Assessment of safety. The Lupron Endometriosis Study Group. *Am J Obstet Gynecol* 1993;169:26–33
10. Dlugi AM, Miller JD, Knittle J. Lupron depot (leuprolide acetate for depot suspension) in the treatment of endometriosis: a randomized, placebo-controlled, double-blind study. Lupron Study Group. *Fertil Steril* 1990;54:419–27
11. Agarwal SK. Comparative effects of GnRH agonist therapy. Review of clinical studies and their implications. *J Reprod Med* 1998;43:293–8
12. Henzl MR, Corson SL, Moghissi K, *et al.* Administration of nasal nafarelin as compared with oral danazol for endometriosis. A multicenter double-blind comparative clinical trial. *N Engl J Med* 1988;318:485–9
13. Cirkel U, Schweppe KW, Ochs H, *et al.* Gonadotropin down-regulation in gynecological practice. In Chada DR, Rolland R, Willemsen WNP, eds. *Effect of LH-RH agonist therapy in the treatment of endometriosis.* New York: A.R. Liss, Inc., 1986:189–99
14. Shaw RW. Current concepts in endometriosis. In Chada DR, Buttram, eds. *Current Concepts in Endometriosis.* New York: A.R. Liss, Inc., 1990:323–83
15. Ranney B. Endometriosis. 3. Complete operations. Reasons, sequelae, treatment. *Am J Obstet Gynecol* 1971;109:1137–44
16. Gray LA. Endometriosis of the bowel: role of bowel resection, superficial excision and oophorectomy in treatment. *Ann Surg* 1973;177: 580–7
17. Hammond CB, Rock JA, Parker RT. Conservative treatment of endometriosis: the effects of limited surgery and hormonal pseudopregnancy. *Fertil Steril* 1976;27:756–66
18. Barbieri RL. Endometriosis and the estrogen threshold theory. Relation to surgical and medical treatment. *J Reprod Med* 1998;43:287–92

Expanding the utility of the GnRH agonists in the treatment of endometriosis 31

M.D. Hornstein

INTRODUCTION

Since their introduction in 1982, the gonadotropin-releasing hormone (GnRH) agonists have been demonstrated to be safe and efficacious in the treatment of endometriosis. They have become the mainstay of medical management of endometriosis-associated pelvic pain in many countries. Their use, however, has generally been limited to a single 6-month course of therapy owing to the drugs' hypoestrogenic side-effects. In fact, in the United States, the Food and Drug Administration (FDA) has limited the use of this class of medications to a single 6-month treatment period owing to concerns over bone density loss. Until recently, it was not clear whether shorter treatment intervals were efficacious and whether they reduced the hypoestrogenic effects of the GnRH agonists. Unfortunately, pain often returns following a single medical treatment for endometriosis. Thus, retreatment would be advantageous, but until recently, there have been no studies to demonstrate the efficacy of retreatment with the GnRH agonists. Although surgery is clearly beneficial to patients suffering from endometriosis-associated pelvic pain, it has been unclear whether medical treatment following laparoscopic surgery would prolong the beneficial effects of surgery. The goals of this chapter are to: (1) assess the efficacy of a shorter course of GnRH agonist therapy; (2) assess the efficacy and safety of retreatment; and (3) determine whether a postoperative course with a GnRH agonist enhances the effects of laparoscopic surgery. This chapter reviews data from three large multicenter prospective randomized controlled trials using nafarelin to attempt to answer these questions.

SHORT-TERM THERAPY

In 1995, Hornstein *et al.*[1] published their findings on the use of the GnRH agonist nafarelin in a 3-month trial. The bone density findings were published separately[2]. In order to enter the study, each patient had to have clinical symptoms presumed to be caused by endometriosis, such as pelvic pain, dysmenorrhea, or dyspareunia. Patients were excluded from the study if they had received hormonal treatment for endometriosis within 3 months preceding study entry; had significant medical illnesses, laboratory test abnormalities, or prior treatment with a GnRH agonist; or were breastfeeding or pregnant. A total of 189 patients were enrolled, but owing to exclusions, data from 183 patients were included in the bone density studies, and 179 patients were included in the efficacy study. The study was carried out by investigators at 15 sites in a double-blind prospective randomized fashion. Patients were randomized to receive 3 months of 200 μg of intranasal nafarelin twice daily followed by 3 months of placebo, or to receive 6 months of nafarelin at the same dosage. Patients were followed for a minimum of 12 months after completion of treatment. Of the 179 patients in the efficacy study, 39 from the 3-month group and 43 from the 6-month group completed the 18-month study without requiring further treatment other than

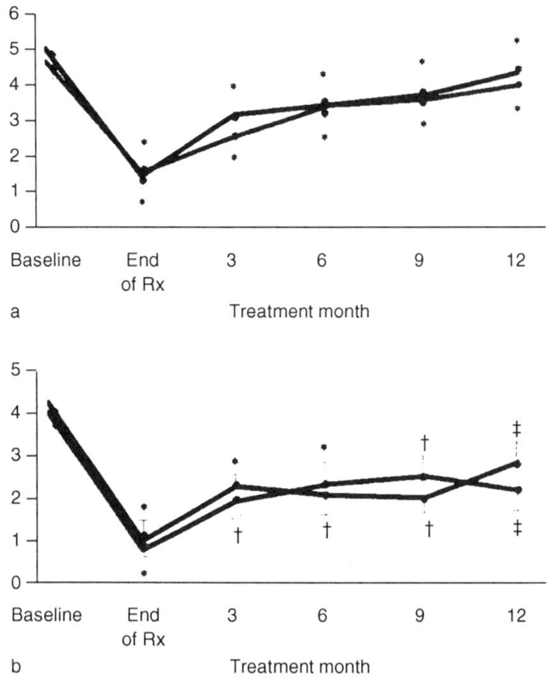

Figure 1 Changes in the mean patient-reported symptom score: (a) intent-to-treat analysis; (b) completed patients' analysis for dysmenorrhea, dyspareunia, and pelvic pain combined at baseline; at end of treatment; and at 3, 6, 9 and 12 months after cessation of treatment. ——, group I, nafarelin 3-month treatment; - - -, group II, nafarelin 6-month treatment. Results reported as means ± SEM. *, $p < 0.0001$; †, $p < 0.01$; ‡, $p < 0.01$ compared with baseline

periodic analgesic medications. The major efficacy endpoints for the study were patient-reported pain symptoms and physician-reported findings on physical examination. For the patient-reported symptoms, the patients completed a pain survey assessing dysmenorrhea, pelvic pain, and dyspareunia on a 0–3 scale developed by Biberoglu & Behrman[3]. In addition, the examining physician completed an assessment based on pelvic examination for tenderness and pelvic induration on a similar 0–3 point scale.

The treatment groups were well matched by age, height, weight, cycle length, mean American Fertility Society Endometriosis score[4] upon entry and ethnic origin. The results were reported as an intent-to-treat analysis and in an analysis of patients completing the study. A total pain index summing the patients' reported pain scores for dysmenorrhea, pelvic pain, and dyspareunia at baseline, at end of treatment, and at 3, 6, 9 and 12 months is seen in Figure 1a. Similarly, pelvic pain scores are reported in Figure 1b for patients who completed the study. As seen in Figure 1, pain and tenderness scores in both groups dropped significantly from the initiation to the end of therapy. After treatment, pain in both the 3- and the 6-month groups increased in a fairly linear fashion until the end of the study. The pain scores remained lower at the end of the study than at study entry, however, at the end of the study they were nearly as high as those at the beginning of the study, suggesting a relatively rapid return of pain symptoms. It was significant that the two treatment groups had nearly identical scores in both the intent-to-treat and the completed patient analyses, thus demonstrating the efficacy of the shorter course of therapy.

The other outcome variable was bone density. The bone loss in the patients treated for the 6-month interval was relatively modest (no greater than 4%) and less in the 3-month group. There was a fairly rapid return toward baseline in both treatment groups, but even 12 months after therapy, there was still some bone loss noted in both groups.

RETREATMENT

As previously noted, GnRH agonists are only approved by the US FDA for a single 6-month course in the treatment of endometriosis owing to concerns about bone density loss. To address these concerns, a second study was undertaken to assess the value of retreatment with a short (3-month) course of nafarelin, in terms of the drug's ability to both induce a second clinical improvement and not cause significant loss in bone density[5].

This study had a multicenter prospective open-label design and included patients who had participated in the comparative trial of 3- and 6-month treatment with nafarelin.

Women who had responded favorably to nafarelin treatment in the previous study and had spinal bone density within 2 standard deviations of the mean for age-matched women or had a decrease in lumbar bone density of less than 2% from baseline in the prior study were eligible to begin retreatment for 3 months. Patients could not be enrolled until at least 6 months had elapsed since GnRH agonist therapy. As in the prior study, patients' self-reported pelvic pain on a 0–3 scale for dysmenorrhea, dyspareunia, and pelvic pain, and physicians reported pelvic tenderness and pelvic induration on physical examination on a similar scale. The study included a bone mineral density assessment by dual X-ray absorptiometry of the lumbar spine within 2 months of starting treatment. Bone density was reassessed 3 months after the cessation of treatment.

Patients in the follow-up study had a mean age of 32.7 years. The mean interval from the last dose of treatment to first dose of retreatment was 10.1 months in patients originally treated for 3 months and 10.8 months in those originally treated for 6 months. On entry, 90% of patients reported moderate or severe dysmenorrhea, only 24% of patients had moderate or severe dyspareunia, and 61% of patients reported moderate or severe pelvic pain. At the end of the 3-month retreatment interval, only 3% of patients had moderate or severe dysmenorrhea, 14% moderate or severe dyspareunia, and 16% moderate or severe pelvic pain. In all, 95% of patients reported moderate or severe symptoms at the beginning of retreatment, and only 29% did so at the end of retreatment. The improvement of endometriosis symptoms over the full 3 month treatment interval is shown in Figure 2.

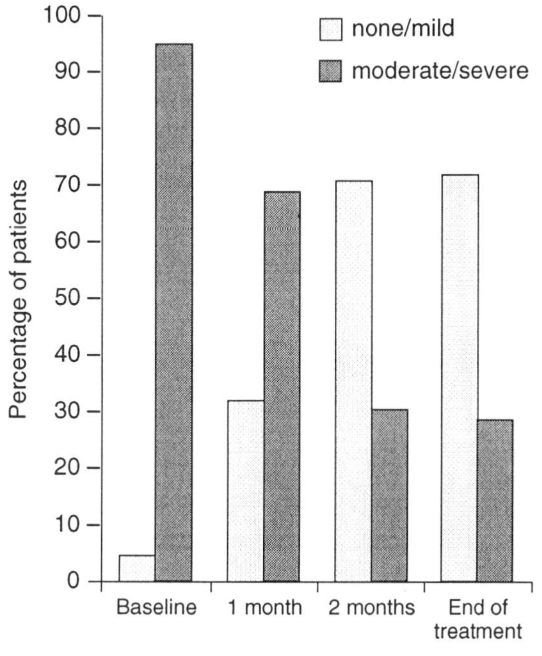

Figure 2 Severity of endometriosis symptoms during retreatment with nafarelin. The total severity score is the sum of the scores for each of five signs or symptoms: dysmenorrhea, dyspareunia, pelvic pain, pelvic tenderness and pelvic induration. Each of the five was scored as follows: 0, absent; 1, mild; 2, moderate; and 3, severe. The total severity score was interpreted as follows: 0, no symptoms; 1 or 2, mild; 3 through 5, moderate; 6 through 10, severe; and 11 through 15, very severe

An important consideration in such a study is whether a significant amount of bone density was lost during retreatment. Patients entering retreatment had lost a mean of 1.43% of bone density compared with values on entry into the original study. Three months after retreatment, they had only lost an additional 0.56% of bone density, not a statistically significant difference. This difference was not significantly different from study entry. Three months after retreatment, the total bone density was only 1.94% lower than at the initiation of the original treatment.

This study demonstrated that 3-month retreatment with a GnRH agonist for recurrent endometriosis symptoms was clearly effective, with significant improvements in pain severity scores from baseline to the end of retreatment for all signs and symptoms. Three months after retreatment, the symptom severity score had increased but was still significantly lower than baseline for several of the symptoms. What is important is that patients had lost only an additional 0.56% of bone mineral density 3 months after retreatment.

In a similar study, Adamson *et al.*[6] evaluated 45 women previously treated for 6 months with nafarelin who had recurrent symptoms and signs of endometriosis. Retreatment of these patients with 400 µg per day of nafarelin intranasally for an additional 3 months alleviated recurrent symptoms and signs of endometriosis. Lumbar bone mineral density decreased but only by a mean of 2% at the end of treatment and was restored within 3–6 months following completion of treatment. This study verified that a short retreatment course (3 months) with a GnRH agonist is both efficacious and safe.

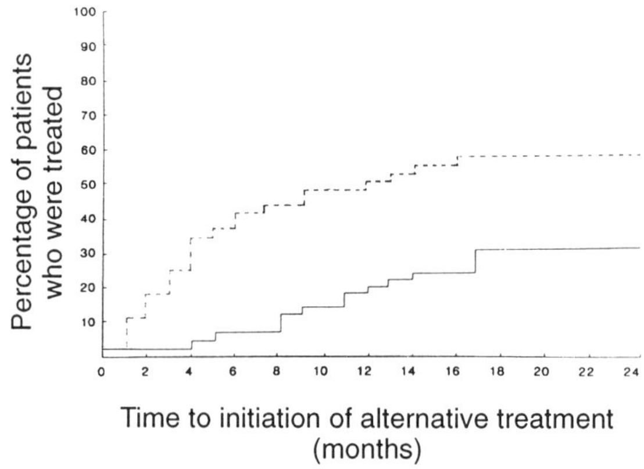

Figure 3 Time to initiation of alternative treatment for patients who were treated postsurgically with nafarelin (——) versus placebo (- - -)

POSTLAPAROSCOPIC TREATMENT

Despite the fact that both laparoscopic surgery and GnRH agonist treatment are known to provide long-term relief for pelvic pain associated with endometriosis, the combination of surgical and medical treatment had been largely unstudied. The purpose of this 6-month study was to evaluate, in a multicenter prospective double-blind trial, the efficacy of a GnRH agonist versus placebo after reductive laparoscopic surgery for endometriosis-associated pelvic pain. The primary endpoint was the time to initiation of alternative treatment for patients treated with nafarelin or a placebo, postsurgically.

One hundred and nine patients at 13 sites were enrolled and randomized in this double-blind study[7]. Following reductive laparoscopy surgery for endometriosis by laser or electrocautery or both, patients were treated for 6 months with nafarelin 200 µg twice daily, or placebo nasal spray and then followed for an additional 18 months. A total of 93 patients were available for analysis.

Patients had clinical symptoms of pelvic pain, dysmenorrhea, or dyspareunia presumed by the investigators to be endometriosis associated and underwent operative laparoscopic surgery for endometriosis in the menstrual cycle preceding study enrollment. Patients treated with danazol, androgen, hormones, or a GnRH agonist within 3 months or with oral contraceptives within 2 months preceding enrollment were excluded. Following reductive laparoscopic surgery, patients began treatment with nafarelin or placebo on day 1 or 2 of their next menstrual cycle. Patients were asked to rate their pelvic pain using the same scale as in previous studies. In addition, physicians recorded their examination findings for pelvic tenderness and induration. The patient and physician scores were summed separately to yield a 'subject summary rating' and a 'physician summary rating'.

The two treatment groups were comparable in age, height, weight, age at menarche, cycle length and the percentage who had moderate or severe pelvic pain on study entry. The median time to initiation of alternative treatment – either surgery or hormonal treatment for endometriosis including oral contraceptives, danazol, or repeat courses of GnRH agonists – was greater than 24 months in the treated group and 11.7 months in the placebo group. Thirty-one per cent of the nafarelin-treated patients required alternative therapy, compared with 57% of the placebo-controlled group (Figure 3). The subject summary rating showed a significant decrease in pain scores in the treated group from baseline to the end of active treatment; although pain scores increased in the 6 months following active treatment, they still remained below those of baseline. The nafarelin-treated patients reported significantly less pain than their placebo-treated counterparts at the end of treatment; however, the difference between the groups disappeared within 6 months following active treatment. The physician summary rating scores dropped significantly in the nafarelin-treated group from baseline to the end of treatment but not in the placebo-treated group. Six months after active treatment, the difference in physician-reported scores between the nafarelin- and placebo-treated patients persisted.

Thus, the major findings of this study were that treatment with a GnRH agonist significantly prolonged the time between surgery and the need for significant additional medical or surgical therapy – more than twice the period for placebo-treated patients. In addition, fewer nafarelin-treated than placebo-treated patients required alternative therapy.

SUMMARY

Taken together, the studies reported here demonstrate that short courses of a GnRH agonist are safe and efficacious. They may be particularly beneficial in patients who either do not desire a standard 6-month course of treatment or cannot tolerate this longer treatment period. Patients can also be safely retreated with GnRH agonist without significant additional bone loss. Such retreatment is both efficacious and safe. Lastly, patients who receive GnRH agonist therapy following laparoscopic surgery have a longer interval before requiring additional therapy for endometriosis. In summary, these studies provide additional flexibility in the prescribing of GnRH agonist for endometriosis-associated pelvic pain.

References

1. Hornstein MD, Yuzpe AA, Burry KA, *et al.* Prospective randomized double-blind trial at 3 versus 6 months of nafarelin therapy for endometriosis associated with pelvic pain. *Fertil Steril* 1995;63:955–62
2. Orwoll ES, Yuzpe AA, Burry KA, *et al.* Nafarelin therapy in endometriosis: long-term effects on bone mineral density. *Am J Obstet Gynecol* 1994; 171:1221–5
3. Biberoglu KO, Behrman SJ. Dosage aspects of danazol therapy in endometriosis: short-term and long-term effectiveness. *Am J Obstet Gynecol* 1981;139:645–54
4. The American Fertility Society. Revised American Fertility Society classification of endometriosis: 1985. *Fertil Steril* 1985;43:351–2
5. Hornstein MD, Yuzpe AA, Burry K, *et al.* Retreatment with nafarelin for recurrent endometriosis symptoms: efficacy, safety, and bone mineral density. *Fertil Steril* 1997;67:1013–18
6. Adamson GD, Heinrichs WL, Henzl MR,*et al.* Therapeutic efficacy and bone mineral density response during and following a three-month retreatment of endometriosis with nafarelin (Synarel). *Am J Obstet Gynecol* 1997;177:1413–18
7. Hornstein MD, Hemmings R, Yuzpe AA, *et al.* Use of nafarelin versus placebo after reductive laparoscopic surgery for endometriosis. *Fertil Steril* 1997;68:860–4

Management of endometriosis: historical background and rationale for the use of steroid hormones

32

G. Benagiano, A. Pera and P. Bianchi

INTRODUCTION

There are several reasons why it is important to revisit the use (and, perhaps also the misuse) of steroid hormones in the management of endometriosis, the first being that many physicians utilize them, in the absence or almost of controlled data.

A second, equally important reason is that a fairly large number of substances, with very different activity and mechanism of action, have been utilized over the last 50 years; by re-evaluating what has been tested and through a critical analysis of all of these treatment regimens, there are still lessons to be learned.

This is particularly true because, one century after the first description of the presence of ectopic endometrium in the pelvis[1] and more than 75 years after Cullen[2] and Sampson[3] identified the disease, the scientific community is still debating the true origin and meaning of endometriosis[4].

This level of uncertainty, probably unequalled in gynecology outside oncology, has had a profound influence on the therapeutic approaches taken for the disease, because treatment is logically the last link in the chain of events leading to the successful management of an illness[5]. As a consequence, no medical treatment ever tested has proven to be superior to expectant management if infertility is associated with endometriosis[6].

The situation is different when considering the symptoms associated with the presence of an ectopic endometrium and in particular with the inflammatory reaction surrounding it. In this case a variety of medical and surgical options exists and hormones and antihormones have been tried with different degrees of success.

HISTORICAL DEVELOPMENTS

The hormonal management of the symptoms associated with endometriosis was made possible, more than 50 years ago, by the availability of synthetic androgens and of diethylstilbestrol. The first attempt in patients with severe endometriosis was made by Hirst[7] in 1943, when – following a suggestion of Salmon & Geist[8] – he reported the results obtained with the use of testosterone propionate in two cases. Treatment resulted in reduction in swelling and relief of pain and Hirst suggested this form of treatment when radical surgical excision was contraindicated or refused[7].

The following year Miller published a case of endometriosis of the rectal wall and ovaries, treated preoperatively with testosterone propionate. He stated: 'testosterone propionate can be used in diminishing the activity and decreasing the size of the lesions in endometriosis so that radical surgery can be performed with less danger'[9].

In commenting on the use of androgens Kistner, some 15 years later, noted that 'androgenic substances, while adequately documented as having produced desirable results in endometriosis, probably exert their effect through inhibition of gonadotrophic substances although direct effect of the substance upon the endometriotic area has been suggested. The undesirable side effects of hirsutism, acne, and deepening of the voice occur sufficiently often to cause the clinician and the patient considerable concern'[10].

The next attempt, still in the 1940s, strange as it might sound today, was to utilize the newly available diethylstilbestrol at high doses. Karnaky, in 1948, reported apparently good results with increasing daily doses of up 100 mg/day to obtain amenorrhea. He concluded that 'endometriosis is not stimulated to grow by large continuous doses of stilbestrol, but small doses of stilbestrol may stimulate it'[11].

In Karnaky's series five patients became pregnant after stilbestrol was discontinued. With today's knowledge, the fact that some endometriosis patients become pregnant, with or without treatment, should surprise no-one.

In spite of the enthusiasm of its proponent, estrogen treatment of endometriosis did not last, and for good reasons, as underlined by Kistner, who wrote: 'the unpredictability of permanent relief in endometriosis following the use of estrogenic substances alone' and the fact that 'estrogen therapy also has the disadvantage of occasionally resulting in rather profuse "break-through" bleeding, endometrial hyperplasia and hypermenorrhea at the time of withdrawal of the hormone'[10], make this treatment unwise.

Indeed, it is today well known that, at the basis of any discussion on steroid treatment there is a fact: endometriosis, although in all likelihood not an endocrine disease, does not appear in the absence of estrogens.

In the case of the disease manifesting itself in post-menopausal women, the latter are usually treated with estrogens[12,13]; in the rare occurrence in non-treated post-menopausal women[13], it is commonly believed that symptoms are the consequence of the progression of the estrogen-independent fibrosis, not of the growth of new foci[14].

At the same time, there is evidence that estrogens are not necessary for the endometrium to implant itself ectopically and indeed, grafting studies in nude mice and, rabbits have shown that estrogen is not necessary for the success of the implantation process[15,16].

In contradistinction to this, the proliferation and growth of ectopic implants need the presence of estrogen. Dizerega and co-workers[15] found, in castrated monkeys, that hyperplastic-decidualized endometrial tissue transplanted into the peritoneum retains viability for more than 4 weeks, even without exogenous hormonal support, but the administration of supplemental estrogen and/or progesterone is required to sustain these endometrial plaques for periods of up to 16 weeks.

In addition, in a rat animal model experimentally implanted with human endometrial cells, following ovariectomy there is a complete regression of the implants, to the point that – two months later – no viable endometrial cells can be detected, even histologically[17].

Figure 1a shows a histological section of the site of the original endometrial graft two months after ovariectomy, and – clearly – there is no evidence of any viable endometrial tissue. Administration of estradiol cypionate to these animals, however, leads to the recurrence of regressed implants, as shown in Figure 1b.

Finally, although endometriosis has been observed in the urinary bladder of men with prostatic carcinoma[18,19], in the case of pure gonadal dysgenesis[20] and Turner's syndrome[21–23] and in a woman with a Rokitansky–Kuster–Hauser syndrome[24], all these patients had endogenous or exogenous estrogens, or were given estrogen–progestogen combinations. Therefore, the concept that estrogens are necessary in order to have active ectopic endometrial foci so far goes unchallenged.

Under the circumstances, a rational approach to the hormonal treatment of endometriosis must involve the use of steroid hormones with an activity capable of either modulating or antagonizing that of endogenous estrogens.

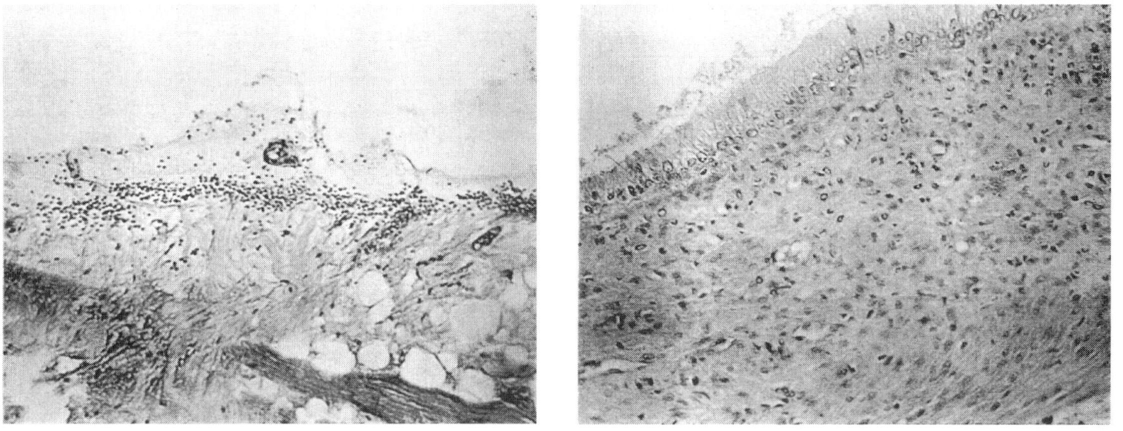

Figure 1 Effect of estrogen in experimental endometriosis. Histological sections of the sites of endometrial grafts in the rat: (a) 2 months after transplant, followed by ovariectomy; notice the complete disappearance of any viable endometrial tissue; (b) one month after the administration of estradiol cypionate to ovariectomized animals; notice the recurrence of the disappeared implants. Reproduced with permission from Rajakumar *et al.*[17]

PSEUDOPREGNANCY AS A THERAPEUTIC REGIMEN

It is fair to state that the first attempt in this direction and the first real advance in the hormonal management of endometriosis came with the advent of the so-called 'pseudo-pregnancy regimen' introduced by Kistner[10] and Andrews[25]. The concept arose from a suggestion made by Meigs[26] who stated: 'It is the author's belief that avoidance of endometriosis through early marriage and frequent childbearing is the most important method of prophylaxis'. Kistner[10] correctly pointed out that 'in many patients with this disease conception is not always possible either because of unknown factors producing infertility or because marriage is not contemplated'. To resolve the impasse, they induced a state of 'pseudopregnancy' in 12 patients by combining large doses of a number of estrogenic compounds (diethylstilbestrol, Estinyl, estradiol valerate) and two progestins (17-hydroxyprogesterone caproate and norethynodrel) in a 'graduate scale' for periods of time up to 7 months and produced amenorrhea as well as a decidual reaction in the endometria of all patients. In general the pseudopregnancy regimen resulted in an improvement of the condition, both subjectively and objectively, except for occasional side-effects like uterine cramps or hypermenorrhea.

A further step ahead was introduced by Andrews and his group[25], when – starting from the same observation of the beneficial effects of pregnancy on endometriosis – they administered Enovid (norethinodrel plus mestranol) to 23 women with endometriosis. Decidual transformation was consistently demonstrated in the endometrial cavity and was present in the ectopic endometrium in all of the five instances in which it was obtained for study. Clinical improvement during therapy was observed in 14 of 17 patients treated because of pain.

To improve the effectiveness of the pseudopregnancy regimen, in 1960 Thomas[27] introduced long-acting steroid hormones and treated 28 women with established endometriosis with an injectable preparation (Delalutin) containing 250 mg of 17-hydroxyprogesterone caproate and 5 mg of estradiol valerate, twice a week for a minimum of 4–6 months. All the patients developed amenorrhea, which persisted throughout the period of hormone administration, and most of the women experienced considerable to complete relief of their symptoms.

Table 1 Major studies reporting on the use of the pseudopregnancy regimen for the management of endometriosis. Reproduced with permission from Moghissi[28]

Investigator	*Combination*	*No. cases*	*Symptomatic relief (%)*	*Pregnancies (%)*
Riva *et al.* (1961)	Norethynodrel and mestranol (2.5 mg)	83	90	10.5
Kistner (1966)	Norethynodrel and mestranol (2.5 mg)	110	79	47.0
Kourides & Kistner (1968)	Norgestrel (0.5 mg) and ethinyl estradiol (0.05 mg)	19	84	54.0
Andrews & Larsen (1974)	Ethynodiol diacetate (1 mg) and Mestranol (0.1 mg)	31	–	25.8

The estrogen–progestogen regimen has been used extensively since then for the treatment of endometriosis, although the last paper on the subject was published in 1975. Symptomatic relief of the disease was reported in a majority of cases; pregnancy rates in women who complained of infertility in addition to endometriosis ranged from 10 to 58%[28]. The principal studies reporting on the pseudo-pregnancy regimen are listed in Table 1, taken from Moghissi[28].

Although extensively utilized, estrogen–progestogen combinations have not been properly tested. Contraceptive pills utilized at present contain low doses of estrogens (30–35 μg daily of ethinyl estradiol) and third generation progestins.

OTHER HORMONAL TREATMENTS

A series of additional hormonal regimens have also been proposed after the pseudo-pregnancy idea gained momentum, the first being to use an antigonadotropic steroid, danazol. It is beyond the scope of this overview to discuss the complex picture created by its introduction for the first time by Greenblatt in 1971[29]. An informative review of the use of danazol in endometriosis has been published by Barbieri[30].

More recently, interesting results have been obtained through the introduction of gestrinone, an antiprogestional steroid. Its effects include androgenic, antiprogestogenic and antiestrogenic activities[31]. Fedele and co-workers[32] have recently compared the clinical effects of gestrinone and danazol and found a significant decrease of pain-related symptoms (dysmenorrhea, pelvic pain, deep dyspareunia) in both groups, without any significant difference. Their data are reported in Figure 2.

The same year Venturini and co-workers[33] showed that gestrinone significantly reduces serum concentrations of total testosterone and SHBG, whereas free testosterone is slightly but significantly increased. Finally, estradiol is not significantly lowered in comparison with pretreatment follicular phase values, as shown in Figure 3.

This brief overview of the spectrum of steroid hormones which have been advocated for the long-term management of endometriosis cannot be completed without mentioning mifepristone[34], also known as RU 486, or the 'abortion pill'. This last epithet is basically the reason why, after very promising early clinical studies, no large-scale experimentation has so far been undertaken. The drug has been officially repudiated by its manufacturer Hoechst-Marion-Roussel and has been the object of a series of complex deals between the Population Council and other recent sponsors. Unless things change dramatically, it is difficult to be optimistic

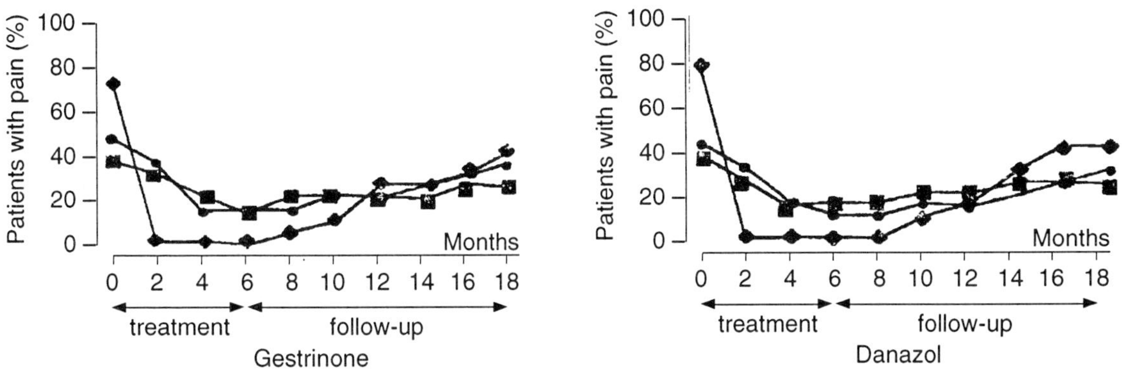

Figure 2 Prevalence of the 'pain symptom' in a comparative clinical study of danazol and gestrinone. The graphs show the situation at time 0 (before treatment), during 6 months of therapy and over the following 12 months, in the two groups. ●-●-● dysmenorrhea; ■-■-■ pelvic pain; ◆-◆-◆ dyspareunia. Reproduced with permission from Fedele *et al.*[32]

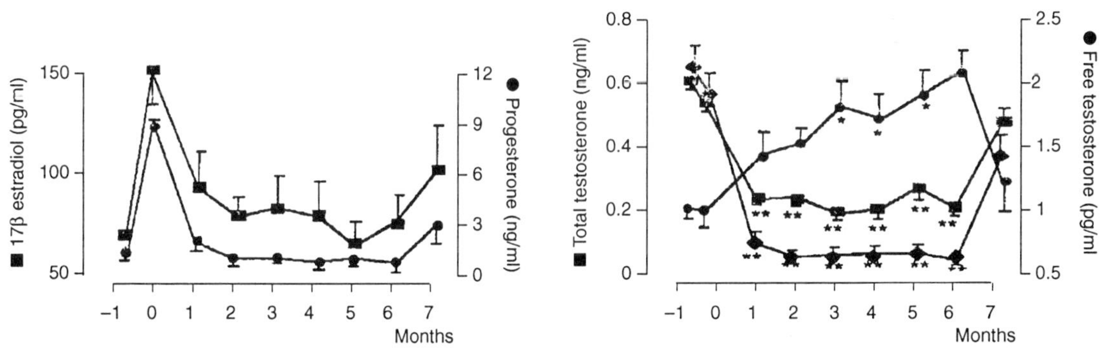

Figure 3 Endocrine effects of gestrinone. Serum levels (mean ± SE) of progesterone, estradiol, total and free testosterone, before, during and after therapy with gestrinone. *, $p < 0.01$; **, $p < 0.001$. Reproduced with permission from Venturini *et al.*[33]

about its availability for clinical testing in the near future. This is very unfortunate because the early studies, conducted by Yen and his group[35, 36] demonstrated a significant improvement not only in pelvic pain and dysmenorrhea but also in the rAFS score, as clearly shown in Figure 4.

RATIONALE FOR THE USE OF ESTROGEN–PROGESTOGEN COMBINATIONS

As already repeatedly stated, there is a solid rationale for the use of estrogen–progestogen combinations and, whereas we have an obvious difficulty in understanding how the administration of an estrogen, especially at high doses, could be beneficial, in particular to patients with advanced endometriosis, the situation is different when we consider the association of an estrogen and a progestogen. In this respect, it is well established that the contemporary administration of an estrogen and a progestogen results in a partially inactive endometrium.

Figure 5a shows the appearance of an endometrial biopsy in a pill-taker: clearly the endometrium is hypoproliferative with a hypotrophic glandular epithelium and

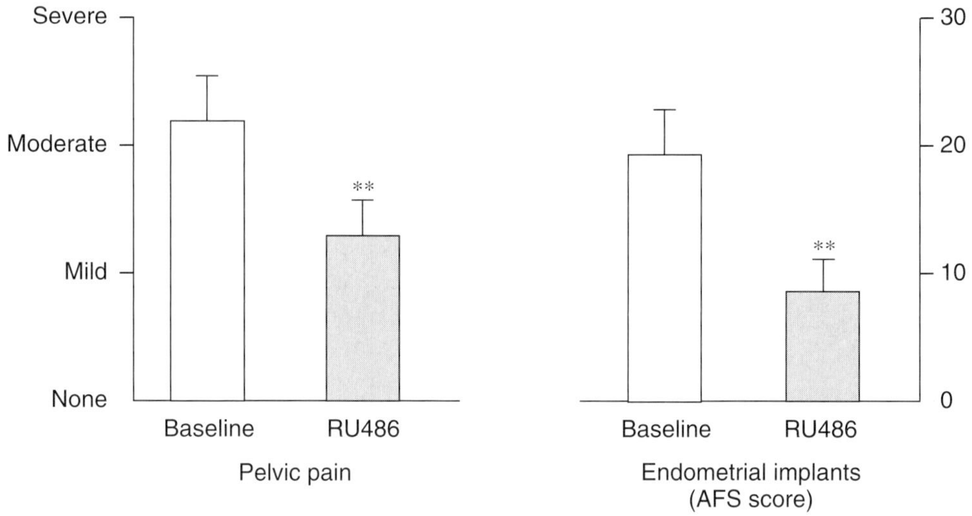

Figure 4 Effect of treatment with mifepristone in patients with endometriosis. Clinical scores for pelvic pain and rAFS scores for endometriotic implants before and after 6 months of treatment with 50 mg/day. **, $p < 0.05$. Reproduced with permission from Yen[36]

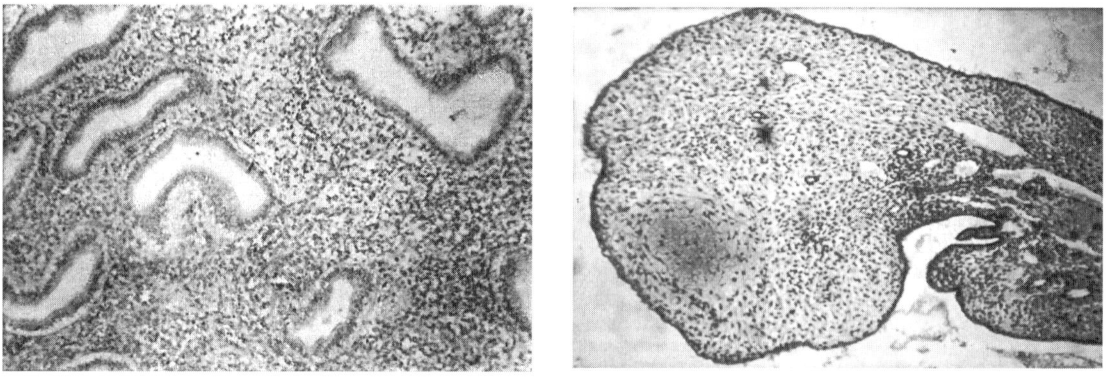

Figure 5 Effects of oral contraceptives on the endometrium. (a) The endometrium is hypoproliferative with hypotrophic glands and pseudo-decidualization of the stroma. (b) The endometrium is in an early secretory phase, the stroma is well represented, with scanty and not well branched glands

pseudo-decidualization of the stroma. In another case, shown in Figure 5b, the endometrium is in an early secretory phase: the stroma is well represented with scanty and not very branched glands.

Although we have ample evidence that ectopic endometrium does not behave in the same way as the eutopic one[37] and that – in the same patient – the two can be out of phase with each other at any given time during the menstrual cycle[38], the basic principle of controlled growth under the combined effect of the estrogen–progestogen combination remains true.

Figure 6 shows the wall of an ovarian endometrioma in a woman treated with a combined pill: glandular structures are not visible and the stroma is pseudo-decidualized under the influence of the oral pill.

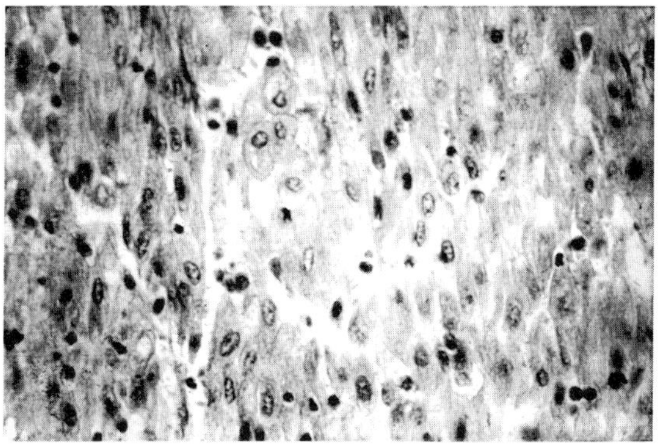

Figure 6 Effect of an oral contraceptive on ovarian endometriosis. Glandular structures are not visible and the stroma is pseudo-decidualized

CONCLUSIONS

In conclusion, there is a sufficient rationale to warrant the use of one of the low-dose contraceptive pills available today on the market for the management of endometriosis patients who do not wish to become pregnant. Therefore, the lack of adequate comparative clinical evaluation of this modality should move us to design proper clinical studies. It is time that we tried to gather the evidence necessary to clearly recommend if, when and for how long a contraceptive pill can be used in the management of endometriosis.

References

1. Russel WW. Aberrant portions of the Müllerian duct found in an ovary. *Johns Hopkins Hosp Bull* 1899;10:8–10
2. Cullen TS. The distribution of adenomyomata containing uterine mucosa. *Am J Obstet Gynecol* 1919;80:130–8
3. Sampson JA. Perforating hemorrhagic (chocolate) cyst of the ovary. *Arch Surg* 1921;3:232–45
4. Benagiano G, Brosens I. The history of endometriosis: identifying the disease. *Hum Reprod* 1991;6:963–8
5. Benagiano G, Bianchi P, Benagiano A. Endometriosis: medical or surgical treatment. In Benagiano G, Mencaglia L, Villani C, *et al.*, eds. *Gynecologic Endoscopic Surgery* . Rome: CIC Edizioni Internazionali, 1994
6. Hughes EG, Fedorkow DM, Collins JA. A quantitative overview of controlled trials in endometriosis-associated infertility. *Fertil Steril* 1993;59:963–70
7. Hirst JC. Favorable response of advanced endometriosis to testosterone propionate therapy. *Am J Obstet Gynecol* 1943;46:97–102
8. Geist SH, Salmon UJ. Androgen therapy in gynecology. *J Am Med Assoc* 1941;117:2207–15
9. Miller JR. Preoperative use of testosterone propionate as an aid to surgical treatment of endometriosis. *J Am Med Assoc* 1944;125:207–8
10. Kistner RW. The use of newer progestins in the treatment of endometriosis. *Am J Obstet Gynecol* 1958;74:264–78
11. Karnaky KJ. The use of stilbestrol for endometriosis. *Southern Med J* 1948;41:1110–1
12. Kempers RD, Dockerty MB, Hunt AB, *et al.* Significant post menopausal endometriosis. *Surg Gynecol Obstet* 1960;111:348–53
13. Legros R, Fain-Giono J. Endomètriose paramènopausique et post-mènopausique. A propos de 20 cas sur 351 d'endomètriose. *Rev Fr Gynècol* 1973;68:25–35
14. Bergqvist IA. Hormonal regulation of endometriosis and the rationales and effects of gonadotrophin-releasing hormone agonist treatment: a review. *Hum Reprod* 1995;10:446–52
15. Dizerega GS, Barber DL, Hodgen GD. Endometriosis: role of ovarian steroids in initiation, maintanance, and suppression. *Fertil Steril* 1980;33:649–53
16. Bergqvist A, Jeppsson S, Kullander S, *et al.* Human uterine endometrium and endometriotic tissue transplanted into nude mice. *Am J Pathol* 1985; 121:337–41
17. Rajkumar K, Schott PW, Simpson CW. The rat as an animal model for endometriosis to examine recurrence of ectopic endometrial tissue after regression. *Fertil Steril* 1990;53:921–5
18. Oliker AJ, Harris AE. Endometriosis of the bladder in a male patient. *J Urol* 1971;106:858–9
19. Pinkert TC, Catlow CE, Straus R. Endometriosis of the urinary bladder in a man with prostatic carcinoma. *Cancer* 1979;43:1562–7
20. Doty DW, Gruber JS, Wolf GC, *et al.* 46xy pure gonadal dysgenesis: report of two unusual cases. *Obstet Gynecol* 1980;55(suppl):61S
21. Peress MR, Sosnowski JR, Mathur RS, *et al.* Pelvic endometriosis and Turner's syndrome. *Am J Obstet Gynecol* 1982;144:474–6
22. Binnis BAO, Banerjee R. Endometriosis with

Turner's syndrome treated with cyclical oestrogen/progestogen: case report. *Brit J Obstet Gynaecol* 1983;90:581–2
23. Bosze P, Gaal M, Toth A, *et al.* Endometriosis and streak gonad syndrome. *Arch Gynecol* 1987;240: 253–4
24. Rosenfeld DL, Lecher BD. Endometriosis in a patient with Rokitansky–Kuster–Hauser syndrome. *Am J Obstet Gynecol* 1981;139:105
25. Andrews MC, Andrews WC, Strauss AF. Effects of progestin-induced pseudopregnancy on endometriosis: clinical and microscopic studies. *Am J Obstet Gynecol* 1959;78:776–85
26. Meigs JV. Endometriosis. Etiologic role of marriage age and parity: conservative treatment. *Obstet Gynecol* 1953;2:46–53
27. Thomas HH. Conservative treatment of endometriosis. Use of long-acting ovarian steroid hormones. *Obstet Gynecol* 1960;15:498–503
28. Moghissi KS. Treatment of endometriosis with estrogen-progestin combination and progestogen alone. *Clin Obstet Gynecol* 1988;31: 823–8
29. Greenblatt RB, Dmowski WP, Mahesh VB, *et al.* Clinical studies with an antigonadotropin–danazol. *Fertil Steril* 1971;22:102–12
30. Barbieri RL. Danazol: molecular, endocrine and clinical pharmacology. *Prog Clin Biol Res* 1990; 323:241–52
31. Worthington M, Irvine LM, Crook D, *et al.* A randomized comparative study of metabolic effects of two regimens of gestrinone in the treatment of endometriosis. *Fertil Steril* 1993;59:522–6
32. Fedele L, Bianchi S, Viezzoli T, *et al.* Gestrinone versus danazol in the treatment of endometriosis. *Fertil Steril* 1989;51:781–5
33. Venturini PL, Bertolini S, Marrè-Bruneghi MC, *et al.* Endocrine, metabolic and clinical effects of gestrinone in women with endometriosis. *Fertil Steril* 1989;52:589–95
34. Ulmann A, Tcutsch G, Philibert D. RU 486. *Sci Am* 1990;262:18–24
35. Kettel ML, Murphy AA, Mortola JF, *et al.* Treatment of endometriosis with the anti-progesterone mifepristone (RU 486). *Fertil Steril* 1996;65:23–8
36. Yen SSC. In Donaldson MS, Dolfinger L, Brown SS, *et al.*, eds. *Clinical Applications of Mifepristone RU486 and Other Antiprogestins.* Washington, DC: National Academy Press, 1993:189
37. Bergqvist A, Ljungberg O, Myhre E. Human endometrium and endometriotic tissue obtained simultaneosly; a comparative histological study. *Int J Gynecol Pathol* 1984;3:135–45
38. Schweppe KW, Wynn RM. Ultrastructural changes in endometriotic implants during the menstrual cycle. *Obstet Gynecol* 1981;58:465–73

The use of estro-progestatives in the management of endometriosis

33

J. Cohen

Since Kistner proposed pseudopregnancy regimens in 1959, pseudopregnancy is commonly used for the treatment of endometriosis. However the efficacy of this regimen is questionable in associated infertility and severe endometriosis. But in mild and moderate endometriosis OC may be proposed as a well tolerated and relatively inexpensive long-term treatment.

ASSOCIATION BETWEEN OC USE AND ENDOMETRIOSIS

Data regarding the possible association between OC use and endometriosis are conflicting.

Biological studies conclude that the risk of the disease is increased with OCs. Dizerega *et al.*[1] showed that either estradiol or progesterone alone or in combination are required for maintenance of 'seeded' endometrium in monkeys. Nisolle-Pochet *et al.*[2] showed that hormonal treatment leads to an incomplete suppression of endometriotic foci.

There is a lack of consensus in the literature on a relationship between oral contraceptives and endometriosis (Table 1). In some studies the risk of developing the disease was reduced by use of the pill[3–5], whereas in others it was increased[6] or not influenced[7,8].

Possible selection bias found in these studies includes:

(1) the difference between current users, recent users and past users is not always known;

(2) different progestagens and different doses have been prescribed;

(3) the duration of use is not always known;

(4) dysmenorrhea is a frequent indication for OC use and also a symptom of endometriosis.

Thus the higher risk for any time users of OC may result from selective mechanisms and indication bias. The lack of a relationship between the total duration of OC use and endo-metriosis and the degree of risk since last use do not support a causal relationship. The risk is reduced only among current or recent OC users.

ESTROGEN/PROGESTAGEN INDUCED PSEUDOPREGNANCY

Different studies[9–11] suggest that oral contraceptive pills may alleviate pelvic pain in patients with endometriosis. Most of the studies were done with high dose preparations that usually caused unpleasant side-effects (weight gain, abdominal swelling, etc.) Vercellini[12] compared a low-dose oral contraceptive containing ethinylestradiol 0.02 mg and desogestrel 0.15 mg per pill to a GnRH agonist (goserelin 3.6 mg per 28 days) during six months in 57 women with moderate or severe pelvic pain and laparoscopically diagnosed endometriosis. It is the only study done with low dose OCs. At 6 months of treatment a significant reduction in deep dyspareunia was observed in both groups, with goserelin superior to the OC at linear analog scale assessment. Non-menstrual pain was diminished on both scales without differences between treatments. Women taking the OC experienced a significant reduction in dysmenorrhea.

Table 1 Main results from selected studies investigating the link between OC use and endometriosis

Authors (country, year)	*Type of study*	*Inclusion criteria*	*No. of cases*	*Relative risk*		
				Current	*Past*	
R.C.G.P. (UK, 1976)	Cohort	Women taking contraceptives	43	0.5	1.4	
Walnut Creek (US, 1981)	Cohort	Women taking contraceptives	104	0.6	1.4	
Strathy *et al.* (US, 1982)	Case-control	Fertile and infertile	25	0.1		
Moen (Norway, 1987)	Prospective	Mostly fertile women asymptomatic	19	NE	0.3†	
Kirshon and Poindexter (US, 1988)	Prospective	Mostly fertile women asymptomatic	42	0.7†	0.7†	
Parazzini *et al.* (Italy, 1989)	Case-control	Histologic diagnosis	114	1.1	2.3	RR for duration of use ≤ 2 years: 1.8; > 2 years: 2.7 RR for time since last use < 5 years: 1.3; ≥ 5 years: 2.2
Mahmood and Templeton (UK, 1991)	Prospective	Fertile + infertile + pain + DUB	227	0.9†		
Moen (Norway, 1991)	Prospective	Mostly fertile women asymptomatic	42	1.0†		
Vessey *et al.* Oxford F.P.A. (UK, 1993)	Cohort	Women taking contraceptives	138	0.4	1.8	Current or stopped in last 12 months Past users are women who stopped pill 2–4 years earlier
Parazzini *et al.* (Italy, 1994)	Case-control	Surgically confirmed	377	0.9	1.7†	
Sangi-Maghpeykat and Poindexter (US, 1995)	Case-control	Multiparae who underwent sterilization	126	0.4†	ND	RR for duration of use ≤ 12 months 1.2; 13–24 months, 0.9; 25–48 months, 1.2

NE, not estimated; DUM, dysfunctional uterine bleeding; RR, relative risk
Table is taken from Chiaffarino F, Parazzini F, *et al.* Oral contraceptive use and benign gynecologic conditions. *Contraception* 1998;57:11–18

Table 2 Pseudopregnancy: clinical results

Author	*No. of patients*	*Medication*	*Clinical improvement %*	*Pregnancy rate %*	*Recurrence rate %*
Andrews *et al.*, 1959	17	Norethynodrel and mestranol	82	25	–
Riva *et al.*, 1962	132	Norethynodrel and mestranol	86	22	12*
Williams, 1967	41	Norethynodrel and mestranol	93	33	–
Kourides & Kistner, 1968	60	3 different products	88	54	23*
Andrews & Larsen, 1974	53	2 different products	82	43	46†
Noble & Letchworth, 1980	23	Noerthynodrel and mestranol	26	36	–
O'Connor, 1987	56	3 different products	'only a few'	14	69‡
Vercellini *et al.*§, 1993	28	Desogestrel 0.15 mg EE 0.02 mg	+++		

From Dmowski *et al.*[11]. *, Within 12–18 months of follow-up; †, 5.5 years of follow-up; ‡, Residual endometriosis; §, OC versus GnRHa

In France, one OC pill containing ethinylestradiol 0.050 mg and 17 ethinyl trienolone 2 mg per pill has received authorization for the treatment of endometriosis from the health authorities. The progestin is a very potent one and there have been studies showing a deep endometrial hypotrophy[13]. Clinicians use it widely, but there is no clinical study published.

There are very few data on the effects of a low-dose cyclic OC on endometriotic lesions. Fedele *et al.*[14] observed an improvement in implants at follow-up laparoscopy after administration of an E-progestin combination, but Dizerega *et al.*[1] have demonstrated that P alone is sufficient for survival of the lesions. One epidemiological study has shown an increased risk of endometriosis in women taking OCs[7], but with a high EE content compared with the preparations now available. Selection and indication biases cannot be excluded because clinical symptoms of endometriosis could *per se* lead to increased OC use. Follow-up laparoscopy in patients with endometriosis undergoing medical therapies is controversial because laparoscopy is usually performed at the end of the treatment when the pelvic vascularization is diminished and the lesions less visible[15].

CLINICAL RESULTS

The symptomatic response to OCs is usually reported to be around 80%, but it may be as low as only a few percent or as high as 93% (Table 2).

The corrected pregnancy rates range between 14% and 54% but it is difficult to draw any conclusions from this in the absence of data concerning the severity of the disease.

The side-effects with high dose OCs are similar to those of pregnancy:

(1) weight gain;

(2) bleeding;

(3) abdominal swelling; and

(4) breast pain and tenderness.

With low dose OCs there are very few side-effects.

The contraindications are the same as for normal use of OCs:

(1) thrombo-embolic and vascular disorders;

(2) impaired liver functions;

(3) neoplasms.

Recurrences[11] range between 16 and 69%.

THE PLACE OF OCS IN THE MANAGEMENT OF ENDOMETRIOSIS

There is no place for OCs in the management of severe endometriosis or infertility with endometriosis.

There is a place for symptomatic mild and moderate endometriosis. The well tolerated, relatively inexpensive long-term treatment with OCs could be proposed to symptomatic patients not desiring offspring. The economical aspect should be considered. If efficacy and tolerance are equivalent one should choose the least expensive treatment.

Figure 1 shows the place of OCs in the management of endometriosis.

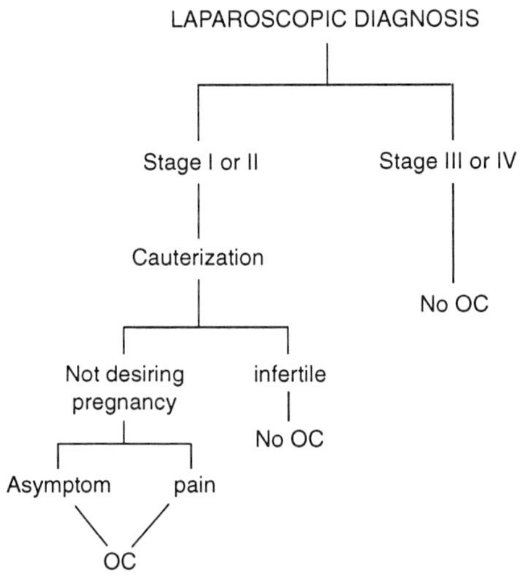

Figure 1 The place of oral contraceptives in the management of endometriosis

CONCLUSION

The risk of endometriosis is reduced among current and recent OC users. Different studies suggest that OC pills may alleviate pelvic pain in patients with endometriosis.

The treatment is indicated only for symptomatic patients with mild or moderate lesions, and not for infertility or severe lesions. It is the least expensive medical long-term treatment.

References

1. Dizerega GS, Barber DL, Hodgen GD. Endometriosis: role of ovarian steroids in initiation, maintenance, and supression. *Fertil Steril* 1980; 33:649–63
2. Nisolle-Pochet M, Casanas Roux F, Donnez J. Histological study of ovarian endometriosis after hormonal therapy. *Fertil Steril* 1988;49:423–6
3. Strathy JH, Molgaard CA, Coulam CB, *et al.* Endometriosis and infertility: a laparoscopic study of endometriosis among fertile and infertile women. *Fertil Steril* 1982;38:667–72
4. Kirshon B, Poindexter AN. Contraception: a risk factor for endometriosis. *Obstet Gynecol* 1988; 71:829–31
5. Mahmood TA, Templeton A. Prevalence and genesis of endometriosis. *Hum Reprod* 1991;6: 544–9
6. Parazzini F, Ferraroni M, Bocciolone L, *et al.* Contraceptive methods and risk of pelvic endometriosis. *Contraception* 1994;49:47–55
7. Parazzini F, La Vecchia C, Franceschi S, *et al.* Risk factors for endometrioid, mucinous and serous benign ovarian cysts. *Int J Epidemiol* 1989;18: 108–12
8. Moen MH. Is a long period without childbirth a risk factor for endometriosis? *Hum Reprod* 1991;6:1404–7
9. Buttram VC, Jr. Endometriosis. In Berhrman SJ,

Kermer RW, Patton GW, eds. *Progress in Infertility: Third Edition*. Little, Brown and Company, 1988;15:273–329

10. Metzger DD, Lucian AA. Hormonal therapy of endometriosis. *Obstet Gynecol Clin N Am* 1989; 16(1)
11. Dmowski WP, Rolland R, Schweppe KW. *Endometriosis. New Treatment Modalities*. Munich: Hoechst education update, 1989
12. Vercellini P, Trespidi L, Vendola N, *et al.* A gonadotropin releasing hormone agonist versus a low dose OC for pelvic pain associated with endometriosis. *Fertil Steril* 1993;60(1):75–9
13. Orcel L, Giorgi H, Dupay A, *et al.* Les modifications endometriales consécutives à l'administration de nouveaux oestro-progestatifs de synthèse. *Rev Franc Gynec* 1974;69(4):229–38
14. Fedele L, Arcaini L, Bianchi S, *et al.* Comparison of cyproterone acetate and danazol in the treatment of pelvic pain associated with endometriosis. *Obstet Gynecol* 1989;73:1000–4
15. Evers JLH. The second-look laparoscopy for evaluation of the result of medical treatment of endometriosis should not be performed during ovarian suppression. *Fertil Steril* 1987;47:502–4

Is there a role for oral contraceptives in endometriosis-associated infertility? 34

S. Daya

INTRODUCTION

Improvements in the ability to diagnose endometriosis have enhanced the understanding of the disease. Before the advent of laparoscopy, only symptomatic disease was treated, but now it is becoming increasingly common to diagnose asymptomatic disease, especially in infertile women. However, because the diagnosis requires an operative procedure, prevalence estimates are biased towards women who have undergone an operation involving the pelvis and do not accurately represent the extent of disease in the general population. Nevertheless, on the basis of observational studies, the association between endometriosis and infertility is now well accepted. It has been reported that 25–50% of infertile women have evidence of the disease, and 30–50% of women with endometriosis have infertility[1]. Despite this association, it is still unclear whether endometriosis is the cause or the result of the lack of child bearing.

In later stages of the disease (i.e. stages III and IV) the presence of endometriosis and/or extensive pelvic adhesions makes it very plausible to implicate the resulting anatomic distortion as a cause of infertility, whereas, in less severe stages (i.e. stages I and II), the anatomic relationship of the pelvic organs is not affected, yet fecundity is reduced. For example, in one study of women undergoing artificial insemination with donor sperm, fecundity was only 2% when endometriosis was present compared with 12% in its absence[2]. Thus, women with endometriosis will require a longer period of time to conceive. In minimal and mild stages of the disease, destruction of the endometriotic implants by electrocautery or laser at the time of laparoscopy significantly improved the cycle fecundity rate[3]. These observations add further support to the notion that infertility may be caused by endometriosis.

POSTULATED MECHANISMS OF INFERTILITY

A variety of mechanisms has been postulated to explain the infertility associated with endometriosis. The disease is one which progresses in severity from the milder categories in which there are a few endometriotic implants, to the more severe categories in which the pelvis may be 'frozen' from extensive adhesions involving the uterus, Fallopian tubes and ovaries. The anatomical disruption that occurs offers the most likely explanation for infertility in the more severe stages of the disease. However, in the less severe stages, in which the normal anatomical relationship of the pelvic organs is intact, other explanations are required.

It has been suggested that corpus luteum deficiency, immunological abnormalities in the peritoneal fluid and alteration in oocyte and embryo quality may all play a role in reducing the chance of pregnancy in women with endometriosis.

Corpus luteum deficiency

The first account of endometriosis-associated luteal phase deficiency (LPD) was published almost 30 years ago in a report of 96 women with endometriosis, 43 of whom had LPD[4]. In a later study, the proportion of out-of-phase endometrial biopsies, dated from the luteinizing hormone (LH) surge, was significantly higher in infertile women with endometriosis compared to those without endometriosis (64% versus 27%, respectively)[5]. Similarly, in a more recent study, women with endemetriosis had a significantly higher prevalence of LPD (29%) compared to those with normal fertility (4.4%), tubal infertility (2.9%), and male factor infertility (7.7%)[6].

Immunological abnormalities in peritoneal fluid

Significant abnormalities in the immune system have been reported by many investigators. These abnormalities include those in the peritoneal cavity (e.g. endometrial stromal cell proliferation, increased macrophage cytotoxicity, increased cytokine levels, and increased natural killer cell activity), and systemic ones (e.g. increased immunoglobulin production, increased T-helper cells, embryo toxicity, suppression of natural killer cell activity, deficient cellular immunity, and abnormal auto-immune function)[7]. These immunological abnormalities may produce infertility by affecting fertilization and implantation. There is also some evidence to suggest that the spontaneous abortion rate is increased in women with earlier stage disease[8].

Oocyte and embryo quality

Despite normal sperm quality in their partners, women with untreated mild endometriosis were found to have significantly lower rates of *in vitro* fertilization compared to those who underwent prior medical therapy for 6 to 9 months or those with infertility resulting from tubal damage[9]. Also, embryo cleavage rates were significantly lower in patients with minimal endometriosis compared to those with tubal disease[10]. Collectively, these observations suggest that the environment created by endometriosis may result in poor quality oocytes that fertilize poorly and produce inferior quality embryos.

TREATMENT OF ENDOMETRIOSIS-ASSOCIATED INFERTILITY

Although all the proposed mechanisms of infertility in early endometriosis emphasize different pathophysiological events, they rely on the presence of ectopic endometriotic implants. Consequently, eradication of the implants would seem to be an appropriate strategy to improve fertility. Supportive evidence for this proposal has been obtained from the recent multicenter, randomized Canadian trial (EndoCan study) in which surgical destruction of the endometrioc implants at the time of a diagnostic laparoscopy was evaluated against no treatment[3]. Stage I or II endometriosis was confirmed at laparoscopy in 348 of the 714 patients who had agreed to participate in the study. Eligibility criteria were verified in 341 patients, of whom 172 were randomized to receive surgical treatment during the laparoscopy, and 169 to receive no treatment. Patients continued to attempt pregnancy over the following 36 weeks. The cumulative probability of pregnancy progressing to 20 weeks' gestation was calculated to be 30.7% in the treated group versus 17.7% in the control group (risk ratio = 1.7; 95% confidence interval 1.2–2.6). The fecundity rate (per 100 person-months) was almost doubled with treatment (4.7 versus 2.4, respectively). Apart from confirming that treatment had a significant therapeutic effect, this study provided very good evidence on the expected probability of pregnancy in the absence of treatment and should form the basis for sample size estimations for subsequent efficacy studies.

Other therapeutic options have involved ovarian suppression with danazol, gonadotropin releasing hormone agonists (GnRHa), and oral contraceptives. The rationale for these options is based on the fact that ectopically located endometrium responds to steroid hormones in a manner similar to eutopic endometrium. Consequently, a hypoestrogenic state should result in atrophy and regression of endometriosis, as has been observed in women who are postmenopausal (both naturally or as a result of surgical castration) and in experimental animals[12].

Oral contraceptives have been used in the treatment of endometriosis for over four decades on the basis of the belief that they are effective. The evidence on which the recommendation for their use has been based will now be reviewed.

Oral contraceptives

The importance of hormonal factors in the pathogenesis of endometriosis is supported by the observations that it has never been detected prior to menarche[13], is rarely diagnosed in amenorrhoeic women[14], occurs only infrequently after menopause, regresses completely and promptly after surgical castration, improves or stabilizes during pregnancy[15], and is relatively infrequent in women with several pregnancies[16]. In contrast, it occurs more commonly in women with uninterrupted cyclic menses[14].

The beneficial changes in areas of endometriosis produced by pregnancy are brought about by the increasing production of placental steroids that stimulate decidual transformation of functioning endometriotic tissue, followed by decidual necrosis and subsequent absorption[17]. Confirmation of the presence of decidua or focal decidual necrosis in the areas of endometriosis has been obtained on biopsy specimens of the endometriotic implants after administration of norethynodrel[18].

The goal of oral contraceptive therapy, therefore, is as a substitute for pregnancy whereby a hormonal environment can be created that is less than ideal to support the ectopically located endometrial tissue, resulting in gradual regression and resorption of the implants. This state of 'pseudo-pregnancy' has been induced by combining large doses of estrogenic and progestogenic hormones in increasing amounts for periods of time varying from 3 to 10 months[18].

The ideal method of evaluating efficacy of such treatment is to compare it with no treatment or with a placebo in a randomized trial with adequate power. In the absence of such large studies, the overall effect of treatment can be estimated by pooling the results from smaller randomized trials using meta-analysis. Unfortunately, to date, there have been no such studies in the use of the combined (estrogen and progestrogen) oral contraceptive for the treatment of endometriosis-associated infertility. However, it should be recognized that the randomized controlled trial was introduced relatively recently into the field of reproductive medicine. In the past, reliance was placed predominantly on expert experience and opinion from which conclusions about efficacy and effectiveness of interventions were drawn. Consequently, in the absence of high quality evidence, one has to resort to reviewing data from comparative studies of one treatment versus another, and reports of case series.

Case series

In general, case series (which are reports of several cases) are not appropriate for evaluating treatment efficacy because of the lack of control groups to account for the effect that would occur without treatment or with a placebo. Occasionally, large and dramatic effects become apparent with treatment (e.g. pregnancy rates with intracytoplasmic sperm injection for male factor infertility) and can be described in case series. However, such situations are relatively infrequent.

The pseudo-pregnancy regimen for endometriosis was first described in 1959 in a group of 24 patients treated for periods of time varying from 3 to 10 months[18]. These patients were assumed, on the basis of the history and pelvic examination, to have endometriosis. In six of these patients, surgery

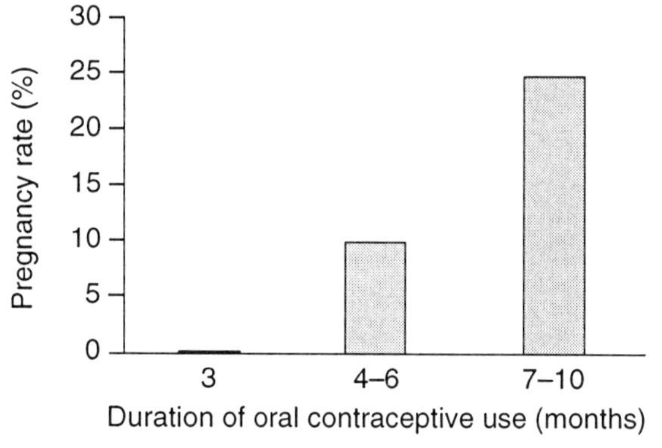

Figure 1 Duration of oral contraceptive use and pregnancy rates[18]

was subsequently required and the diagnosis of endometriosis was confirmed in all of them. Treatment was with Enovid (norethynodrel and ethinyl estradiol) at an initial dose of 10mg daily, and increased by 10mg every 2 weeks, to a maximum dose of 40–50mg. In 10 patients, the treatment duration was 3 months; in another 10 patients, treatment continued for 4–6 months; and in four patients, treatment was extended to 7–10 months. There were only two pregnancies in this group. As shown in Figure 1, pregnancy appeared more likely when the duration of treatment was for 7 or more months. This approach then became the standard of care for the treatment of endometriosis-associated infertility, despite the high rate of side-effects such as nausea, breast soreness, vaginal discharge and fluid retention.

Over the ensuing two decades, several publications of case series, reporting the use of different oral contraceptive preparations, appeared in the literature[19–25]. The pregnancy rates ranged from 16% to 100%, but despite the fact that the sample sizes on which these estimates were based were very small (varying from 4 to 49) (Table 1), the use of oral contraceptives continued as the mainstay of treatment for this disorder.

There are many issues that arise in relying on this quality of evidence to evaluate the efficacy of oral contraceptives. First, the method of diagnosis was not standardized, but was based on a variety of methods, including history and physical examination, culdoscopy, colpotomy and laparotomy. Clearly, using this approach, the asymptomatic cases of endometriosis were unlikely to have been identified to receive such therapy. Second, there was no uniform method of quantifying the extent of the endometriosis in each patient. Based on the diagnostic approach, it seems reasonable to assume that women with more severe disease were offered treatment. Thus, it is difficult to evaluate the role of oral contraceptives in milder disease. Third, the effect of known prognostic factors, such as female age, duration of infertility and presence of other infertility factors, was not addressed in the studies. Since these factors have only come to light more recently, it is understandable that they were not taken into account when therapy was suggested to the patients. Fourth, and of most importance, is the lack of control groups and randomization which are prerequisites for evaluating efficacy.

Controlled trials

A search of the literature failed to identify any controlled trials comparing oral contraceptives with no treatment to improve pregnancy rates in endometriosis-associated infertility.

Pseudo-pregnancy versus danazol

Although estrogen/progesterone combinations had been in use for some time, there was no consensus regarding the choice or dose of the preparation that should be used. Side-effects were particularly troublesome and, as discussed above, the value of the treatment was difficult to assess. The availability of danazol (an anabolic, weakly androgenic, non-progestagenic and non-estrogenic, synthetic hormone), which suppresses ovarian steroid secretion and causes endometrial atrophy, made it possible to undertake a comparative study with the pseudo-pregnancy regimen.

Table 1 Pregnancy rates with pseudopregnancy regimen using oral contraceptive

Authors	*Treatment*	*Duration of treatment*	*Pregnancy*	
			proportion	*%*
Andrews *et al.*, 1959[19]	Norethynodrel and ethinyl estradiol	14–22 weeks	1/4	25
Riva *et al.*, 1962[20]	Norethynodrel and ethinyl estradiol	2–12 months (average 6.1 mths)	8/49	16
Kistner, 1965[21]	Megestrol acetate and ethinyl estradiol	1½–14 months	4/5	80
	Ethynodiol diacetate and mestranol	3–18 months	3/12	25
	Chlorimadinone and mestranol	4–14 months	4/4	100
Williams, 1967[22]	Norethynodrel	2–4 months	8/16	50
Kourides & Kistner, 1968[23]	Norethindrone acetate and ethinyl estradiol	3–12 months	7/11	64
	Lynestrenol and mestranol	3–12 months (average 6 mths)	5/11	45
	Norgestrel and ethinyl estradiol	3–12 months	7/13	54
Andrews & Larsen, 1974[24]	Ethynodiol diacetate and mestranol or Norethynodrel and mestranol	≥ 4 months (average 6 mths)	8/34	24
Hammond *et al.*, 1976[25]	Norethynodrel and ethinyl estradiol	6–9 months	7/23	30

Patients with endometriosis, confirmed and staged at laparotomy or laparoscopy, were allocated using a quasi-random method involving case note numbers to either danazol (odd numbers) or Enavid (a combination of norethynodrel and mestranol) (even numbers)[26]. Treatment was started with a low dose (100 mg danazol twice daily or 5 mg Enavid twice daily) and the dose was progressively increased until amenorrhoea was established. Although the intention was to continue treatment for 6 months, premature discontinuation of Enavid became necessary in seven patients because of severe side-effects. A second-look laparoscopy was performed after 6 months to evaluate the extent of disease.

In the danazol treated group, 44% experienced side-effects compared to 87% ($p = 0.005$) in the Enavid group. Complete resolution or improvement in signs of disease was evident in 23/27 (85%) patients receiving danazol compared with 6/23 (26%) patients receiving Enavid (p=0.0001). Among the patients with infertility (together with endometriosis), 9/16 (56%) became pregnant with danazol compared with 4/11 (29%) with Enavid ($p = 0.53$).

Thus, from the results of this study, it can be concluded that the pseudo-pregnancy regimen is not very effective in eradicating endometriosis, is associated with side-effects in the majority of patients, and has a low probability of achieving pregnancy in women with infertility.

Danazol versus gestrinone

Since its introduction in 1975, danazol became widely used in the treatment of endometriosis. In 1990, gestrinone (13β-ethyl-17-α-ethinyl-17-hydroxygona-4,9,11-triene-3-one), a 19-nortestosterone derivative, became available. It has both agonist and antagonist effects on the progesterone receptor and, like danazol, decreases gonadotropin secretion with marked reduction in levels of estradiol and progesterone. Preliminary studies of the value of gestrinone in the treatment of endometriosis led to its comparison with danazol in a large, double-blind, multicenter, randomized trial[27].

Patients with endometriosis, confirmed and staged by laparoscopy or laparotomy, were allocated at random to receive either gestrinone (2.5 mg twice weekly, $n = 132$) or danazol (200 mg twice daily, $n = 137$) for 6 months. Treatment was allocated using a double-blind, double-dummy method (i.e. patients received two sets of capsules, one containing the active drug, the other containing placebo). The placebo capsules given to the gestrinone patients were identical to danazol capsules and vice versa. Following treatment, a second laparoscopy was performed, and patients were followed for a further 12 months.

There were no significant differences between the two groups in the endometriosis score at baseline and at the end of treatment. Among those who wished to become pregnant, a significantly higher proportion was successful with gestrinone (43.5% versus 27.3% with danazol, $p = 0.035$).

In a second randomized study of 39 nulliparous, infertile women with laparoscopically confirmed diagnosis of endometriosis, 6 months of treatment with danazol (600 mg daily) or gestrinone (25 mg twice a week) were compared[28]. The doses were increased, respectively, to 800 mg/day and 25 mg three times a week if an amenorrhoea was not achieved after 1 month of treatment. All patients were followed for at least 12 months from the end of treatment.

Among those who agreed to have a second laparoscopy one month after the end of treatment, a significant reduction in the endometriosis score was observed in each of the two groups, but there was no difference between the two groups. There was no significant difference in the pregnancy rate at 18 months from the commencement of treatment (6/19 [31.6%] with gestrinone versus 7/19 [36.8%] with danazol, $p = 0.73$).

Thus, the results of these two well conducted studies demonstrate that the probability of pregnancy with treatment in women with endometriosis-associated infertility is similar (i.e. approximately 30% in each group).

Gestrinone versus placebo

The importance of placebo as control in evaluating the efficacy of any treatment that is believed to improve pregnancy rates cannot be emphasized enough. In this context, the value of gestrinone was assessed in a randomized, double-blind, placebo controlled trial in infertile women with asymptomatic endometriosis, diagnosed and staged at laparoscopy[29]. Patients were allocated at random to either placebo or gestrinone (2.5 mg twice weekly) for 24 weeks. A repeat laparoscopy was performed in the final week of treatment to evaluate the response.

Complete elimination of endometriosis occurred in 12/20 (60%) patients receiving gestrinone compared with 4/17 (24%) in the placebo group ($p = 0.058$). The respective pregnancy rates after 12 months follow-up were 5/20 (25%) and 4/17 (24%) ($p = 1.00$).

Thus, although the sample size was quite small, this placebo-controlled study demonstrated that the pregnancy rate in untreated women with endometriosis-associated infertility is similar to that observed in the EndoCan study[3] (i.e. approximately 20–25%). Furthermore, gestrinone does not appear to significantly improve the chance of pregnancy.

CONCLUSIONS

The pseudo-pregnancy regimen for the treatment of endometriosis by using oral contraceptives to simulate pregnancy was first described in 1959 and has been in use ever since. However, the evidence on which the recommendations were made was of extremely poor quality, gleaned predominantly from uncontrolled observations reported in case series. Especially noteworthy is the fact that the untreated probability of pregnancy after 9–12 months is approximately 20–25%. Although surgical eradication of minimal and mild endometriosis has been demonstrated to be efficacious, similar studies on the value of oral contraceptives, unfortunately, have not been performed. Therefore, the efficacy of oral contraceptives in the treatment of endometriosis-associated infertility remains untested and unproven. In light of the beneficial effect of surgical treatment, undertaken at the time of diagnostic laparoscopy, the wisdom of conducting a proper placebo-controlled trial of oral contraceptives in this area is questionable. Consequently, based on the evidence to date, the only conclusion one can draw is that oral contraceptives do not appear to have a beneficial role in treating infertility resulting from endometriosis. Whether they have a role in the prevention of infertility in young women diagnosed with endometriosis remains to be determined.

References

1. Glass RH. Infertility. In Yen SSC, Jaffe RB, eds. *Reproductive Endocrinology*, edn 2. Philadelphia: WB Saunders, 1986:571–613
2. Jansen RPS. Minimal endometriosis and reduced fecundability. Prospective evidence from an artificial insemination by donor program. *Fertil Steril* 1986;46:141–3
3. Marcoux S, Maheux R, Bérubé S, and the Canadian Collaborative Group on Endometriosis. Laparoscopic surgery in infertile women with minimal or mild endometriosis. *N Eng J Med* 1997;97:212–22
4. Grant A. Additional sterility factors in endometriosis. *Fertil Steril* 1966;17:514–19
5. Cheesman KL, Cheesman SD, Chatterton RT, *et al.* Alterations in progesterone metabolism and luteal function in infertile women with endometriosis. *Fertil Steril* 1983;40:590–5
6. Li TC, Dockery P, Cooke ID. Endometrial development in the luteal phase of women with various types of infertility: comparison with women of normal fertility. *Hum Reprod* 1991;6:325–30
7. Gleicher N, Pratt D. Abnormal (auto)immunity and endometriosis. *Int J Gynecol Obstet* 1993; 40(Suppl):21–7
8. Daya S. Endometriosis and spontaneous abortion. *Infert Reprod Med Clin N Amer* 1996; 7:759–73
9. Wardle PG, Foster PA, Mitchell JD, *et al.* Endometriosis and IVF: effect of prior therapy. *Lancet* 1986;i:276–7
10. Tanbo T, Omland A, Dale PO, *et al. In vitro* fertilization/embryo transfer in unexplained infertility and minimal peritoneal endometriosis. *Acta Obstet Gynecol Scand* 1995;74:539–43
11. Wardle PG, McLaughlin EA, McDermott A, *et al.* Endometriosis and ovulatory disorder : reduced fertilization *in vitro* compared with tubal and unexplained infertility. *Lancet* 1995;ii:236–9
12. DiZerega GS, Barber DL, Hodgen GD. Endometriosis: role of ovarian steroids in initiation, maintenance and suppression. *Fertil Steril* 1980;33:649–53
13. Huffman JW. Endometriosis in young teenage girls. *Pediatr Ann* 1981;10:44–9
14. Cramer DW, Wilson E, Stillman RJ, *et al.* The relation of endometriosis to menstrual characteristics, smoking and exercise. *J Am Med Assoc* 1986;255:1904–8
15. Schenken RS, Williams RF, Hodgen GD. Effect of pregnancy on surgically induced endometriosis in cynomolgus monkeys. *Am J Obstet Gynecol* 1987;157:1392–6
16. Meigs JV. Endometriosis: etiologic role of marriage, age and parity: conservative treatment. *Obstet Gynecol* 1953;2:46–53
17. Kistner RW. The use of newer progestins in the treatment of endometriosis. *Am J Obstet Gynecol* 1958;75:264–78
18. Kistner RW. The treatment of endometriosis by inducing pseudopregnancy with ovarian hormones. A report of fifty-eight cases. *Fertil Steril* 1959;10:539–56
19. Andrews MC, Andrews WC, Strauss AF. Effects of progestin-induced pseudopregnancy on endometriosis: clinical and microscopic studies. *Am J Obstet Gynecol* 1959;78:776–85
20. Riva HL, Kawasaki DM, Messinger AJ. Further experience with norethynodrel in treatment of endometriosis. *Obstet Gynecol* 1962;19:111–17
21. Kistner RW. The effects of new synthetic progestogens on endometriosis in the human female. *Fertil Steril* 1965;16:61–80
22. Williams BFP. Conservative management of endometriosis: follow-up observations of

progestin therapy. *Obstet Gynecol* 1967;30:76–82

23. Kourides IA, Kistner RW. Three new synthetic progestins in the treatment of endometriosis. *Obstet Gynecol* 1968;31:821–8
24. Andrews WC, Larsen GD. Endometriosis: treatment with hormonal pseudopregnancy and/or operation. *Am J Obstet Gynecol* 1974;118:643–51
25. Hammond CB, Rock JA, Parker RT. Conservative treatment of endometriosis: the effects of limited surgery and hormonal pseudopregnancy. *Fertil Steril* 1976;27:756–66
26. Noble AD, Letchworth AT. Treatment of endometriosis : a study of medical management. *Br J Obstet Gynaecol* 1980;87:726–8
27. Bromham DR, Booker MW, Rose GL, *et al.* Updating the clinical experience in endometriosis – the European perspective. *Br J Obstet Gynaecol* 1995;102 (Suppl):12–16
28. Fedele L, Bianchi S, Viezzoli T, *et al.* Gestrinone versus danazol in the treatment of endometriosis. *Fertil Steril* 1989;51:781–5
29. Thomas EJ, Cooke ID. Successful treatment of asymptomatic endometriosis: does it benefit infertile women? *Br Med J* 1987;294:1117–19

Recurrent or persistent endometriosis? 35

D.C. Martin

INTRODUCTION

Until we have a technique for identifying all endometriosis in every situation, we have no way of knowing what we are leaving behind at the time of the first surgery. Therefore any endometriosis seen at a second operation may be persistent rather than recurrent. This is true for superficial peritoneal lesions as they may have been microscopic at the first operation and it is true for deep lesions as they may have been retroperitoneal and hidden.

RECOGNITION

Endometriosis is a difficult disease to recognize. From 31% to 40% of endometriosis that is sent to the pathology lab is not documented at the time of surgery. An additional 36% to 39% of patients who are diagnosed with endometriosis are not confirmed by the pathologist[1,2]. Although dark lesions are easy to see and document[3–6], these are not the most common lesions or the most common source of difficulty. Subtle forms are more common[5,7,8], hidden retroperitoneal disease can be missed at laparoscopy[9–12], bowel disease can be hidden from view[13], and microscopic disease can be missed even with close observation at laparoscopy[14–17]. Fibrotic lesions in the uterosacrals can be obscured as their fibrotic appearance is similar to that of the uterosacrals[18].

Detection and resolution have been adequate for histologic confirmation of red lesions as small as 400 μm[4], clear lesions as small as 180 μm[5], and carbon particles as small as 40 μm. But Redwine has documented an undetected probable endometriotic lesion of 120 μm[14] while lesions of 168 μm and 350 μm were not detected in baboons[17]. An undetected lesion of 400 μm in what appeared to be normal peritoneum at the base of pelvic pockets has also been noted[19]. At present, clinical resolution appears to be limited to 180 to 400 μm for endometriosis at laparoscopy.

In addition, up to 59% may not be documented owing to coexistent disease, intratubal position, mesenteric involvement, appendiceal disease, obscuring adhesions, or lack of attempt to observe endometriosis[1,2,20–22]. The distribution of the penetration depth of lesions in 10 patients who had laparotomy for bowel endometriosis (6–30 mm) and the laparoscopic appearance of the other 18 patients with proven, probable, or possible bowel involvement suggest that some of these 18 patients had deep penetration not recognized at laparoscopy[18].

Protocols using biochemical markers are useful in some treatment monitoring studies. However, even with deep infiltrating endometriosis, the sensitivity of CA-125 is only 26% and the specificity 87%[23]. Ongoing study of markers, MRI and other technology may help in determining the presence of endometriosis and/or the completeness of surgery[23–29].

AGE DEPENDENCY

The chance that endometriosis will be found at a second operation is age dependent. Almost all teenagers who have laparoscopies repeated have evidence of endometriosis. This is generally the clear, pink and red lesions associated with early endometriosis[7,30–32]. When these clear, pink and red lesions are seen at second surgery, they may be growth from previous microscopic lesions or may be new implants; there are no published markers

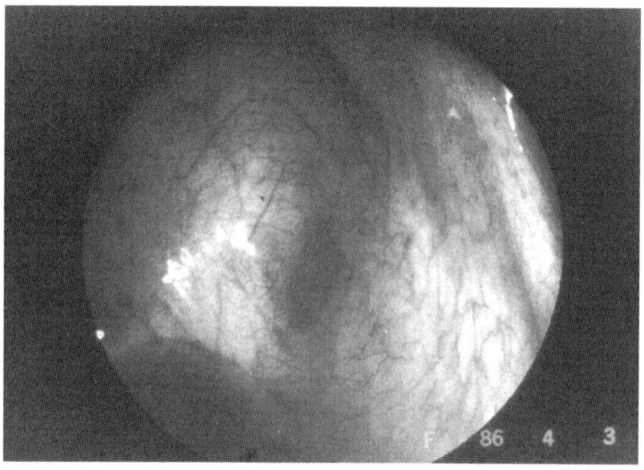

Figure 3 Reddish coloration in the right cul-de-sac medial to the uterosacral ligament is seen in a patient at age 14

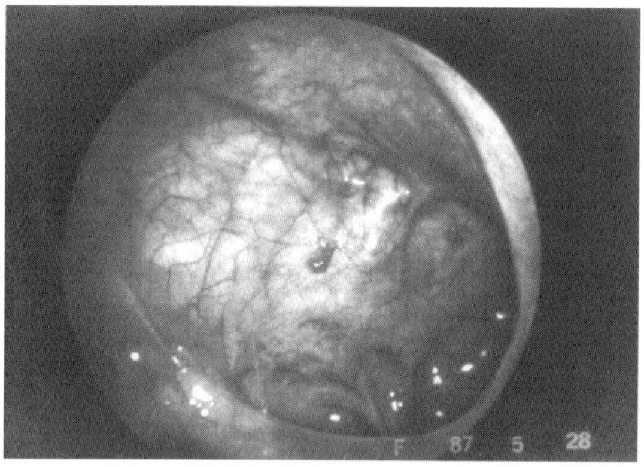

Figure 4 Pockets and red lesions in the same area as Figure 3 were seen at second look operation at age 15 years

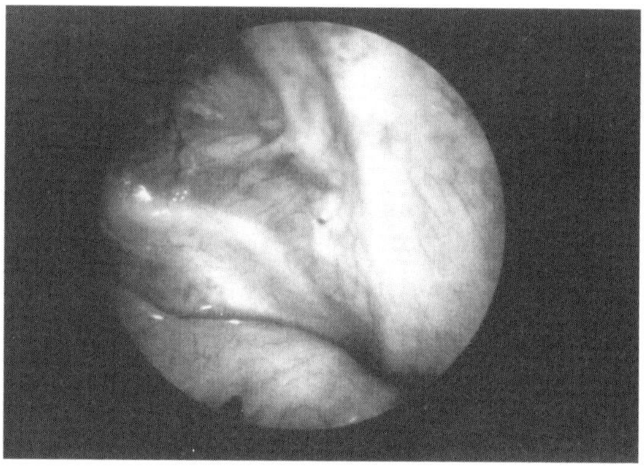

Figure 5 Right cul-de-sac with a dark lesion immediately above the entrance to a pocket

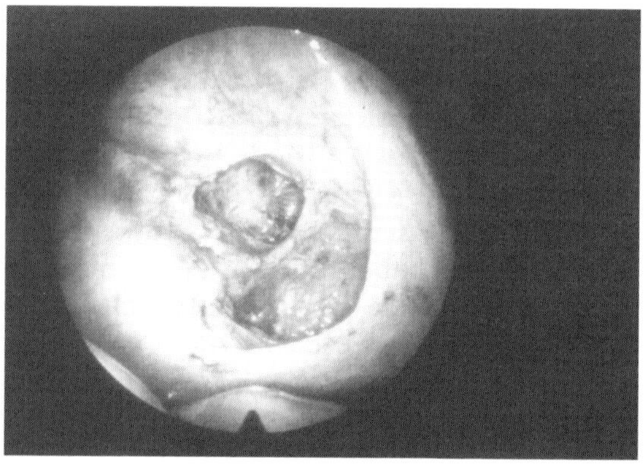

Figure 6 Area after the lower pocket has been exposed and the upper pocket found by accident in resecting the lesion seen in Figure 5

Case 2

The difficulty with determining whether deep hidden lesions are related to a retroperitoneal origin or peritonealization of pockets or lesions is demonstrated in one young patient in whom the original appearance was one of an anatomically symmetrical pelvis with a reddish blush to the surface in the right cul-de-sac (Figure 3). At second operation, pockets and superficial endometriotic nodules are easily seen (Figure 4). This patient demonstrates the occurrence of pockets developing associated with endometriosis with the first surgery done at age 14 and the second at age 15. These lesions were biopsied at the first operation and the development of the pockets may be related to the biopsy and/or endometriosis. In either situation, they developed over time and not congenital.

Case 3

This patient demonstrates what may be the result of a process similar to Case 2. In this patient, the entrance to one pocket was noted directly beneath a dark lesion (Figure 5). When this pocket was expanded, endometriosis was seen within the peritoneal pocket. When the lesion itself was excised, a second pocket was noted (Figure 6). No

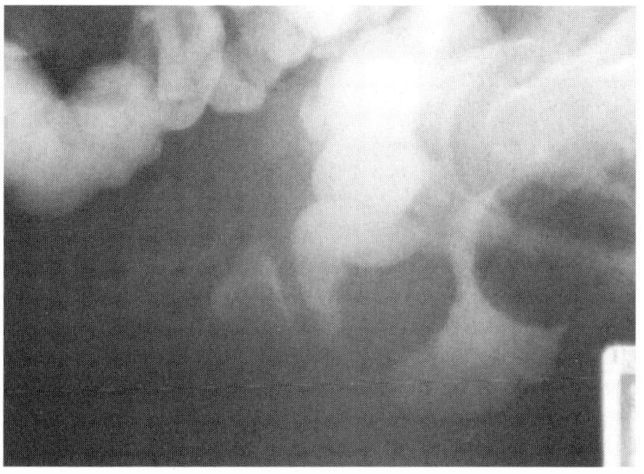

Figure 7 Napkin ring lesion of the sigmoid colon

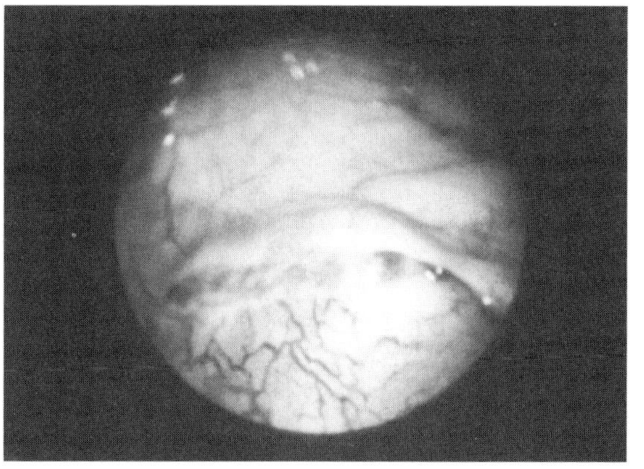

Figure 8 Dark scarred lesion following menstruation in a Rhesus monkey (*Macaca mulatta*). There had been an open red area during menstruation

entrance to the second pocket had been noted and this was found only after resecting the dark lesion. Although this pocket may have been a Müllerian rest occurring behind superficial peritoneal endometriosis, it would appear at least as likely that this was developmentally related to the large dark lesion.

Case 4

This barium enema of a napkin ring lesion (Figure 7) demonstrates a patient similar to those of Moore who were difficult to diagnose and difficult to treat[9]. This patient had her deep bowel endometriosis missed by the radiologist who took this film, by the first gynecologist who did a laparoscopy, by a second gynecologist who did a laparotomy and it was finally picked up by the radiologist on a repeat barium enema almost two years later. I was referred the case because of what was said to be rapid development of bowel endometriosis. It instead ended up being a delayed diagnosis of retroperitoneal and intramuscular bowel endometriosis. Comparing the two barium enemas, the napkin ring lesion was unchanged over the time the patient had twice undergone surgery.

Case 5

In a study of dioxin in Rhesus monkeys[55], one monkey had conversion from a deep encapsulated lesion to a surface hemorrhagic lesion with menses. The lesion appeared to invaginate and become a dark scarred lesion after menstruation ceased (Figure 8).

CONCLUSIONS

At present, there appears to be no readily acceptable fashion in which to determine whether disease seen at a second surgery is persistent or recurrent. Until we have techniques for identifying all endometriosis in all situations, we can only draw tentative conclusions.

Endometriosis occurring after pregnancy, medical therapy or menopause is persistent in most situations. Superficial clear, pink or red lesions may be either persistent or recurrent. Fibrotic dark lesions and deep infiltration found within 3 years of previous surgery are likely to be persistent.

Resection appears to be associated with an increase resolution of endometriosis. However, resection increases the difficulty of the procedure, the time of the operation and the cost.

References

1. Scott RB, TeLinde RW. External endometriosis – the scourge of the private patient. *Ann Surg* 1950;131:697–720
2. Martin DC, Ahmic R, El-Zeky FA,*et al.* Increased histologic confirmation of endometriosis. *J Gynecol Surg* 1990;6:275–9
3. Jansen RPS, Russell P. Nonpigmented endometriosis: clinical, laparoscopic, and pathologic definition. *Am J Obstet Gynecol* 1986;155:1154–9
4. Stripling MC, Martin DC, Chatman DL, *et al.* Subtle appearance of pelvic endometriosis. *Fertil Steril* 1988;49:427–31
5. Martin DC, Hubert GD, Vander Zwaag R, *et al.* Laparoscopic appearances of peritoneal endometriosis. *Fertil Steril* 1989;51:63–7
6. Moen MH, Halvorsen TB. Histologic confirmation of endometriosis in different peritoneal lesions. *Acta Obstet Gynecol Scand* 1992;71:337–42
7. Redwine DB. Age-related evolution in color appearance of endometriosis. *Fertil Steril* 1987; 48:1062–3
8. Davis GD, Brooks RA. Excision of pelvic endometriosis with the carbon dioxide laser laparoscope. *Obstet Gynecol* 1988;72:816–19
9. Moore JG, Binstock MA, Growdon WA. The clinical implications of retroperitoneal endometriosis. *Am J Obstet Gynecol* 1988;158:1291–8
10. Koninckx PR, Martin DC. Deep endometriosis: a consequence of infiltration or retraction or possibly adenomyosis externa? *Fertil Steril* 1992; 58:924–8
11. Martin DC. *Atlas of Endometriosis.*London: Gower Medical Publishing, 1993
12. Fedele L, Piazzola E, Raffaelli R, Bianchi S. Bladder endometriosis:deep infiltrating endometriosis or adenomyosis? *Fertil Steril* 1998;69: 972–5
13. Weed JC, Ray JE. Endometriosis of the bowel. *Obstet Gynecol* 1987;69:727–30
14. Redwine DB, Yocum LB. A serial section study of visually normal pelvic peritoneum in patients with endometriosis. *Fertil Steril* 1990;54:648–51
15. Nisolle M, Paindaveine B, Bourdon A, *et al.* Histologic study of peritoneal endometriosis in infertile women. *Fertil Steril* 1990;53:984–8
16. Martin DC. Laparoscopic excision of infiltrating pelvic endometriosis. In Levensohn A, ed. *OB-GYN Illustrated.* Slingerlands, New York: LTI Medica (Upjohn), 1992
17. D'Hooghe TM, Bambra CS, De Jonge I, *et al.* A serial section study of visually normal posterior pelvic peritoneum from baboons (*Papio cynocephalus, Papio anubis*) with and without spontaneous minimal endometriosis. *Fertil Steril* 1995;63:1322–5
18. Martin DC, Hubert GD, Levy BS. Depth of infiltration of endometriosis. *J Gynecol Surg* 1989;5:55–60
19. Martin DC. *Laparoscopic Appearance of Endometriosis. First Revision. Color Atlas.* (Second ed.) Memphis: Resurge Press, 1991
20. Pittaway DE. Appendectomy in the surgical treatment of endometriosis. *Obstet Gynecol* 1983;61:421
21. Martin DC. Laparoscopic treatment of advanced endometriosis. In Sutton C, Diamond M, eds. *Endoscopic surgery for gynaecologists.* London: W.B. Saunders Company Ltd, 1993: 239–7
22. Martin DC. Surgical treatment of endometriosis. *Clin Consul Obstet Gynecol* 1995;7:190–9
23. Koninckx PR, Muyldermans M, Meuleman C, *et al.* CA 125 in the management of endometriosis. *Eur J Obstet Gynaecol Reprod Biol* 1993;49:109–13
24. Koninckx PR, Ruttinen L, Seppala M, *et al.* CA-125 and placental protein 14 concentrations in plasma and peritoneal fluid of women with deeply infiltrating pelvic endometriosis. *Fertil Steril* 1992;57:523–30
25. Bateman BG, Kolp LA, Mills S. Endoscopic versus laparotomy management of endometriomas. *Fertil Steril* 1994;62:690–5
26. Myers TJ, Arena B, Granai CO. Pelvic endometriosis mimicking advanced ovarian cancer: presentation with pleural effusion, ascites, and elevated serum CA 125 level. *Am J Obstet Gynecol* 1995;173:966–7
27. Pittaway DE, Rondinone D, Miller KA, *et al.* Clinical evaluation of CA-125 concentrations as a prognostic factor for pregnancy in infertile women with surgically treated endometriosis. *Fertil Steril* 1995;64:321–4
28. Koninckx PR, Meuleman C, Oosterlynck D, *et al.* Diagnosis of deep endometriosis by clinical examination during menstruation and plasma CA-125 concentrations. *Fertil Steril* 1996;65:280–7
29. Guzick DS, Silliman NP, Adamson GD, *et al.* Prediction of pregnancy in infertile women based on the American Society for Reproductive Medicine's revised classification of endometriosis. *Fertil Steril* 1997;67:822–9
30. Karnaky KJ. Theories and known observations about hormonal treatment of endometriosis-in-situ, and endometriosis at the enzyme level. *Arizona Med* 1969;January:37–41
31. Koninckx PR, Meuleman C, Demeyere S, *et al.* Suggestive evidence that pelvic endometriosis is a progressive disease, whereas deeply infiltrating endometriosis is associated with pelvic pain. *Fertil Steril* 1991;55:759–65

32. Davis GD, Thillet E, Lindemann J. Clinical characteristics of adolescent endometriosis. *J Adolesc Health* 1993;14:362–8
33. Sampson JA. Perforating hemorrhagic (chocolate) cysts of the ovary. Their importance and especially their relation to pelvic adenomas of the endometrial type ("adenomyoma" of the uterus, rectovaginal septum, sigmoid, etc.). *Arch Surg* 1921;3:245–323
34. Redwine DB. Conservative laparoscopic excision of endometriosis by sharp dissection: life table analysis of reoperation and persistent or recurrent disease. *Fertil Steril* 1991;56:628–34
35. Wheeler JM, Malinak LR. Recurrent endometriosis. *Contr Gynecol Obstet* 1987;16:13–21
36. Evers JLH, Dunselman GAH, Land JA, *et al.* Is there a solution for recurrent endometriosis? *Brit J Clin Pract* (Suppl 72) 1991;72:45–50
37. Sampson JA. Ovarian hematomas of endometrial type (perforating hemorrhagic cysts of the ovary) and implantation adenomas of endometrial type. *Boston Med Surg J* 1922;186:445
38. Jacobson VC. The autotransplantation of endometrial tissue in the rabbit. *Arch Surg* 1922;5:281–300
39. Sampson JA. Peritoneal endometriosis due to menstrual dissemination of endometrial tissue into the peritoneal cavity. *Am J Obstet Gynecol* 1927;14:422–69
40. Martin DC. Laparoscopic and vaginal colpotomy for the excision of infiltrating cul-de-sac endometriosis. *J Reprod Med* 1988;33:806–8
41. Donnez J, Nisolle M, Smoes P, *et al.* Peritoneal endometriosis and endometriotic nodules of the rectovaginal septum are two different entities. *Fertil Steril* 1996;66:362–8
42. Nisolle M, Donnez J. Peritoneal endometriosis, ovarian endometriosis, and adenomyotic nodules of the rectovaginal septum are three different entities. *Fertil Steril* 1997;68(4):585–96
43. Russell WW. Aberrant portions of the Müllerian duct found in an ovary. *Johns Hopkins Hosp Bul* 1899;94–96(January, February, March):8–10
44. Gruenwald P. Origin of endometriosis from the mesenchyme of the celomic walls. *Am J Obstet Gynecol* 1942;44:470–4
45. Damario MA, Horowitz IR, Rock JA. The role of uterosacral ligament resection in conservative operation for recurrent endometriosis. *J Gynecol Surg* 1994;10:57–61
46. Martin DC, Koninckx PR, Batt RE, *et al.* Deep endometriosis. In Minaguchi H, Sugimoto O, eds. *Endometriosis Today: Advances in Research and Practice.* Carnforth, UK: Parthenon Publishing Group, 1997: 50–7
47. Martin DC. *Laparoscopic Appearance of Endometriosis Color Atlas.* (2nd edn.) Memphis: Resurge Press, 1990
48. Hoshiai H, Ishikawa M, Sawatari Y, *et al.* Laparoscopic evaluation of the onset and progression of endometriosis. *Am J Obstet Gynecol* 1993;169:714–19
49. D'Hooghe TM, Bambra CS, Raeymaekers B, *et al.* Serial laparoscopies over 30 months show that endometriosis in captive baboons (*Papio anubis, Papio cynocephalus*) is a progressive disease. *Fertil Steril* 1996;65:645–9
50. D'Hooghe TM. Clinical relevance of the baboon as a model for the study of endometriosis. *Fertil Steril* 1997;68:613–25
51. Steingold KA, Cedars M, Lu JKH, *et al.* Treatment of endometriosis with a long-acting gonadotropin-releasing hormone agonist. *Obstet Gynecol* 1987;69:403–11
52. Vessey MP, Villard-Mackintosh L, Painter R. Epidemiology of endometriosis in women attending family planning clinics. *Br Med J* 1993;306:182–4
53. Wheeler J, Malinak LR. Recurrent endometriosis; incidence, management, and prognosis. *Am J Obstet Gynecol* 1983;146:247–53
54. Kempers RD, Dockerty MB, Hunt AB, *et al.* Significant postmenopausal endometriosis. *Surg Gynecol Obstet* 1960;111(Sept):348–56
55. Rier S, Martin DC, Bowman RE, *et al.* Endometriosis in rhesus monkeys (*Macaca mulatta*) following chronic exposure to 2,3,7,8-tetrachlorodibenzo-p-dioxin. *Fundamental Appl Toxicol* 1993;21:433–41

Recurrent pain following hysterectomy may be due to persistent endometriosis in the uterosacral ligaments

36

I.R. Horowitz, A.B. Namnoum and J.A. Rock

INTRODUCTION

Over the last two decades an increase of retroperitoneal disease has been reported. Prior to this observation, hysterectomy was performed with or without ovarian conservation. Recurrence rates for pain were not insignificant in either case. Our group addresses a possible explanation for this observed inconsistency.

BACKGROUND

Pelvic pain was documented following hysterectomy with and without ovarian conservation by Namnoum and colleagues in 1995[1]. Twenty-nine women had a hysterectomy with some ovarian tissue preserved, while 109 had all their ovarian tissue preserved. Uterosacral ligaments were not routinely resected at the time of hysterectomy. Compared with women who had oophorectomy, women who underwent hysterectomy with preservation of ovaries had a 6.1-fold greater risk of developing pain and an 8.1-fold greater risk of reoperation.

Symptom recurrence was also documented following hysterectomy with oophorectomy and estrogen replacement. Hickman *et al.*[2] performed a retrospective cohort study of 95 women who underwent total abdominal hysterectomy with bilateral salpingo-oophorectomy for endometriosis and subsequently received estrogen replacement therapy. The mean length of follow-up was 57 months. Those women who started estrogen replacement therapy had a relative risk of 5.7 for pain recurrence.

Damario *et al.*[3] noted that the gross appearance of the uterosacral ligaments may not be reliable in determining microscopic presence of endometriosis. In 50% of their cases histologic involvement would not have been detected if the authors had relied solely on their clinical findings. Horowitz *et al.*[4] presented data at the Sixth World Congress on Endometriosis pertaining to the conservative management of endometriosis through radical resection. The authors retrospectively reviewed 92 patients who had undergone conservative surgery for endometriosis. Bilateral ureterolysis and resection of uterosacral ligaments were performed. Fifty-three per cent reported no pain and 22% reported decreased pain after surgery. The remaining 25% (20.7% no change; 4.3% increased pain) presented with postoperative pain atypical of their initial presentation. This pain was more charac-teristic of symptoms associated with irritable bowel syndrome. The authors also looked at the volume of tissue resected from the uterosacral ligaments but found no significant correlations with postoperative pain.

DISCUSSION

Over the past several decades, the treatment of endometriosis has evolved through several generations of medical therapy as well as surgical techniques. Conservative therapy in symptomatic women has a significant recurrence rate of approximately 50% 5 years after medical therapy and 40% after surgical therapy. The increasing age of our patients and their desire to maintain fertility have encouraged clinicians to re-evaluate the surgical techniques utilized for the treatment of these patients.

Initially the role of uterosacral ligament resection in the conservative management of recurrent endometriosis was controversial. It has been accepted knowledge that those uterosacral ligaments that are grossly affected with endometriosis should be either ablated or resected. Damario *et al.*[3] demonstrated that approximately 50% of their cases did not have gross evidence of disease prior to resection. In addition to the marked endometriosis, a significant fibrosis exists in uterosacral ligaments resected in the patient with severe endometriosis. It is quite possible that the incidence of endometriosis present in uterosacral ligaments would be increased if sampling of the fibrotic uterosacral ligaments was more extensive[4]. Horowitz and colleagues[4], in their conservative management of endometriosis, routinely resected the uterosacral ligament. Many patients who did not have gross disease on the peritoneal surface did in fact have deep retroperitoneal invasion of the uterosacral ligament, at times extending towards the sacrum. Seventy-five per cent of their patients reported decreased or no abdominal discomfort upon completion of this procedure. The remaining 25% had the same or increased pain, which appears to be most probably secondary to irritable bowel syndrome rather than endometriosis. In the light of the change in the character of this pain, it appears that the radical resection of the uterosacral ligaments was successful in decreasing pain secondary to invasive endometriosis. This study, however, includes only preliminary data. A prospective study with pain scores and long-term follow-up is needed to further test the hypothesis that resection of uterosacral ligaments will decrease pain and recurrence of endometriosis in patients undergoing conservative management.

Fedele *et al.*[5] used transrectal ultrasonography to assess invasion of the rectovaginal septum and uterosacrum by endometriosis in 140 women. Rectovaginal septum involvement was present in 34 (specificity 97% (127/130); sensitivity 96%). Uterosacral involvement was identified with a sensitivity of 80% (8/10) and specificity of 97%. Transrectal ultrasonography may assist the surgeon to identify patients with deeply invasive disease that will require radical retroperitoneal dissection and possible bowel resection. Ohba *et al.*[6] have successfully utilized transrectal ultrasonography to quantitate the amount of endometriosis infiltration of the uterosacral ligaments. We concur with Querleu[7] in recommending that resection of invasive endometriosis (described above) be performed by surgeons with skills in oncologic dissection. Although the authors believe radical resection of retroperitoneal endometriosis is most successful via a laparotomy, Chapron *et al.*[8] advocate laparoscopic resection of deep endometriosis. This technique also requires considerable expertise.

Namnoum *et al.*[1] showed that patients who underwent hysterectomy with ovarian conservation had 6.1-fold greater risk of developing recurrent pain and 8.1-fold greater risk of reoperation compared with patients who had oophorectomy. These results once again challenge the clinician in treating patients with severe endometriosis who do not desire conservative therapy. This greater risk of developing recurrent pain may be secondary to continued stimulation of microscopic endometriosis that was not identified during the surgical procedure or it could be that retroperitoneal endometriosis was present at the time of the hysterectomy and was not identified. It may not be possible to evaluate the presence of deep endometriosis by laparoscopic examination or palpation depending on its location. If deep endometriosis is present away from the cuff in areas palpated on bimanual examination, the patient may suffer from chronic pain without a definitive diagnosis being made. At the present time our study group evaluates this group of patients with two approaches. The first is hormonal testing to ensure that ovarian remnants are not present. The patient is taken off all hormone replacement therapies and 4–6 weeks later measurements of estradiol, luteinizing hormone (LH) and follicle-stimulating hormone (FSH) are obtained. The second approach, if the physical examination is unremarkable, is to use magnetic resonance imaging in the hope of identifying retroperitoneal endometriosis. Although the authors have been successful in using the latter procedure, disease is often not identified. It is unfortunate that this group of patients may continue to experience severe pain without a definitive diagnosis. Empiric treatment with gonadotropin-releasing hormone (GnRH) analogs, progestational agents or Danocrine® (Sanofi, New York, USA) is not appropriate in the majority of these patients. Reoperation was necessary 8.1 times more often than in those without ovarian preservation. Patients who undergo a simple hysterectomy or radical hysterectomy with ovarian conservation may require reoperation secondary to pelvic pain or ovarian neoplasms. Ovarian function can also be decreased in patients who undergo a hysterectomy with ovarian conservation. Finan *et al.*[9] reported increased morbidity when removing ovaries in patients who had previously undergone hysterectomy for endometriosis. In addition to dense adhesions, two patients required enterotomy repair and four required bowel resection and anastomosis. Fifteen of the 27 patients had an objective finding of a pelvic mass or nodularity.

In Hickman and colleagues'[2], retrospective cohort study, patients subsequently received estrogen replacement therapy after undergoing total abdominal hysterectomy with bilateral salpingo-oophorectomy. The data suggested that the time of initiating estrogen replacement therapy was correlated with its success. Of 60 women who began estrogen replacement therapy in the immediate postoperative period, four had recurrent pain, whereas of 35 women who began more than six weeks postoperatively seven (20%) experienced recurrent pain. In their analysis the crude rate of symptom recurrence was not statistically significant ($p = 0.09$). However, when controlling length of patient follow-up and adjusting for covariates of stage, age and postoperative hydroxyprogesterone therapy, those who started replacement therapy more than six weeks postoperatively had a relative risk of 5.7 (95% confidence interval 1.3–25.2) for pain recurrence. Although the small numbers in this study prevented it being statistically significant, the findings do suggest that immediate treatment with hormones does not present a greater risk for recurrent pain than for those who have therapy initiated six weeks postoperatively. In fact, it appears that those who were started later have a higher relative risk for pain recurrence.

CONCLUSION

The authors have been involved in several studies looking at the role of uterosacral ligament resection, hysterectomy and oophorectomy in patients with endometriosis. The data appear to be compelling evidence that deep endometriosis of the uterosacral ligaments may be one of the primary etiologies of pelvic pain in these patients. Hysterectomy failure may be secondary to not resecting the uterosacral ligaments at the time of initial surgery. At present, the authors resect uterosacral ligaments of patients undergoing hysterectomy for severe endometriosis. Also of note is the role of estrogen supplement in those who have undergone bilateral oophorectomy.

References

1. Namnoum AB, Hickman TN, Goodman SB, *et al.* Incidence of symptom recurrence after hysterectomy for endometriosis. *Fertil Steril* 1995;64:898–902

2. Hickman TN, Namnoum AB, Hinton EL, *et al.* Timing of estrogen replacement therapy following hysterectomy with oophorectomy for endometriosis. *Obstet Gynecol* 1998;91:673–7
3. Damario MA, Horowitz IR, Rock JA. The role of uterosacral ligament resection in conservative operations for recurrent endometriosis. *J Gynecol Surg* 1994;57–61
4. Horowitz IR, Scarbrough GL, Rock RA. Conservative management of endometriosis through radical resection. *Proceedings VI World Congress on Endometriosis*, Quebec City, Canada, 1998
5. Fedele L, Bianchi S, Portuese A, *et al.* Transrectal ultrasonography in the assessment of rectovaginal endometriosis. *Obstet Gynecol* 1998;91:444–8
6. Ohba T, Mizutani H, Maeda T, *et al.* Evaluation of endometriosis in uterosacral ligaments by transrectal ultrasonography. *Hum Reprod* 1996;11:2014–17
7. Querleu D. Pelvic pain and external endometriosis. Physiopathology and treatment. [French] *Contracept Fertil Sex* 1995;23:29–36
8. Chapron C, Dubuisson JB, Tardif D, *et al.* Retroperitoneal endometriosis and pelvic pain: results of laparoscopic uterosacral ligament resection according to the rAFS classification and histopathologic results. *J Gynecol Surg* 1998;14:51–8
9. Finan MA, Kwark JA, Joseph GF, *et al.* Surgical resection of endometriosis after prior hysterectomy. *J Louisiana State Med Soc* 1997;149:32–5

Recurrent ovarian endometrioma

37

M. Canis, R. Botchorishvili, L. Schindler, G. Durruty, J.L. Pouly, A. Wattiez, G. Mage, H. Manhes and M.A. Bruhat

Endometriosis is generally decribed as an enigmatic disease, mainly because of the risk of 'recurrence'. However the incidence and clinical relevance of this problem are difficult to assess. Obviously, there is a confusion in the literature between the need for a second treatment and the recurrence rate of the disease. Indeed the 'recurrence' of an endometrioma after a medical treatment is not a recurrence but a persistence since we do know that endometriomas include a lot of fibrosis which cannot be effectively treated with GnRH analogs or contraceptive pills.

To discuss the incidence of a recurrent ovarian endometrioma after a laparoscopic treatment[1,2] we will present the results of three studies.

The first was performed in 1992 and included patients treated for ovarian endometriosis whatever the diameter of the cyst and the surgical technique used, the mean follow-up being short (less than 2 years); the second study, performed in 1996, included 45 patients treated by laparoscopy for a cyst ≥ 3 cm in diameter who subsequently had a transvaginal ultrasonographic ovocyte pick up; the third study, performed in 1996, included patients from our database about adnexal masses, treated for a cyst > 3 cm, with a mean follow-up > 4 years.

MATERIAL AND METHODS

The management of ovarian endometriomas was similar to that used for any adnexal masses in premenopausal patients[3,4]. After a peritoneal cytology and a careful inspection of the ovary and of the entire peritoneal cavity, adnexal masses were punctured and/or ruptured only when assumed to be benign. Endometriomas were often ruptured and emptied while freeing the ovary from the broad ligament. After the rupture a careful lavage was required to remove the 'chocolate' fluid and to inspect the internal cyst wall. If signs of malignancy were found a vertical midline laparotomy was performed.

Whenever the diagnosis of ovarian endometrioma was confirmed, the treatment was peformed by laparoscopy. The techniques used were as described below.

Small cysts, < 3 cm in diameter, were treated by drainage, biopsy and ablation of the internal cyst wall using a CO_2 laser or bipolar coagulation.

Large cysts, ≥ 3 cm, were treated by intraperitoneal cystectomy whenever technically feasible. Three second puncture trocars were inserted in the suprapubic area. As recurrence of adhesion is very common after treatment of dense ovarian adhesions[2], endometriomas were drained by freeing their anterior surface from the broad ligament rather than by puncturing their posterior surface. The cystectomy was performed using the incision induced by the adhesiolysis. However, this incision was enlarged to identify the cleavage plane, which is generally difficult to identify on the site of the rupture. If the cyst was not ruptured during the adhesiolysis, it was punctured on the antimesenteric surface of the ovary.

A careful inspection of the ovarian incision allowed the identification of the cleavage plane. The cyst wall and the ovarian cortex were grasped with atraumatic forceps. The dissection plane was then developed using two grasping forceps pulling slowly in opposite directions. The forceps were frequently drawn down towards the cleavage plane to allow permanent visual control of the dissection. Hemostasis was achieved with bipolar coagulation.

The final step of the dissection of an ovarian endometrioma close to the ovarian hilum was often difficult because of the fibrosis induced by the endometrioma. This step was initiated by the surgeon when red fibers on the outer surface of the cyst wall were seen. Then two grasping forceps were used to expose the cleavage plane and a third instrument, generally a bipolar coagulation forceps, was used to dissect the right plane, which was found close to the cyst wall rather than in the remaining ovarian tissue. Working in another plane, away from the cyst wall, would induce unnecessary trauma to the ovary and to the ovarian vessels. The ovarian capsule was generally left open, however, when the shape of the ovary is not satisfactory, it should be repaired. However, the ovarian cortex should only be approximated using intra-ovarian sutures. When the cystectomy was too difficult, the remaining part of the cyst wall was treated with CO_2 laser or bipolar coagulation.

One patient was reoperated on 18 months later, for an abdominal wall endometrioma located on one of the suprapubic trocar sites[3]. It is essential to avoid abdominal wall contamination when removing an endometrioma[4].

A 3 months postoperative medical treatment was used in infertile patients referred to IVF and in a patient who did not wish to be pregnant.

Definitions

To discuss the problem of recurrent ovarian endometria, definitions are necessary. By including only cysts, whose diagnosis would be confirmed by a pathologic examination, one would clearly underesti-mate the number of patients who will be diagnosed and/or treated for an adnexal cystic mass after the laparoscopic treatment of an ovarian endometrioma. Therefore in the three following studies, the 'recurrent' cyst was diagnosed as:

(1) an endometrioma after a pathologic examination, or when 'chocolate' fluid was found during an ovocyte pick up;
(2) a benign organic ovarian cyst after a pathologic examination;
(3) a functional cyst, if an entirely cystic mass disappeared with treatment by contraceptive pill;
(4) a cyst of unknown diagnosis, if an entirely cystic mass could not be treated successfully with an hormonal treatment.

Except in study 2, follow-up data were obtained by mail and/or by reviewing the charts of the patients.

RESULTS

Study 1

One hundred and sixty-three patients treated between January 1986 and December 1990 were included. These patients were treated for 199 endometriomas whose diameter ranged from 2 to 12 cm. The mean age was 34.7 ± 7.3 years, 74 patients (45.4%) had R-AFS stage III endometriosis, 89 (54.6%) R-AFS stage IV. All these patients had a follow-up > 12 months.

The recurrence rates are presented in Table 1. There were no significant differences according to the diameter of the cyst, the surgical technique used or the R-AFS stage. The recurrence rate was significantly higher on the treated adnexae than on the contralateral adnexae. However the recurrence rate was the same in these two groups when excluding the recurrences observed during the first postoperative year, suggesting that during the first postoperative year, recurrences occurred mainly on the treated adnexae as a consequence of an incomplete treatment (Figure 1).

Study 2

Forty-five patients were included, the mean age being 30.4 ± 4.1 (range 24–42) years old.

Table 1 Recurrence rates in study 1

		Pathologic diagnosis of the recurrent cyst			
		Endometrioma	*Functional*	*?*	*Total*
All patients	163	26 (15.9)	7 (4.3)	7 (4.3)	40 (24.5)
Patients with					
unilateral cyst	127	18 (14.2)	7 (5.5)	6 (4.7)	31 (24.4)
bilateral cyst	36	8 (22.0)	0 (0.0)	1 (2.8)	9 (25.0)
All adnexae	326	22 (13.0)	9 (4.1)	7 (3.1)	38 (11.7)
Ipsilateral (all)	199	25 (12.6)	7 (2.5)	5 (2.5)	37 (18.5)
Controlateral	127	7 (5.5)	2 (1.6)	2 (1.6)	11 (8.6)
Ipsilateral (> 1 year)	199	5 (7.5)	–	2 (1.6)	7 (3.5)
Cystectomy	133	17 (12.7)	4 (3.0)	4 (3.0)	25 (18.7)
Ablation	42	6 (14.3)	1 (2.4)	0 (0.0)	7 (16.7)

Seventeen patients had moderate endometriosis (37.8%), 28 severe endometriosis (62.2%), including 21 extensive endometriosis (R-AFS score > 70) (46.6%). Thirty-three patients had a unilateral endometrioma and 12 had bilateral cysts including seven with 2 cysts > 3 cm in diameter.

The recurrence rates are presented in Table 2. Because of the design of this study, all the cysts encountered in this group are reported as endometriomas, and functional and organic ovarian cysts are not reported. Among the recurrences two were diagnosed only by the presence of 'chocolate' fluid during the ovocyte pick up although there was no abnormality at ultrasound. Among the 10 remaining cases, the diameter ranged from 2 cm to 5 cm. In this study, 5 of the 12 patients (41.6%) with a recurrence and 19 of the 33 patients without recurrence (57.7%) had a baby after IVF, 16 of these deliveries occurred after the first cycle. The mean delay between the laparoscopic treatment and the recurrence was 21.4 ± 18.4 months, whereas the delay between the treatment and the last normal ovocyte pick up in patients without recurrence was 21.2 ± 16.4 months; 9 of the 12 recurrences were diagnosed during the first attempt.

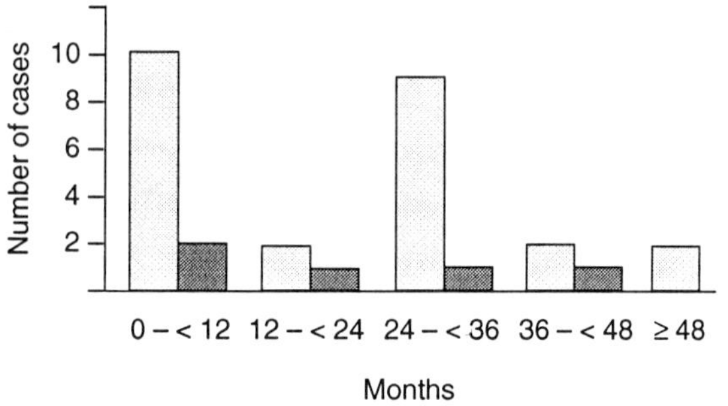

Figure 1 Ipsilateral recurrences in study 1; 199 treated adnexae. □, endometrioma; ■, pathology ?

Table 2 Recurrence rates in study 2

		Recurrent endometrioma *n* (%)
All patients	45	12 (26.6)
Patients with		
Stage III	17	3 (17.7)
Stage IV	28	9 (32.2)
Bilateral	12	2 (16.7)
Unilateral	33	10 (30.3)
Adnexae		
All	90	16 (17.7)
Cystectomy*	44	10 (22.7)
Ablation*	13	2 (15.4)
Ipsilateral†	52	10 (19.2)
Controlateral	38	6 (15.8)

*, Including all the cysts treated whatever the diameter; †, On an adnexa treated for a cyst of more than 3 cm in diameter

Table 3 Recurrence rates in study 3

		Pathologic diagnosis of the recurrent cyst			
		Endometrioma	*Functional*	*?*	*Organic benign*
All patients	172	20 (11.6)	14(8.1)	2 (1.1)	3 (1.7)
Age at treatment					
< 30	46	6 (13.0)			
30–35	41	5 (12.2)			
35–40	37	4 (10.8)			
> 40	48	5 (10.84)			
Treatment					
Cystectomy	143	14 (9.8)	10 (7.0)	2 (1.4)	3 (2.1)
Ablation	29	6 (20.7)	4 (13.8)	0 (0.0)	0 (0.0)

Study 3

Among 193 patients treated for an endometrioma > 3 cm, 172 treated conservatively (preserving the ovary) were included in the study. The mean age was 34.7 ± 7.2 years, the duration of follow-up was 51.1 ± 34.6 months. The recurrence rates are presented in Table 3. The recurrence rate was 11.6% per patient and 6.9 per cyst. Among 20 recurrent endometriomas, 8 were diagnosed on the contralateral adnexa and 12 on the treated adnexa.

Among the patients followed, the risk of recurrence per year is presented in Figure 2. Some late recurrences occurred. Beyond 6 years, results should be interpreted cautiously as only 34 patients were followed.

Obviously the ultrasonographic follow-up of the patients included in study 2 was much more aggressive. Moreover the recurrence rate may have been overestimated since the diagnosis of endometrioma was not confirmed by pathologic examination. However most of these recurrent cysts were confirmed by several ultrasound guided punctures.

The clinical risk of recurrence is probably lower, closer to that observed in study 3, which included only recurrent endometrioma treated by surgery. Surprisingly, recurrent endometrioma was not related to the parameters studied. The higher incidence of recurrence after ablation was not statistically significant, suggesting that when adequately used ablation is an effective treatment.

DISCUSSION

From these studies, recurrent ovarian endometrioma appeared a common problem. However, the incidence depends on the technique used to assess the ovary. The recurrence rate per patient ranged from 11.6% in study 3 to 15.9% in study 1 and 22.6% in study 2; whereas the recurrence rate per cyst ranged from 6.9% in study 3 to 12.6% in study 1 and to 17.5% in study 2. Similarly in the literature, the incidence of recurrent endometrioma ranged from 8% in a study by Donnez *et al.*[5] to 20% in a study by Koninckx[6].

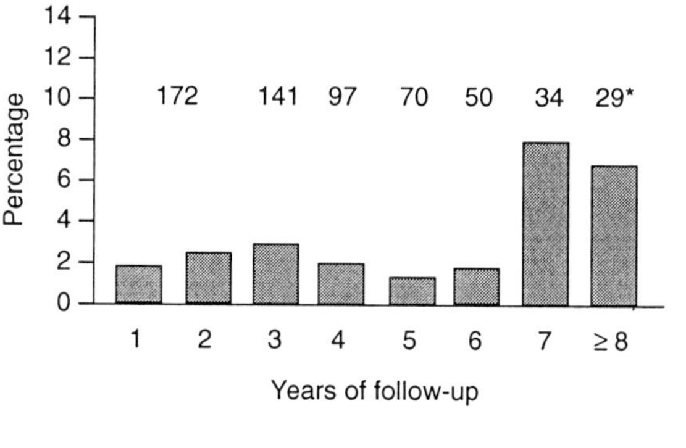

Figure 2 Study 3: Recurrence rate/year. *Number of patients followed-up to the end of this year

Obviously there are early recurrences, which may be related to an inadequate surgical procedure. Two mistakes are possible: an inadequate treatment of the cyst, and an inadequate assessment of the treated and of the contralateral ovary, implying that a second or third endometrioma is not diagnosed. This problem is more common in patients with extensive adhesions. All enlarged ovaries should be punctured[7]. If a small (< 3 cm) endometrioma is found, it should be treated immediately after the diagnosis, since, when the ovary is enlarged by several cysts and or traumatized by several incisions, it may be difficult to find the lesion again several minutes after the drainage.

As we stated before the laparoscopic treatment should be a microsurgical procedure[2]. The cystectomy should be meticulous, with careful hemostasis, gentle tissue handling, slow movements of the instruments and permanent visual control. It is essential to avoid damage to the ovary and to the ovarian vessels. In a young patient, it is better to treat a recurrence than a menopause induced by surgery. In older patients (> 40) an aggressive approach and even an oophorectomy may be used. Among 21 patients treated by oophorectomy in study 3, only one had a recurrence (5%).

Interestingly, there were also late recurrences, more than 8 years after the laparoscopic treatment, probably related to the natural history of the disease. The problem of recurrences should not be overestimated, since in study 3, the risk per year was below 5 %. Therefore a routine ultrasound follow-up is not necessary, as many small endometriomas which are not clinically relevant and/or many functional cysts would be identified, inducing unnecessary stress, ultrasonographic examinations, medical treatments and surgical procedures.

The management of a recurrent cyst depends on the age of the patient, the diameter of the cyst, the clinical problem (pain, infertility, none), and the spontaneous evolution of the cyst.

(1) Small cysts of less than 2 cm should only be followed by ultrasound.

(2) Recurrent cysts in patients included in an IVF program should be operated on only when ≥ 5 cm in diamter.

(3) Recurrent cysts (> 3 cm) in young patients may be treated surgically.

(4) In young patients, vaporization of the cyst wall with a CO_2 laser is probably the best approach. It seems worthwhile to refer these patients to a center where a CO_2 laser is available. An ultrasonographic drainage followed by a medical treatment may be proposed to decrease the surgical trauma. However this approach has to be evaluated prospectively.

(5) In patients over 40, the treatment should be complete, using a cystectomy and an excision whenever necessary. An adnexectomy should be discussed when the treatment is too difficult. When performing an adnexectomy to treat an endometrioma, it is often necessary to excise all the peritoneum of the broad ligament, with a complete dissection of the ureter, to avoid the problems related to ovarian remnants.

References

1. Canis M, Mage G, Manhes H, *et al.* Laparoscopic treatment of endometriosis. *Acta Obstet Gynecol Scand* 1989;150(Suppl):15–20
2. Canis M, Mage G, Wattiez A, *et al.* Second look laparoscopy after laparoscopic cystectomy of large ovarian endometriomas. *Fertil Steril* 1992;58:617–19
3. Canis M, Mage G, Pouly JL, *et al.* Laparoscopic diagnosis of adnexal cystic masses: a 12 year experience with long term follow up. *Obstet Gynecol* 1994;83:707–12
4. Canis M, Pouly JL, Wattiez A, *et al.* Laparoscopic management of adnexal masses suspicious at ultrasound. *Obstet Gynecol* 1997;89:679–83

5. Donnez J, Nisolle M, Gillet N, *et al.* Large ovarian endometrioma. *Hum Reprod* 1996;11:641–6
6. Koninckx P. Recurrence rates of deep endometriosis. Presented at the VIth World congress on endometriosis. Quebec June 30 – July 4th. Abstract 81
7. Candiani GB, Vercellini P, Fedele L. Laparoscopic ovarian puncture for correct staging of endometriosis. *Fertil Steril* 1990;53:994–7

Recurrence rate of deep endometriosis 38

P.R. Koninckx

INTRODUCTION

The pathophysiology of endometriosis is poorly understood, but the prevailing concept is that following implantation[1,2] or metaplasia[3], the disease progresses inevitably to a more severe condition, albeit at a variable speed. The endometriotic disease theory[4] on the contrary, holds the view that implantation and minimal disease are physiologic conditions occurring intermittently in all women[5] and that this does not necessarily progress to a more severe condition; according to this theory severe endometriosis is caused by cellular changes such as a mutation similar to those found in benign tumors (Figure 1). The key event in the pathophysiology of severe endometriosis is thus no longer the implantation of menstrual cells or the metaplasia of cells, but the incident in the endometriotic cell which changes its behavior, and leads to proliferation, invasion or adhesion formation. The type of cellular or genomic modification, together with the local microenvironment, will determine whether the disease will be expressed as cystic ovarian endometriosis or as deep endometriosis, whether the disease will be accompanied by adhesion formation, and whether the morphology will be endometrium-like, cystic with 'chocolate' fluid or adenomyosis externa[4]. The words 'classic endometriosis' will be used to indicate the traditional implantation and progression theory whereas 'endometriotic disease-endo' will be used to designate the endometriotic disease concept.

Recurrence rates of classic endometriosis are poorly documented for obvious ethical reasons since this requires a repeat laparoscopy, which cannot be done without

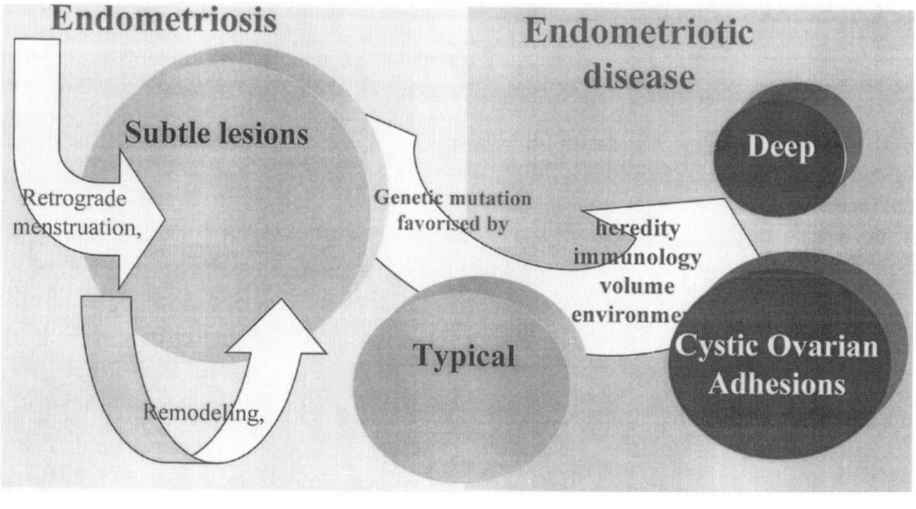

Figure 1 The endometriotic disease theory, according to which the crucial event in the development of severe endometriosis is not the implantation but the cellular event changing the behavior of the endometrial cell

medical indication. During repeat laparoscopy following surgical treatment of cystic ovarian endometriosis recurrence rates of between 3% and 20% were reported[6–9]. The recurrence rate of minimal and mild endometriosis is equally poorly documented[10–13]. Specific data of recurrence rates of deep disease are not available. We therefore reviewed the recurrence of deep endometriotic disease in our database.

MATERIALS AND METHODS

The Leuven database

Since 1986 all women treated for infertility and/or pelvic pain in the division of endoscopic surgery were entered prospectively into a database immediately following surgery[14]. All data are purely descriptive and for each endometriosis lesion and adhesion the appearance, the size, the depth of infiltration and the localization were entered. Simultaneously other variables such as patient characteristics, type, severity and duration of pain and infertility, peritoneal fluid volume and color were recorded.

This database was subsequently used to contact intermittently patients either by mail or by telephone to document follow-up, which comprised pregnancies and outcome, pain using visual analog scales, and subsequent treatments and/or surgery. Pain was scored on a 0 to 5 scale, and pain intensity was recorded for dysmenorrhea, deep dyspareunia and chronic pelvic pain together with the pain radiation in the lower abdomen, in the lower back, to the perineum or during defecation.

The database contains information on 2482 women with infertility ($n = 1297$), pain ($n = 918$) and infertility and pain ($n = 267$). Over the period 1986 to 1998 the main indication shifted progressively from infertility to pain. The prevalence of classic endometriosis remained constant over the years at around 60% for women with infertility or pain and 80% in women with infertility and pain. The severity of the disease increased progressively from 20% to 35% stages III and IV of the revised AFS classification and from 5% to nearly 40% for deep endometriosis, especially for the most severe forms (Figure 2).

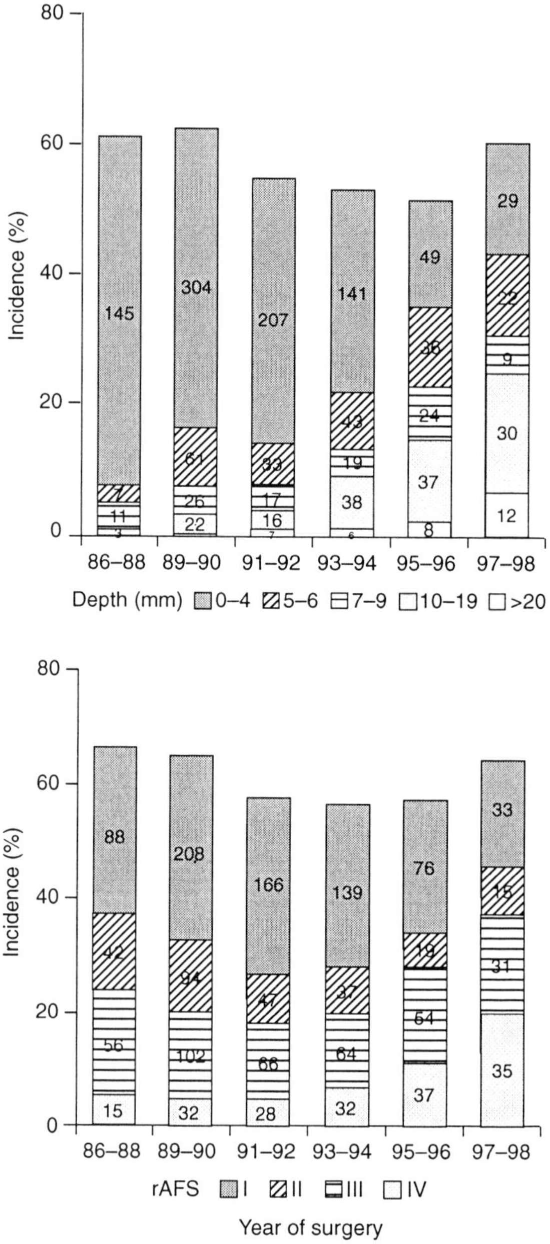

Figure 2 Evolution of severity of endometriosis registered in the Leuven database between 1986 and 1998. The prevalence of endometriosis is shown, broken down by rAFS class (lower graph) or by the depth of infiltration (upper graph)

Recurrences were evaluated as follows. Recurrences were originally registered either as repeat surgery in Leuven or repeat surgery elsewhere when informed of the latter. A second series of data was obtained from a questionnaire mailed to all women with deep or cystic endometriosis, asking for details of recurrences of pain and its treatment. At the moment of analysis 512 responses were available (68%). We are currently checking the surgery and pathology reports of the women who have been reoperated on for a recurrence of pain.

The Leuven adaptation of the revised American fertility society (rAFS)[15] classification (L-AFS)

Deep endometriosis is a severe form of endometriosis but most women were classified in the rAFS classes I and II (Figure 3). Deep endometriosis and cystic ovarian endometriosis are different entities. Therefore women with deep endometriosis – defined as endometriosis infiltrating deeper than 5 mm – were classified separately, leaving for analysis women without deep lesions with rAFS endometriosis stage I ($n = 603$), II ($n = 148$), III ($n = 272$) and IV ($n = 99$), to women with deep endometriosis ($n = 258$) and to women with deep and cystic ovarian endometriosis ($n = 117$).

Data analysis and statistics

As reported before[14], for each endometriotic lesion the pelvic area and volume were calculated assuming typical and deep lesions as cylinders and ovarian endometriosis as spheres. From the pain scales the maximal pain and the mean pain scores were calculated from the scores of hypogastric, perineal, lower back and dyschezia pain scores. This was done for deep dyspareunia, chronic pain and dysmenorrhea, together with a separate total pain score. Maximal pain scores will be used throughout this manuscript, unless stated otherwise.

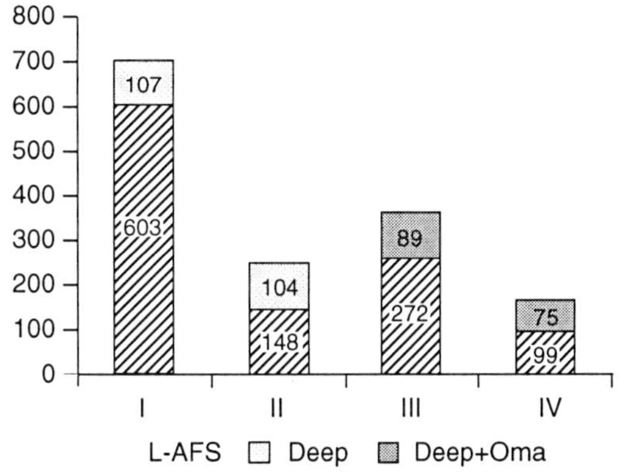

Figure 3 The Leuven adaptation of the rAFS classification where women with deep lesions of classes I+II and III+IV are classified separately as deep and as deep+oma respectively

Statistical analysis was done using the SAS program, using Wilcoxon and Chi- square tests, Spearman correlation, and analysis of variance when appropriate.

RESULTS

The severity of endometriosis evaluated by the rAFS classification correlated weakly with the pain score of dysmenorrhea ($p = 0.05$) and not with the pain score of dyspareunia or chronic pain (Figure 4). Using the L-AFS classification (Figure 5), no differences were found between the pain scores of L-AFS 1 and L-AFS 2. Women with deep, with cystic (Leuven AFS III and IV) or with deep and cystic endometriosis had higher (Wilcoxon) total pain scores than women with L-AFS I or II ($p =$ 0.005; 0.0001 and 0.0002 respectively), higher scores for dysmenorrhea ($p = 0.01$, 0.0002 and 0.0002 respectively), for deep dyspareunia ($p = 0.01$, 0.0001 and 0.0002 respectively) and for chronic pain ($p = 0.02$, 0.003 and 0.01 respectively). Similar results were obtained for mean pain scores. In the women with L-AFS-deep, total pain scores correlated with the depth and volume ($p = 0.002$) of deep lesions. In the women with L-AFS III+IV, pain scores did not correlate significantly with the volume of cystic ovarian endometriosis.

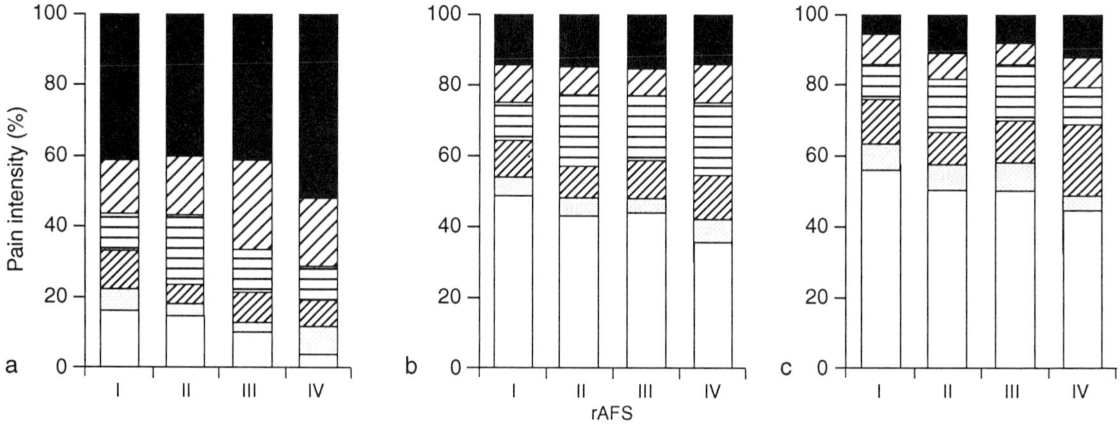

Figure 4 Pain intensity (0 to 5, □ □ ▨ ⊟ ▨ ■) of (a) dysmenorrhea, (b) deep dyspareunia and (c) chronic pain respectively in women with endometriosis rAFS class I to IV

Following surgery total pain scores decreased immediately and with a follow-up of 5 years, no global recurrences of pain were seen (Figure 6).

The incidence of a previous pregnancy is higher than 50% in women over 40 years old with deep or cystic endometriosis (Figure 7). The severity of pain did not correlate with a previous pregnancy, either before or after surgery.

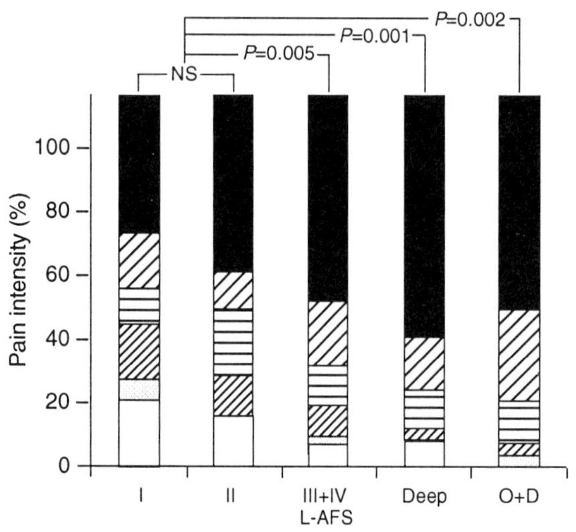

Figure 5 Pain intensity (0 to 5, □ □ ▨ ⊟ ▨ ■) in women with endometriosis, classified according to the Leuven adaptation of the rAFS classification

According to the database (Figure 8), four women had a recurrence of cystic ovarian endometriosis and 11 women had a recurrence of deep endometriosis. In five of these women the deep lesion or part of it had manifestly been missed at the first surgery, in two excision had been done incompletely and only four had a true recurrence.

Answers to the postal questionnaire revealed that 43% of those women who responded had some recurrence of pain, of whom 32% had cystic ovarian endometriosis and 46% had deep endometriosis. This pain required drug treatment in 5%, repeat surgery in 13% and a hysterectomy in 12%. An incomplete review of the pathology found during subsequent surgery shows that true recurrences of deep or cystic endometriosis were rare.

DISCUSSION AND CONCLUSIONS

It should be emphasized that the results reported are a first and incomplete analysis of the follow-up of pain following surgery and of the recurrence of deep and cystic endometriosis. The data, however, support the concept of the endometriotic disease theory, which considers severe endometriosis to be comparable to a benign tumor.

Pelvic pain is clearly related to deep endo-

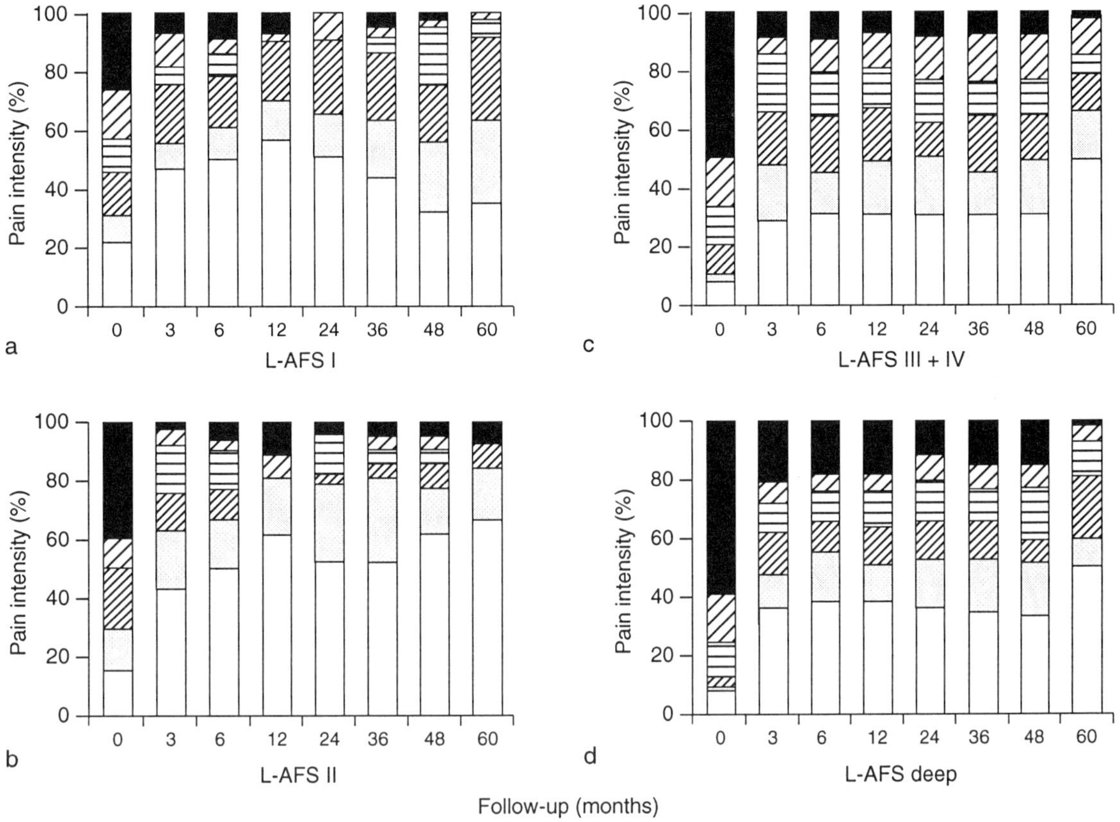

Figure 6 Pain intensity (0 to 5, □□▨▤▧■) following surgery in women with endometriosis. The L-AFS classes, (a) I, (b) II, (c) III+IV and (d) deep endometriosis are listed

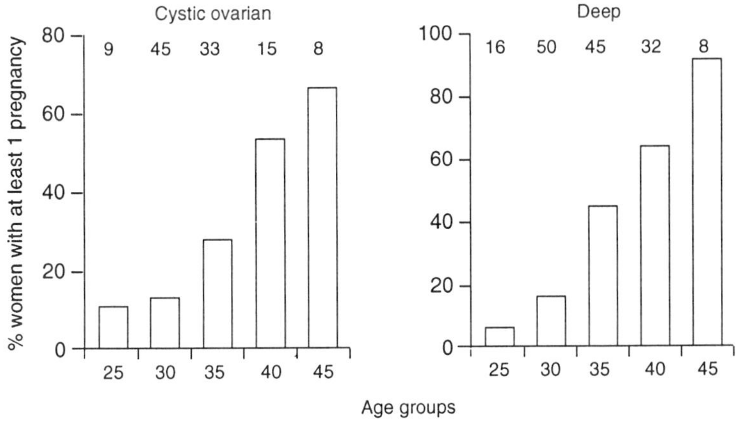

Figure 7 The percentage of women who had been pregnant at the moment of surgery for deep or cystic ovarian endometriosis

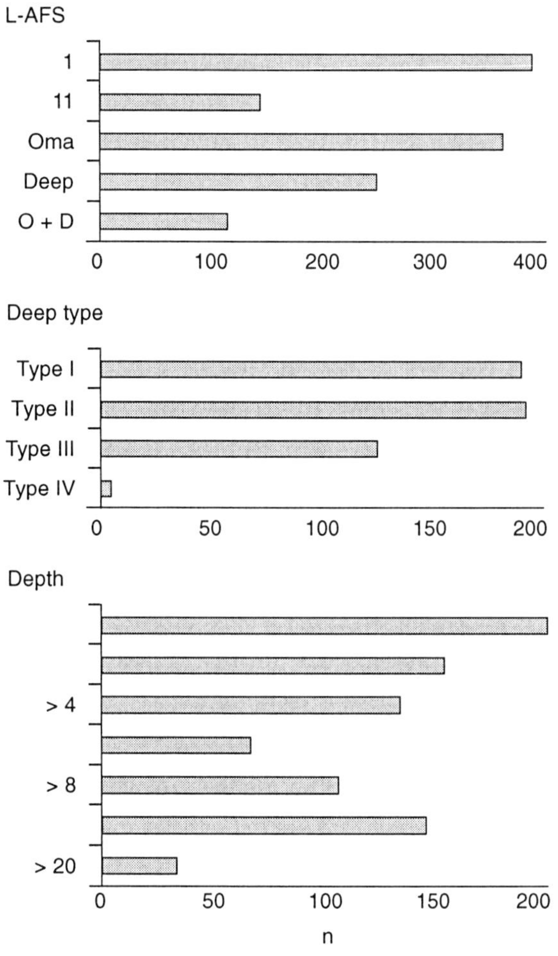

Figure 8 The number of women with deep endometriosis and the frequency distribution according to type of deep endometriosis and to the depth of infiltration

metriosis and to cystic ovarian endometriosis[14–15], whereas women with minimal and mild endometriosis (Leuven AFS class I and II) have much less pain, half of them being practically pain free and those with pain reporting mainly dysmenorrhea. As shown by these data, the rAFS classification[16] is not suited for evaluation of the relationship between pelvic pain and the severity of endometriosis since the correlation between severity of disease and severity of pain will depend on the incidence of deep endometriosis in the rAFS classes I and II. The L-AFS, the Leuven modification of the rAFS, groups the women with deep endometriosis from rAFS I and rAFS II and from rAFS III and rAFS IV into two separate classes and thereby eliminates this problem. These data clearly show that using the L-AFS modification, it becomes apparent that cystic ovarian and deep endometriosis are the main causes of pain, and that pain intensity increases with the severity of the lesions, at least the deep lesions. The L-AFS modification thus is superior to the rAFS classification for the evaluation of pelvic pain. It should moreover be realized that almost all women in the L-AFS classes III and IV have cystic ovarian endometriosis as shown before[14]. It is beyond the scope of this manuscript to discuss whether it could be advantageous to redefine rAFS classes III and IV simply as applying to women with a cystic ovarian endometriosis. This simplification would affect the classification of some 5% of women only, i.e. those with cystic ovarian endometriosis without adhesions and those with mild endometriosis and severe adhesions, often for non-endometriotic related reasons. Such a modification would have the advantage that these stages of endometriosis would harbor pathophysiologically homogenous groups. For the results of pain analysis, the conclusions would, however, remain the same because of the small number of women affected by this simplification of classification. In order to make it more obvious for the reader that L-AFS III and IV contain almost exclusively women with cystic ovarian endometriosis, this has been indicated in the legends of the figures.

The recurrence rate of pelvic pain requires additional in-depth analysis, since 43% of women reported a recurrence of pain which is not apparent from the pain scores they reported. This discrepancy could be explained by the fact that the women with the most severe pain had been reoperated on or hysterectomized thus leaving only those with less pain in the follow-up group. Although life table analysis will be required to confirm or eliminate this possibility, the data show that almost all repeat surgery was performed within 2 years after the first surgery. Since there is no marked recurrence of pain over a period of 5 years we expect this possibility not to be true. The data rather suggest that complete surgery removes the endometriotic disease permanently, as is the case for most benign tumors, whereas incomplete surgery or surgery for endometriosis which was not the cause of the pelvic pain leads to a rapid recurrence of pain as can be expected. Another possibility to explain the discrepancy between the reported recurrence of pain and the actual pain scores could be the occurrence of pelvic adhesions, causing some discomfort which does not require treatment. This is supported by the fact that 68% of the women who reported a pain recurrence did not require any treatment. Taken together, these data highlight the difficulty in assessing pain, which remains a subjective experience.

Our observed recurrence rate of cystic ovarian endometriosis within 5 years is lower than 1%. This is probably an underestimation of reality, but our available data, after reviewing the surgical findings and pathology reports during repeat surgery outside Leuven, do not show a high number of recurrent cystic ovarian endometriosis. To interpret the discrepancy between this very low recurrence rate and those reported previously, it should be taken into account that reports of recurrence rates are not strictly comparable. The 11% to 19% recurrence rate of Bateman[7] was the incidence of an endometrioma in the other ovary following ovariectomy. This is the risk of missing a (small) endometrioma or the risk of *de novo* formation of an endometrioma in the other ovary. The 15% recurrence rate reported by Wood *et al.*[17] actually represents a recurrence rate of less than 7% since it is the recurrence rate of endometriosis in the 50% of patients with persistent infertility or pain. The 7% recurrence rate reported by Canis[6] was observed during repeat laparoscopy following excision of endometriomas larger than 3 cm in diameter. The surgical technique is most comparable with our data, where all cystic endometriosis less than 5 cm in diameter were removed by stripping of the cyst wall or, for larger endometriotic cysts, by focal treatment followed by either stripping the cyst wall or removal of the remaining endometriosis during a second procedure. Since our results do not take into account those women without complaints or in whom a recurrence was not clinically detected, and thus include only those patients with repeat surgery, the data are most comparable with those of Ahmed *et al.*[9], reporting a recurrence rate of 3.2%. Although the data are not entirely comparable, Candiani *et al.*[18] reported a 14% incidence of a third intervention after a second conservative surgery for endometriosis. The 19% reoperation rate of Redwine[11] includes all endometriosis, making it unwise to draw conclusions on the specific recurrence rate of cystic ovarian endometriosis. For all reports using pain as an indication for repeat surgery, it is, moreover, unclear whether the endometriosis found at repeat laparoscopy and the pain were causally related[19] (for review[20]).

For deep endometriosis the recurrence rate is extremely low. In five women the diagnosis was missed during the first laparoscopy. In two women the diagnosis was made later by a menstrual clinical examination and in three women the diagnosis of sigmoid endometriosis had been missed and was diagnosed soon after the first surgery, since persistence of pain prompted additional investigations. In two women sigmoid endometriosis had been incompletely removed for technical reasons, and in two women the sigmoid endometriosis was not treated during the first laparoscopy since, during surgery, it was judged that the pain symptoms had been sufficiently treated by the concurrent treatment of deep or cystic ovarian endometriosis. Interestingly, all four subsequently required a partial rectal resection up to 3 years later, and one woman needed reanastomosis. In two women the vaginal extension of deep endometriosis was probably missed during the first surgery, since recurrence of symptoms and diagnosis by inspection and menstrual clinical examination was made within a few months. Taken together, the real recurrences rate was less than 1%, and it is unclear whether these recurrences are true recur-rences or the result of incomplete surgery.

Widely accepted concepts are that pregnancy is favorable for endometriosis, whereas those with endometriosis are subfertile. The observation that in older age groups the majority of women with cystic or deep endometriosis had one or more children challenges these concepts. It is at present unclear whether women with endometriotic disease have a reduced monthly conception rate but ultimately become pregnant, or whether in these women the onset of endometriotic disease occurs at a later age. The observation, however, that a large number of women had a pregnancy shortly before the diagnosis of endometriotic disease together with three women who became pregnant on the waiting list with an immediate recurrence of symptoms and the surgical removal of a deep endometriosis after delivery rather support the concept of a benign tumor, which can decrease but not prevent the probability of conception and which is relatively unaffected by the pregnancy itself.

In conclusion, the recurrence rate of endometriotic disease, both deep endometriosis and cystic ovarian endometriosis, seems to be very low. Bearing in mind that we favor the endometriotic disease theory, which considers endometriotic disease as a benign tumor, we even speculate that all recurrences of endometriotic disease may arise from either missed diagnosis, or incomplete surgery, whereas *de novo* recurrence of endometriotic disease is probably rare. A second conclusion is that pregnancy does not prevent or cure endometriotic disease. Finally the rAFS classification is clearly not adequate to evaluate pelvic pain. Considering the results obtained with our Leuven AFS adaptation, which groups women with deep endometriosis separately, we suggest an adaptation of the rAFS classification, in which women with deep endometriosis and cystic ovarian endometriosis are grouped separately.

ACKNOWLEDGEMENTS

Professor David Barlow and Mr Stephen Kennedy, Nuffield Department of Obstetrics and Gynaecology, Oxford, UK, are thanked for the many fruitful discussions, generating many of the ideas expressed. We thank the co-workers and assistants in training for their effort to enter the data of surgery immediately after the intervention into the database. Mr Benijts and Dr Lempereur, Ipsen NV, Belgium are thanked for their generous support which has been essential to develop and maintain the database. Mrs Diane Wolput is thanked for taking care of the database and for typing this manuscript. This manuscript was partially supported by FWD grant number 1.5.436.97.

References

1. Sampson JA. Peritoneal endometriosis due to the menstrual dissemination of endometrial tissue into the peritoneal cavity. *Am J Obstet Gynecol* 1927; 14:422–69
2. Sampson JA. The development of the implantation theory for the development of endometriosis. *Am J Obstet Gynecol* 1940;40:549–57
3. Gruenwald P. Origin of endometriosis from the mesenchyme of the celomic walls. *Am J Obstet Gynecol* 1942;44:470–4
4. Koninckx PR, Kennedy SH, Barlow DH. Endometrium and endometriosis: the role of peritoneal fluid. *Human Reprod* 1998;in press
5. Koninckx PR, Oosterlynck D, D'Hooghe T, *et al.* Deeply infiltrating endometriosis is a disease whereas mild endometriosis could be considered a non-disease. *Ann NY Acad Sci* 1994;734:333–41
6. Canis M, Mage G, Wattiez A, *et al.* Second-look laparoscopy after laparoscopic cystectomy of large ovarian endometriomas [see comments]. *Fertil Steril* 1992;58:617–19
7. Bateman BG, Kolp LA, Mills S. Endoscopic versus laparotomy management of endometriomas. *Fertil Steril* 1994;62:690–5

8. Wood C, Maher P, Hill D. Diagnosis and surgical management of endometriomas. *Aust NZ J Obstet Gynaecol* 1992;32:161–3
9. Ahmed MS, Barbieri RL. Reoperation rates for recurrent ovarian endometriomas after surgical excision. *Gynecol Obstet Invest* 1997;43:53–4
10. Wheeler JM, Malinak LR. Recurrent endometriosis: incidence, management, and prognosis. *Am J Obstet Gynecol* 1983;146:247–53
11. Redwine DB. Conservative laparoscopic excision of endometriosis by sharp dissection: life table analysis of reoperation and persistent or recurrent disease. *Fertil Steril* 1991;56:628–34
12. Crosignani PG, Vercellini P. Conservative surgery for severe endometriosis: should laparotomy be abandoned definitively? *Hum Reprod* 1995;10: 2412–18
13. Wheeler JM, Russel Malinak L. Recurrent endometriosis. *Contrib Gynecol Obstet* 1987;16: 13–21
14. Koninckx PR, Meuleman C, Demeyere S, *et al.* Suggestive evidence that pelvic endometriosis is a progressive disease, whereas deeply infiltrating endometriosis is associated with pelvic pain. *Fertil Steril* 1991;55:759–65
15. Cornillie FJ, Oosterlynck D, Lauweryns JM, *et al.* Deeply infiltrating pelvic endometriosis: histology and clinical significance. *Fertil Steril* 1990;53:978–83
16. Revised American Fertility Society classification of endometriosis: 1985. *Fertil Steril* 1985;43: 351–2
17. Wood C, Maher P, Hill D. Diagnosis and surgical management of endometriomas. *Aust NZ J Obstet Gynaecol* 1992;32:161–3
18. Candiani GB, Fedele L, Vercellini P, *et al.* Repetitive conservative surgery for recurrence of endometriosis. *Obstet Gynecol* 1991;77:421–4
19. Damario MA, Rock JA. Pain recurrence: a quality of life issue in endometriosis. *Int J Gynaecol Obstet* 1995;50(Suppl 1):S27–42
20. Revelli A, Modotti M, Ansaldi C, *et al.* Recurrent endometriosis: a review of biological and clinical aspects. *Obstet Gynecol Surv* 1995;50:747–54

Prevention of recurrences by postoperative medical treatment

39

P. Vercellini, O. De Giorgi, A. Pesole, B. Zaina, A. Pisacreta and P.G. Crosignani

INTRODUCTION

The management of endometriosis has recently undergone major modifications based on several advances in surgical, medical and alternative treatments. The introduction of safe and effective endoscopic techniques for debulking or radical conservative surgery of the disease has almost relegated diagnostic laparoscopy to the history of medicine[1,2]. Nowadays it is standard practice to eliminate or reduce visible lesions on the same occasion as visual confirmation[3]. This has both scientific and clinical consequences. First, until a valid and reliable method for the nonsurgical diagnosis of endometriosis is found, probably no more studies will be conducted on hormonal treatments as first-line therapy for the disease. In fact, as randomized, double-blind controlled trials have demonstrated the efficacy of endometriosis ablation in increasing the pregnancy rate in infertile women[4] and in reducing pelvic pain in symptomatic patients[5,6], it may be considered hardly ethical to refrain from surgery in the presence of a laparoscopic diagnosis solely with the aim of evaluating the effects of new drugs on non-treated disease. Accordingly, gynecologists will use hormones as isolated therapies mainly for recurrent endometriosis and will have to redefine indications, type of drugs and schedules[7]. Thus, assessment of the efficacy of medical treatment alone has lost much of its original interest, especially in infertile women. Previously untreated disease will be eradicated immediately after diagnosis, and women with persistent infertility after surgery will probably be better off with assisted reproductive technologies. As a result of the increasing surgical approach to endometriosis, the combination of postoperative medical treatment with laparoscopic procedures represents a growing field of application of drugs[8,9]. Unfortunately, little information is available on the potential benefits of hormonal treatments in combination with conservative surgery for endometriosis[10–12]. The main purpose of the present review was to assess the effects of administering drugs after the intervention on postoperative pregnancy rate, endometriosis-associated pelvic pain and disease recurrence rate, and to compare them with those of surgery alone.

RATIONALE FOR THE USE OF POSTOPERATIVE MEDICAL TREATMENT

The notion that hormonal therapies after conservative surgery for endometriosis reduce the risk of recurrence should be based on knowledge of both the natural history of the disease and the mechanism of action of administered drugs. A distinction should be made between simple persistence of implants and *de novo* development of foci[13]. Persistence may be the result of incomplete operations because it was deemed impossible or inopportune to remove all the lesions. The missed recognition of atypical endometriotic papules, small deep ovarian endometriomas, retroperitoneal nodules and microscopic implants may give a false impression of disease recurrence when it is actually disease persistence. On the other hand, after radical surgical ablation, the reappearance of endometriosis should follow the same pathogenetic pathways hypothesized for the original forms. Because hormonal drugs do not cause degeneration and resorption of ectopic endometrial cells but only their temporary hypotrophy[14,15], it is probable that their use in women with 'persistence' would not modify the eventual healing of lesions. Moreover, it has been repeatedly demonstrated that only a minority of implants actually undergoes progression[6,16–18]. Accordingly, only adequately designed studies with systematic long-term second-look laparoscopy can demonstrate an effect of postoperative medical treatment on the number and pathologic aspects of persistent lesions. The administration of hormonal drugs after radical conservative surgery would not act on ectopic endometrial cells *per se* but on risk factors for disease recurrence. Most of the available experimental, epidemiologic and clinical evidence suggests that menstruation and ovulation constitute a *sine qua non* for the development of implants[19–21]. Furthermore, it has been demonstrated that female monkeys and women with endometriosis, respectively, experience more frequent retrograde menstruations and more abundant menstrual flows than controls without the disease[19,22]. If this is true, long-term ovulation inhibition and/or suppression or reduction of menstrual flow after endometriosis has been completely excised should limit the risk of disease recurrence as long as medical therapy is continued. Several drugs are indeed effective in inducing anovulation and amenorrhea. However, it is well known that androgens (danazol and gestrinone) induce profound metabolic alterations and GnRH agonists cause bone resorption[23]. Moreover, both treatments are associated with major side-effects, are costly, and cannot usually be prescribed for more than a few months. Such a short period of treatment would be very unlikely to influence the natural history of the disease. Progestins may induce anovulation, hypoestrogenism and amenorrhea according to their dosage, and they provoke marked decidualization and acyclicity of eutopic and ectopic endometrium[24,25]. These hormones are characterized by side-effects of relatively limited clinical importance, good overall tolerability, and low cost. Either alone or combined with estrogens as in birth control pills, progestins might constitute an optimal choice for long-term (even years) post-operative medical treatment in selected women with endometriosis who do not want children[26]. Unfortunately, data on this potentially prophylactic use of progestogens and estrogen–progestogen combinations are lacking, and the epidemiological evidence for a possible relation between previous oral contraceptive use and endometriosis development is inconsistent[27] mainly because of confounding factors. In fact, 'the pill' is very often prescribed for severe dysmenorrhea without further diagnostic procedures, that is, when endometriosis is probably already there.

THE DEFINITION OF ENDOMETRIOSIS RECURRENCE

It has been definitively proven that medical treatments for endometriosis are not cytoreductive and cause only temporary quiescence of foci[14,15]. Consequently, results from trials on drug-only regimens are not useful for studying the long-term behavior of the disease in terms of tendency to reappear and progress. In fact, mainly endometriosis persistence would be observed and not real recurrence. Accordingly, only findings in women who underwent radical lesion ablation and were followed for an adequately prolonged period are of use in disentangling the issue. Data from large series have demonstrated that the 5-year cumulative recurrence rate is approximately 20% after conservative surgery at both laparoscopy and laparotomy[28,29]. However, these estimates were based on events such as the reappearance of pelvic pain or number of reinterventions, which may not accurately reflect the real incidence of recurrence. This aspect is directly related to the diagnostic modalities of recurrent endometriosis which may not differ greatly from the accepted criteria for first-line diagnosis, i.e. visual or histologic confirmation. In this respect, the figures available in the literature may well be underestimates because they do not take into account recurrent asymptomatic disease, especially peritoneal or superficial implants, which, unlike ovarian cysts, are not detected by pelvic ultrasonography. Ideally, a cohort of women operated on conservatively should undergo serial follow-up laparoscopies over a 5- to 10-year time span. Only such a study, which is obviously unethical and of doubtful clinical value, would offer reliable estimates on the incidence of real endometriosis recurrence. An alternative would be the periodical performance of a highly sensitive and specific non invasive test which, unfortunately, is not yet available. The definition of endometriosis recurrence is vague at the moment in both the scientific literature and clinical practice. Consequently, in the present review we deal with the possibility that postoperative medical treatments influence 'recurrent manifestations' of endometriosis (i.e. infertility, pain, ultrasonographic evidence of ovarian endometriomas, and need for reoperation) and do not consider recurrence from a pathologic point of view because reliable data on this aspect are almost non-existent.

RESULTS

The articles included in this review are randomized and non-randomized controlled clinical studies published in the last decade in English-language medical papers on the efficacy of medical treatments after conservative surgery for endometriosis. We conducted a MEDLINE search from 1987 to 1997 using relevant medical subject heading terms (endometriosis, surgery, medical therapy, infertility, pelvic pain, dysmenorrhea, dyspareunia), identified additional reports by reviewing all references from retrieved papers, and consulted books and monographs on endometriosis published in the last 10 years.

The initial screening yielded seven citations for further assessment. Of these, we excluded one because it is unclear if laparoscopy performed before danazol treatment was ablative or simply diagnostic[30], one with a misleading title because the effects of gestrinone were evaluated without prior surgical debulking[31], and one because the outcomes of interest were not included in the results[32]. Data on the effect of postoperative medical treatment were extracted from the remaining four articles[7,17,33,34]. One study[7] reported exclusively variations of symptoms and it was included only in the evaluation of the effect on pain, and in Parazzino *et al.*s' study[34] it was not possible to extrapolate the absolute numbers of non-responders after the intervention, as the effect of treatments was expressed in terms of median reduction of pain scores. The effect on conception was assessed by evaluating studies by Telimaa *et al.*[17], Chong *et al.*[33] and Parazzini *et al.*[34], which were published in full in peer-reviewed journals. However, Chong *et al.*[33] reported the results of a retrospective cohort study without untreated controls. The main characteristics and details of the four studies considered are shown in Tables 1 and 2. Two studies evaluated drug therapy after microsurgery at laparotomy, and two after operative laparoscopy. Three trials were placebo-controlled, but the method of randomization was defined only for one of them. A preplanned calculation of the sample size based on the expected difference in the main outcome measure was not reported in the considered articles. Moreover, specific protocol objectives were not identified in Telimaa *et al.*s' study[17]. The mean number of patients included was 91 and endometriosis was always staged according to the revised American Fertility Society (AFS) classification[35]. One study included subjects with disease at all stages[17], one only at stage I[33], and one only at stages III and IV[34], whereas in Hornstein *et al.*s' study[7] only mean scores are indicated with no stage attribution.

Table 1 Main characteristics of studies on medical treatment after conservative surgery for endometriosis: literature data, 1987–1997

Source	*Origin, year*	*Type of study*	*Type of randomization*	*Surgical modality*	*Treatment schedule*	*Control*	*Life-table analysis*
Telimaa *et al.*[17]	Finland, 1987	RCT	nr	Laparotomy	Oral danazol 600 mg/day for 6 months, oral MPA† 100 mg/day for 6 months	Placebo	no
Chong *et al.*[33]	USA, 1990	retro-spective	na	Laparoscopy	Oral danazol 600–800 mg/day for 4 months	Surgery or danazol only	no
Parazzini *et al.*[34]	Italy, 1994	RCT	Computer-generated list, centralized allocation by phone	Laparotomy	Nasal nafarelin 400 μg/day for 3 months	Placebo	no
Hornstein *et al.*[7]	USA and Canada, 1997	RCT	nr	Laparoscopy	Nasal nafarelin 400 μg/day for 6 months	Placebo	yes

RCT, randomized controled trial; nr, not reported; na, not applicable; †MPA, medroxyprogesterone acetate

Table 2 Details of patients enrolled in studies on medical treatment after conservative surgery for endometriosis: literature data, 1987–1997

Source	*Sample size*	*Mean age* (years)	*Endometriosis stage*	*No. of women with infertility at entry (n)*	*Infertility factors other than endo-metriosis*	*No. of women with pain at entry (n)*	*Months of follow-up*
Telimaa *et al.*[17]	60	30	AFS, all stages	22	nr	nr	6
Chong *et al.*[33]	167	31	Revised AFS stage I	167	yes	nr	12
Parazzini *et al.*[34]	75	< 38	Revised AFS stages III and IV	75	no	60	12
Hornstein *et al.*[7]	109	31	Revised AFS†	na	na	109	18

AFS, American Fertility Society classification; †Only mean scores are available with no stratification by stage; na, not applicable; nr, not reported

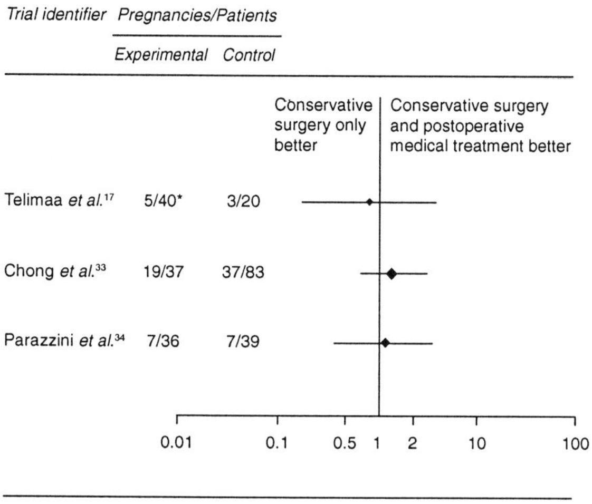

*Including subjects allocated to both danazol and medroxyprogesterone acetate treatment

Figure 1 Overview of studies comparing conservative surgery for endometriosis with or without postoperative medical treatment. Diamonds represent odds ratio of conception and horizontal lines are 95% confidence intervals

Effect on fertility

Assessment of effect in terms of postoperative conception rate at the end of follow-up of the three studies identified is shown in Figure 1. A total of 264 women were evaluated. Medical treatment schedules varied among studies: one used a gonadotropin releasing hormone (GnRH) agonist given intranasally for 3 months[34], one oral danazol for 4 months[33], and one either oral medroxyprogesterone acetate (MPA) or danazol for 6 months[17]. The odds ratio (OR) of conception in the trials considered ranged from 0.81 to 1.31, all with 95% confidence intervals (CI) including unity, suggesting that the treatment effects of surgery plus postoperative medical therapy or surgery alone were equivalent. Clinical heterogeneity between studies is inevitable as different interventions were used for comparison.

Effect on pain

In Telimaa *et al.*s' study[17], MPA and danazol given postoperatively reduced pelvic pain scores more effectively than placebo, the difference being significant at 6 months of therapy. It is unclear if the difference in symptomatic relief persisted also after the withdrawal of medical therapy. Moreover, absolute numbers of responders/non-responders were not indicated, a limitation also of Parazzini *et al.*s' trial[34]. The latter assessed the antalgic effect of nasal nafarelin for 3 months after surgery using a seven-point multidimensional verbal rating scale and a ten-point linear analog scale. At 12 month follow-up, the mean reduction of the multidimensional score was 3.6 in the women allocated to nafarelin and 4.0 in those given placebo, and the mean reductions of the ten-point linear scale score were 7.0 and 6.9, respectively. These differences were not statistically significant.

Effect on disease recurrence

Very limited information is available in the literature on the long-term effect of postoperative medical treatments on endometriosis recurrence rates. Consequently, we decided to analyse our surgical series to verify if the incidence of disease reappearance differs according to the use of hormonal drugs after the intervention. In the period 1990–1997, 954 patients underwent first-line conservative surgery at laparoscopy or laparotomy at our institution, 729 of whom have been followed with serial clinical and sonographic evaluations. The diagnosis of endometriosis recurrence was based on the observation of ovarian endometriomas at pelvic ultrasonography[36,37] or on visual and histologic findings at subsequent surgical explorations. Cox's proportional hazards model was adopted to test the influence of several variables of interest on disease recurrence, including postoperative medical treatment. Three hundred and twenty-eight subjects received 6 month adjuvant therapy after surgery (estrogen–progestogen, $n = 180$; GnRH agonists, $n = 112$; progestogen, $n = 22$; danazol, $n = 14$) and 401 did not. A total of 69 recurrences were diagnosed (9.5%) during a follow-up period ranging from 1 to 8 years. According to multivariate analysis, postoperative medical treatment was significantly associated with a higher frequency of disease recurrence ($p = 0.0006$), the relative risk being 2.58 (95% CI, 1.50–4.42). Interestingly, we detected only a trend towards increasing incidence of endometriosis reappearance according to revised AFS stage at first-line surgery ($p = 0.073$; relative risk = 1.50; 95% CI, 0.96–2.34).

DISCUSSION

Enthusiasm for adjuvant drug therapy after conservative interventions for endometriosis increased after publication of Wheeler and Malinak's retrospective study[38] reporting a pregnancy rate of 79% (15/19) after combined surgery and postoperative danazol therapy compared with 30% (36/119) after surgery alone. The hypothetical advantages of postoperative medical treatment include resorption of residual visible lesions whose surgical removal was considered inopportune or not possible, 'sterilization' of microscopic implants, and reduction in the risk of disease dissemination when endometriomas rupture during mobilization. This should increase the postoperative pregnancy rate and reduce the recurrence rate[8,10–12]. However, the major misunderstanding undermining the entire concept of medical therapy of endometriosis lies in the conviction that ectopic implants may regress, degenerate and ultimately disappear owing to an unfavorable hormonal milieu. This erroneous belief has been largely supported by findings at follow-up laparoscopies which were performed with the patients still under the effect of treatment and showed reductions in the AFS scores. However, it is now evident that the difference in the aspect of lesions before and at the end of treatment is not definitive. In fact, implants undergo simple modification of their appearance with just partial and temporary regression but no resorption or healing[14,15,39]. Ectopic endometrium is still there, ready to re-grow with metabolic activity no different than before treatment and, most importantly, independently of the type and dosage of the drug used[26,40,41]. The problem is that drugs suppressing ovulation do not constitute a cure for endometriosis in terms of healing processes and resorption. Unfortunately, the lesson learned with medical therapies when used alone, obviously applies also to postoperative treatments. Furthermore, medical treatment might prevent a pregnancy just when a conception may be more likely, i.e. in the immediate postoperative period. However, this last supposition has never been confirmed formally.

The effect of drug therapy after surgery can be assessed with confidence as data from three true randomized controlled trials are available[7,17,34]. The results of the present review do not support the notion that suppressing ovarian activity postoperatively increases the long-term pregnancy rate. As far as pelvic pain is concerned, more data are needed to verify the reduced symptoms recurrence rate found in one trial[7] in women allocated to postoperative medical therapy, particularly in view of the different results obtained by Parazzini *et al.*[34]. Finally, the analysis of our large case series did not demonstrate a protective effect of postoperative medical therapies on the incidence of recurrence after conservative surgery. More data are needed to verify if prolonged treatments (more than 1 year) with oral contraceptives or progestogens alone can influence this variable in women not wanting children immediately.

References

1. Crosignani PG, Vercellini P. Conservative surgery for severe endometriosis: should laparotomy be abandoned definitively? *Hum Reprod* 1995;10: 2412–18
2. Crosignani PG, Vercellini P, Biffignandi F, *et al.* Laparoscopy versus laparotomy in conservative surgical treatment for severe endometriosis. *Fertil Steril* 1996;66:706–11
3. Gambone JC, DeCherney AH. Surgical treatment of minimal endometriosis. *N Engl J Med* 1997; 337:269–70
4. Marcoux S, Maheau R, Bérubé S, *et al.* Laparoscopic surgery in infertile women with minimal or mild endometriosis. *N Engl J Med* 1997;337:217–22
5. Sutton CJG, Ewen SP, Whitelow N, *et al.* Prospective, randomized, double-blind controlled trial of laser laparoscopy in the treatment of pelvic pain associated with minimal, mild, and moderate endometriosis. *Fertil Steril* 1994;62: 696–700
6. Sutton CJG, Pooley AS, Ewen SP, *et al.* Follow-up report on a randomized controlled trial of laser laparoscopy in the treatment of pelvic pain associated with minimal to moderate endometriosis. *Fertil Steril* 1997;68:1070–4
7. Hornstein MD, Hemmings R, Yuzpe AA, *et al.* Use of nafarelin versus placebo after reductive laparoscopic surgery for endometriosis. *Fertil Steril* 1997;68:860–4
8. Thomas EJ. Combining medical and surgical treatment for endometriosis: the best of both worlds? *Br J Obstet Gynaecol* 1992;99:5–8
9. Malinak LR. Surgical treatment and adjunct therapy of endometriosis. *Int J Gynecol Obstet* 1993; 40 (Suppl):S43–7
10. Kaplan RC, Schenken RS. Combination medical and surgical treatment. In Schenken RS, ed. *Endometriosis: Contemporary Concepts in Clinical Management.* Philadelphia, USA: J.B. Lippincott Company, 1989;279–92
11. Kettel LM, Murphy AA. Combination medical and surgical therapy for infertile patients with endometriosis. *Obstet Gynecol Clin North Am* 1989;16:167–77
12. Malinak LR, Wheeler JM. Combination medical-surgical therapy for endometriosis. In Shaw RW, ed. *Endometriosis.* Carnforth, UK: The Parthenon Publishing Group, 1990:85–91
13. Evers JHL, Dunselman GAH, Land JA, *et al.* Is there a solution for recurrent endometriosis? *Br J Clin Pract* 1991;45(Suppl 72):45–50
14. Brosens IA, Verleyen A, Cornillie F. The morphologic effect of short-term medical therapy of endometriosis. *Am J Obstet Gynecol* 1987;157:1215–21
15. Nisolle-Pochet M, Casanas-Roux F, Donnez J. Histologic study of ovarian endometriosis after hormonal therapy. *Fertil Steril* 1988;49:423–6
16. Thomas EJ, Cooke ID. Impact of gestrinone on the course of asymptomatic endometriosis. *Br Med J* 1997;294:272–4
17. Telimaa S, Ronnberg L, Kauppila A. Placebo-controlled comparison of danazol and high-dose medroxyprogesterone acetate in the treatment of endometriosis after conservative surgery. *Gynecol Endocrinol* 1987;1:363–71
18. Mahamood TA, Templeton A. The impact of treatment on the natural history of endometriosis. *Hum Reprod* 1990;5:965–70
19. D'Hooghe TM. Clinical relevance of the baboon as a model for the study of endometriosis. *Fertil Steril* 1997;68:613–25
20. Eskenazi B, Warner ML. Epidemiology of endometriosis. *Obstet Gynecol Clin North Am* 1997;24:235–58
21. Vercellini P, Aimer G, De Giorgi O, *et al.* Is cystic ovarian endometriosis an asymmetric disease? *Br J Obstet Gynaecol* 1998;105:1018–21
22. Vercellini P, De Giorgi O, Aimo G, *et al.* Menstrual characteristics in women with and without endometriosis. *Obstet Gynecol* 1997;90:264–8
23. Berga SL. A skeleton in the closet? Bone health and therapy for endometriosis revisited. *Fertil Steril* 1996;65:702–3
24. Moghissi KS, Boyce CR. Management of endometriosis with oral medroxyprogesterone acetate. *Obstet Gynecol* 1976;47:265–7
25. Luciano AA, Turksoy RN, Carleo J. Evaluation of oral medroxyprogesterone acetate in the treatment of endometriosis. *Obstet Gynecol* 1988;72:323–7
26. Vercellini P, Cortesi I, Crosignani PG. Progestins for symptomatic endometriosis: a critical analysis of the evidence. *Fertil Steril* 1997;68:393–401
27. Vercellini P, Ragni G, Trespìdi L, *et al.* Does contraception modify the risk of endometriosis? *Hum Reprod* 1993;8:547–51
28. Wheeler JM, Malinak LR. Recurrent endometriosis. *Contrib Gynecol Obstet* 1987;16:13–21
29. Redwine DB. Conservative laparoscopic excision of endometriosis by sharp dissection: life table analysis of reoperation and persistent or recurrent disease. *Fertil Steril* 1991;56:628–34
30. Soong YK, Chang FH, Chou HH, *et al.* Life table analysis of pregnancy rates in women with moderate or severe endometriosis comparing danazol therapy after carbon dioxide laser

laparoscopy plus electrocoagulation or laparotomy plus electrocoagulation versus danazol therapy only. *J Am Assoc Gynecol Laparosc* 1997;4:225–30
31. Nieto A, Tacuri C, Serra M, *et al.* Evaluation of gestrinone after surgery in treatment of endometriosis. *Gynecol Obstet Invest* 1997;43:192–4
32. Vercellini P, Ventola N, Bocciolone L, *et al.* Laparoscopic aspiration of ovarian endometriomas: effect with postoperative gonadotropin releasing hormone agonist treatment. *J Reprod Med* 1992;37:577–80
33. Chong AP, Keene ME, Thornton NL. Comparison of three modes of treatment for infertility patients with minimal pelvic endometriosis. *Fertil Steril* 1990;53:407–10
34. Parazzini F, Fedele L, Busecca M, *et al.* Postsurgical medical treatment of advanced endometriosis: results of a randomized clinical trial. *Am J Obstet Gynecol* 1994;171:1205–7
35. American Fertility Society. Revised American Fertility Society classification of endometriosis. *Fertil Steril* 1985;43:351–2
36. Mais V, Guerriero S, Ajossa S, *et al.* The efficiency of transvaginal ultrasonography in the diagnosis of endometrioma. *Fertil Steril* 1993;60:776–80
37. Kurjak A, Kupesic S. Scoring system for prediction of ovarian endometriosis based on transvaginal color and pulsed Doppler sonography. *Fertil Steril* 1994;62:81–8
38. Wheeler JM, Malinak LR. Postoperative danazol therapy in infertility patients with severe endometriosis. *Fertil Steril* 1981;36:460–3
39. Evers JLH. The second-look laparoscopy for evaluation of the result of medical treatment of endometriosis should not be performed during ovarian suppression. *Fertil Steril* 1987;47:502–4
40. Candiani GB, Vercellini P, Fedele L, *et al.* Medical treatment of mild endometriosis in infertile women: analysis of a failure. *Hum Reprod* 1990; 5:901–5
41. Vercellini P, Crosignani PG. Minimal and mild endometriosis. Is there anything new under the sun? *J Reprod Med* 1993;38:49–52

Index